# PROGRESS IN CLINICAL AND BIOLOGICAL RESEARCH

## 1983 TITLES

Please contact the publisher for previous titles in this series

# 13th International Cancer Congress, Part D

# RESEARCH AND TREATMENT

# 13th International Cancer Congress, Part D

# RESEARCH AND TREATMENT

**Proceedings of the 13th International Cancer Congress
September 8–15, 1982
Seattle, Washington**

**Editors**

**Edwin A. Mirand** ⅄
Roswell Park Memorial Institute
Buffalo, New York

**William B. Hutchinson**
Fred Hutchinson Cancer Research Center
Seattle, Washington

**Enrico Mihich**
Roswell Park Memorial Institute
Buffalo, New York

**ALAN R. LISS, INC. • NEW YORK**

Address all Inquiries to the Publisher
Alan R. Liss, Inc., 150 Fifth Avenue, New York, NY 10011

Library of Congress Cataloging in Publication Data

International Cancer Congress (13th : 1982 : Seattle, Wash.)
13th International Cancer Congress.

(Progress in clinical and biological research ; 132)
Includes bibliographies and indexes.
Contents: pt. A. Current perspectives in cancer -- pt. B. Biology of cancer (1) -- pt. C. Biology of cancer (2) -- pt. D. Research and treatment -- pt. E. Cancer management.
1. Cancer--Congresses. I. Mirand, Edwin A., 1926– . II. Hutchinson, William B. III. Mihich, Enrico. IV. Title. V. Title: Thirteenth International Cancer Congress. VI. Series. [DNLM: 1. Medical oncology--Congresses. W1 PR668E v.132 / QZ 200 I604 1982z]
RC261.A2I56 1982a      616.99'4      83-48399
ISBN 0-8451-0132-3 (set)
ISBN 0-8451-0132-3 (pt. D)

# Contents

## I. PAIN CONTROL IN THE MANAGEMENT OF THE CANCER PATIENT

## II. LIVER AND PANCREATIC NEOPLASIA

# Contributors

Giorgio Arcangeli, Division of Radiation Therapy, Istituto Medico e di Ricerca Scientifica, Rome, Italy [217]

Hassan K. Awwad, Radiotherapy Department, National Cancer Institute, Cairo University, Cairo, Egypt [305]

Robert L. Baehner, Department of Pediatric Hematology/Oncology, James Whitcomb Riley Hospital for Children, Indiana University School of Medicine, Indianapolis, IN [179]

H. Abd El Baki, Radiotherapy Department, National Cancer Institute, Cairo University, Cairo, Egypt, [305]

Marcelle Bertrand, Department of Medical Oncology, City of Hope National Medical Center, Duarte, CA [329]

Haim I. Bicher, Western Tumor Medical Group, Hyperthermia Clinic, Valley Cancer Institute, Van Nuys, CA [235]

Baruch S. Blumberg, Institute for Cancer Research, Fox Chase Cancer Center, Philadelphia, PA; and University of Pennsylvania, Philadelphia, PA [77]

Erik Boijsen, Department of Diagnostic Radiology, University Hospital, Lund, Sweden [373]

Susan S. Bond, Life Sciences Department, Midwest Research Institute, Kansas City, MO [33]

John J. Bonica, Department of Anesthesiology, University of Washington, Seattle, WA [3]

C. Brechot, Unité de Recombinaison et Expression Génétique, Institut Pasteur, Paris, France [495]

W. Robert Bruce, Ludwig Institute for Cancer Research, Toronto Branch; and Department of Medical Biophysics, University of Toronto, Toronto, Ontario, Canada [131]

Joseph A. Buckwalter, Department of Orthopedics, University of Iowa School of Medicine, University of Iowa, Iowa City, IA [399]

J. Gregory Cairncross, Ontario Cancer Treatment and Research Foundation, London Clinic, London, Ontario, Canada [319]

Jacques Camonis, Institut du Cancer de Montréal, Centre Hospitalier Notre-Dame, Montréal, Québec, Canada [431]

Federico Caligaris Cappio, Istituto Medicina Interna, I Cattedra Patologia Speciale Medica, Università di Torino, Turin, Italy [431]

Stephen K. Carter, Northern California Cancer Program, Palo Alto, CA [279]

Ronald A. Castellino, Division of Diagnostic Radiology, Stanford University School of Medicine, Palo Alto, CA [365]

Joseph R. Castro, Radiotherapy Section, Department of Radiation Oncology, University of California Lawrence Berkeley Laboratory, Berkeley, CA [279]

The number in brackets is the opening page number of the contributor's article.

**Devron Char,** Department of Ophthalmology, University of California, San Francisco, CA **[279]**

**George T.Y. Chen,** Radiotherapy Section, Lawrence Berkeley Laboratory, Berkeley, CA **[279]**

**Malcolm B. Clague,** Nutritional Support Services, St. Luke's Episcopal Hospital; and M.D. Anderson Hospital and Tumor Institute, Houston, TX **[161]**

**Thomas D. Coates,** Department of Pediatric Hematology/Oncology, James Whitcomb Riley Hospital for Children, Indiana University School of Medicine, Indianapolis, IN **[179]**

**Harvey Cohen,** Life Sciences Department, Midwest Research Institute, Kansas City, MO **[33]**

**J. Michael Collier,** Radiotherapy Section, Lawrence Berkeley Laboratory, Berkeley, CA **[279]**

**Mary R. Cook,** Life Sciences Department, Midwest Research Institute, Kansas City, MO **[33]**

**Charles W. Cummings,** Department of Otolaryngology, University of Washington, Seattle, WA **[407]**

**Franco De Conno,** Division of Pain Therapy, Istituto Nazionale per lo Studio e la Cura dei Tumori, Milan, Italy **[17]**

**A. Dejean,** Unité de Recombinaison et Expression Génétique, Institut Pasteur, Paris, France **[495]**

**Stanley Dische,** Marie Curie Research Wing for Oncology, Regional Radiotherapy Center, Mount Vernon Hospital, Northwood, Middlesex, England **[293]**

**J.B. Dubois,** Department of Radiotherapy, Cancer Institute, Centre Paul Lamarque, Cliniques St. Eloi, Montpellier Cedex, France **[171]**

**Stanley J. Dudrick,** Nutritional Support Services, St. Luke's Episcopal Hospital; and M.D. Anderson Hospital and Tumor Institute, Houston, TX **[161]**

**William Duncan,** Department of Clinical Oncology, University of Edinburgh, Western General Hospital, Edinburgh, Scotland **[261]**

**Horatio T. Enterline,** Department(s) of Pathology and Laboratory Medicine, University of Pennsylvania School of Medicine, Philadelphia, PA **[117]**

**H.I. Farag,** Radiotherapy Department, National Cancer Institute, Cairo University, Cairo, Egypt **[305]**

**Manlio Ferrarini,** Cattedra Immunologia, Università di Genova, Genoa, Italy **[431]**

**S.B. Field,** MRC Cyclotron Unit, Hammersmith Hospital, London, England **[195]**

**Gilbert H. Fletcher,** Department of Radiotherapy, University of Texas System Cancer Center, M.D. Anderson Hospital and Tumor Institute, Houston, TX **[267]**

**Robin Foa,** Istituto Medicina Interna, I Cattedra Patologia Speciale Medica, Università di Torino, Turin, Italy **[431]**

**Sophia S. Fotopoulos,** Life Sciences Department, Midwest Research Institute, Kansas City, MO **[33]**

**John F. Fowler,** Gray Laboratory of the Cancer Research Campaign, Mount Vernon Hospital, Northwood, Middlesex, England **[249]**

**Felice Gavosto,** Istituto Medicina Interna, I Cattedra Patologia Speciale Medica, Università di Torino, Turin, Italy **[431]**

**Mary Gerkovich,** Life Sciences Department, Midwest Research Institute, Kansas City, MO **[33]**

**Charles Graham,** Life Sciences Department, Midwest Research Institute, Kansas City, MO **[33]**

**Ranu Grewal-Bahl,** Department of Radiation Oncology, Letterman Army Hospital, Presidio, San Francisco, CA **[279]**

**Jay L. Grosfeld,** Department of Pediatric Surgery, James Whitcomb Riley Hospital for Children, Indiana University School of Medicine, Indianapolis, IN **[179]**

**M. Hadchouel,** Unité de Recherche d'Hépatologie Infantile, Clinique Pédiatrique, Hôpital d'Enfants, Le Kremlin Bicêtre, France **[495]**

**Frederick Hausheer,** Department of Medicine, University of Missouri, Columbia, MO **[347]**

**Günter Henze,** Children's University Hospital; and Department of Pediatrics, University of West Berlin, West Berlin, Federal Republic of Germany **[445]**

**David H. Hussey,** Department of Radiotherapy, University of Texas System Cancer Center, M.D. Anderson Hospital and Tumor Institute, Houston, TX **[267]**

**William B. Hutchinson,** Fred Hutchinson Cancer Research Center, Seattle, WA **[89]**

**Marian Isaacs,** Department of Medicine, Memorial Sloan-Kettering Cancer Center, New York, NY **[337]**

**Ole M. Jensen,** Danish Cancer Registry, Copenhagen, Denmark **[151]**

**H. Joyeux,** Department of Nutrition and Cancer Surgery, Cancer Institute, Centre Paul Lamarque, Cliniques St. Eloi, Montpellier Cedex, France **[171]**

**Henry S. Kaplan,** Department of Radiology, Cancer Biology Research Laboratory, Stanford University School of Medicine, Stanford, CA **[471]**

**Humphrey E.M. Kay,** Department of Haematology, Institute of Cancer Research, London, United Kingdom **[451]**

**Allegria Kessous,** Institut du Cancer de Montréal, Centre Hospitalier Notre-Dame, Montréal, Québec, Canada **[461]**

**Leonard Klein,** Department of Medical Oncology, City of Hope National Medical Center, Duarte, CA **[329]**

**Theodore Knapp,** Life Sciences Department, Midwest Research Institute, Kansas City, MO **[33]**

**Fritz Lampert,** Children's University Hospital; and Department of Pediatrics, University of Giessen, Giessen, Federal Republic of Germany **[445]**

**Hans Joachim Langermann,** Children's University Hospital; and Department of Pediatrics, University of West Berlin, West Berlin, Federal Republic of Germany **[445]**

**Károly Lapis,** Institute of Pathology and Experimental Cancer Research, Semmelweis Medical University, Budapest, Hungary **[67]**

**David L. Larson,** Department of Head and Neck Surgery, University of Texas System Cancer Center, M.D. Anderson Hospital and Tumor Institute, Houston, TX **[421]**

**John T. Lyman,** Radiotherapy Section, Lawrence Berkeley Laboratory, Berkeley, CA **[279]**

**Michael Mansour,** Institut du Cancer de Montréal, Centre Hospitalier Notre-Dame, Montréal, Québec, Canada **[461]**

**Moshe H. Maor,** Department of Radiotherapy, University of Texas System Cancer Center, M.D. Anderson Hospital and Tumor Institute, Houston, TX **[267]**

**Giampiero di Mayorca,** Department of Microbiology, UMDNJ, New Jersey Medical School, Newark, NJ **[485]**

**M. El Merzabani,** Radiotherapy Department, National Cancer Institute, Cairo University, Cairo, Egypt **[305]**

**Hanno Millesi,** Department of Plastic and Reconstructive Surgery, 1st Surgical University Clinic, University of Vienna Medical School; and Ludwig Boltzmann Institute for Experimental Plastic Surgery, Vienna, Austria **[387]**

**H. Abd El Moneim,** Radiotherapy Department, National Cancer Institute, Cairo University, Cairo, Egypt **[305]**

**W.P. Laird Myers,** Department of Medicine, Memorial Sloan-Kettering Cancer Center, New York, NY **[337]**

**Kyoichi Nakamura,** Department of Pathology, Tsukuba University, Ibaraki, Japan; and Cancer Institute, Tokyo, Japan **[107]**

**Guy R. Newell,** Department of Cancer Prevention, The University of Texas System Cancer Center, M.D. Anderson Hospital and Tumor Institute, Houston, TX **[141]**

**Joseph J. O'Donnell,** Nutritional Support Services, St. Luke's Episcopal Hospital; and M.D. Anderson Hospital and Tumor Institute, Houston, TX **[161]**

**S. Omar,** Department of Surgery, National Cancer Institute, Cairo University, Cairo, Egypt **[305]**

**J. Odo Op den Orth,** Department of Radiology, St. Elisabeth's of Groote Gasthuis, Haarlem, The Netherlands **[363]**

**Jens Overgaard,** The Institute of Cancer Research, Radiumstationen, Aarhus C, Denmark **[205]**

**Alan Pater,** Department of Microbiology, UMDNJ, New Jersey Medical School, Newark, NJ **[485]**

**Mary M. Pater,** Department of Microbiology, UMDNJ, New Jersey Medical School, Newark, NJ **[485]**

**Carlos A. Perez,** Washington University School of Medicine; and Mallinckrodt Institute of Radiology, St. Louis, MO **[329]**

**Theodore L. Phillips,** Radiation Oncology, University of California School of Medicine, San Francisco, CA **[279]**

**Enrico Pietrojusti,** Division of Pain Therapy, Istituto Nazionale per lo Studio e la Cura dei Tumori, Milan, Italy **[17]**

**C. Pourcel,** Unité de Recombinaison et Expression Génétique, Institut Pasteur, Paris, France **[495]**

**Noemi Prajda,** Laboratory for Clinical Experimentation, National Institute of Oncology, Budapest, Hungary; and Laboratory for Experimental Oncology, Indiana University School of Medicine, Indianapolis, IN **[79]**

**Cary A. Presant,** Department of Medical Oncology, City of Hope National Medical Center, Duarte, CA; and Wilshire Oncology Medical Group, Inc., West Covina, CA **[329]**

**Arthur J. Provisor,** Department of Pediatric Hematology/Oncology, James Whitcomb Riley Hospital for Children, Indiana University School of Medicine, Indianapolis, IN **[179]**

**H. Pujol,** Department of Surgery, Cancer Institute, Centre Paul Lamarque, Cliniques St. Eloi, Montpellier Cedex, France **[171]**

**William E. Rawls,** Department of Pathology, McMaster University, Hamilton, Ontario, Canada **[461]**

**Karyl A. Rickard,** Departments of Pediatric Nutrition and Dietetics, James Whitcomb Riley Hospital for Children, Indiana University School of Medicine, Indianapolis, IN **[179]**

Hans-Jörg Riehm, Children's University Hospital; and Department of Pediatrics, University of West Berlin, West Berlin, Federal Republic of Germany [445]

Franco Rilke, Division of Pathology, Istituto Nazionale per lo Studio e la Cura dei Tumori, Milan, Italy [99]

Hubert L. Rosomoff, Department of Neurological Surgery, University of Miami, School of Medicine, Miami, FL [27]

William M. Saunders, Radiotherapy Section, Lawrence Berkeley Laboratory, Berkeley, CA [279]

Günther Schellong, Children's University Hospital; and Department of Pediatrics, University of Münster, Münster, Federal Republic of Germany [445]

J. Scotto, Unité de Recherche d'Hépatologie Infantile, Clinique Pédiatrique, Hôpital d'Enfants, Le Kremlin Bicêtre, France [495]

Rene Simard, Institut du Cancer de Montréal, Centre Hospitalier Notre-Dame, Montréal, Québec, Canada [461]

C. Solassol, Department of Nutrition and Cancer Surgery, Cancer Institute, Centre Paul Lamarque, Cliniques St. Eloi, Montpellier Cedex, France [171]

Haruo Sugano, Cancer Institute, Tokyo, Japan [107]

Marcello Tamburini, Division of Pain Therapy, Istituto Nazionale per lo Studio e la Cura dei Tumori, Milan, Italy [17]

P. Tiollais, Unité de Recombinaison et Expression Génétique, Institut Pasteur, Paris, France [495]

Cornelius A. Tobias, Biology and Medicine Division, Lawrence Berkeley Laboratory, Berkeley, CA [279]

Sun Tsung-tang, Department of Immunology, Cancer Institute, Chinese Academy of Medical Sciences, Beijing, China [57]

Vittorio Ventafridda, Division of Pain Therapy, Istituto Nazionale per lo Studio e la Cura dei Tumori, Milan, Italy [17]

Donald E. Wagner, Fred Huchinson Cancer Research Center, Seattle, WA [89]

S. Wain-Hobson, Unité de Recombinaison et Expression Génétique, Institut Pasteur, Paris, France [495]

Robert M. Weetman, Department of Pediatric Hematology/Oncology, James Whitcomb Riley Hospital for Children, Indiana University School of Medicine, Indianapolis, IN [179]

Kay H. Woodruff, Radiotherapy Section, Lawrence Berkeley Laboratory, Berkeley, CA [279]

Huang Xing-yao, Department of Surgery, Qidong Cancer Institute, Qidong, Kiangsu, China [57]

J.W. Yarbro, Department of Medicine, University of Missouri, Columbia, MO [347]

# Foreword

The papers presented in the Plenary Lectures and the Congress Symposia at the 13th International Cancer Congress, September 8–15, 1982, Seattle, Washington, are included in these volumes. The United States was the official host of the Congress, which was held under the auspices of the International Union Against Cancer (UICC), and the Fred Hutchinson Cancer Research Center, Seattle, Washington was the host institution.

Dr. William B. Hutchinson of the Fred Hutchinson Cancer Research Center was the Congress President and Dr. Edwin A. Mirand of Roswell Park Memorial Institute, Buffalo, New York, was the Secretary-General.

The scientific program of the Congress contained over 4,000 presentations. The National Program Committee, chaired by Dr. Enrico Mihich of Roswell Park Memorial Institute, felt that it would be appropriate to include only the papers from the Plenary Lectures and the Congress Symposia to keep the number of volumes at a reasonable level. These papers are presented in five volumes.

*Volume A* — Final Report of the Secretary-General that includes the organizational details of the scientific program
            — Plenary Lectures

*Volumes B & C* — Basic science topics in oncology

*Volumes D & E* — Clinical oncology topics

Since it would be impossible to cover all the areas of oncology presented at the Congress, by presenting the plenary and symposia sessions, we attempted to select the most rapidly advancing and promising areas of clinical and basic research. A good index of the growth in the field of oncology can be obtained by comparing the publications of this meeting with the last cancer congress publications (12th International Cancer Congress) held in Buenos Aires from October 5–10, 1978.

Looking over the topics covered herein, one can only marvel at the tremendous rate of progress and the increase in interest in oncology in the past four years. This reflects the developments in molecular biology as it relates to cancer viral and chemical carcinogenesis, in the design and evaluation of clinical trials, biological response modifiers, cancer nursing, psychosocial aspects of cancer, etc.

On behalf of the Congress officers, we wish to express our gratitude to the National Program Committee and to all the scientists, physicians, dentists, nurses, and other participants engaged in oncology who attended this Congress and who made it a success. I am sure that both the scientific and social interchange which was experienced at the Seattle meeting will have a positive, lasting effect on our lives. We hope to see you at the 14th International Cancer Congress to be held in Budapest, Hungary in 1986 to further the scientific and social interaction.

The editors are deeply indebted to all the authors for their outstanding contributions to these volumes.

We wish to express thanks and appreciation to Catherine O'Leary, Lisa Barone, Linda Beverage, Kevin Craig, Ann M. Gannon, Ramon Melendez, Amy Mirand and Lucy Mirand, all of whom aided in various ways in the preparation of these volumes.

Finally, we wish to acknowledge the support of the National Cancer Institute, American Cancer Society, Pacific Northwest Regional Commission for their generous support of the 13th International Cancer Congress.

**Edwin A. Mirand**

# Preface to Part D

What is the most effective treatment for liver cancer? Is nutritional debility a serious problem in cancer patients? What constitutes an "oncologic emergency?" What is the relationship between lifestyle and carcinogenesis? Has science detected any links between retroviruses and human leukemias? What new cancer treatments show the most promise?

As disparate and diverse as these issues may appear, they have been identified and addressed by clinical investigators worldwide. The link between the scientist and the public, the clinician plays the primary role in the development, assimilation, application, and dissemination of new information concerning cancer detection, diagnosis, treatment, management and cure. This volume highlights the work of these investigators. Emphasizing major advances made in clinical investigation and practice within the last decade, internationally renowned experts from many disciplines discuss their research and elucidate the implications this research has on the future direction of the cancer problem.

**Edwin A. Mirand**

CONGRESS SYMPOSIA


PAIN CONTROL IN THE MANAGEMENT OF THE CANCER
PATIENT Bunyaratavej, C., Thailand, Chairman;
Houde, R., USA, Co-Chairman; Rainier Room

Management of Cancer Pain - Importance of the
Problem. *Bonica, J. J., Seattle, WA USA.

Multimodal Approach in Management of Cancer Pain.
*Ventafridda, V. and De Conno, F., Milan, Italy.

Controversies in the Use of Analgesics in the
Management of Cancer Pain. *Foley, K. M., New York,
NY USA. (By Title Only)

Surgical Approaches to Pain Control.
*Rosomoff, H. L., Miami, FL USA.

Cancer Pain: Evaluation of Electromyographic
and Electrodermal Feedback. *Fotopoulos, S. S.,
Cook, M. R., Graham, C., Gerkovich, M. M. and
Cohen, H., Kansas City, MO USA.

Please note: Papers that are listed as "By Title
Only" were presented at the 13th International
Cancer Congress, but are not included in these
volumes.

13th International Cancer Congress, Part D
Research and Treatment, pages 3–16

MANAGEMENT OF CANCER PAIN - IMPORTANCE OF THE PROBLEM

John J. Bonica, MD, DSc, FFARCS

Department of Anesthesiology, RN-10, University
of Washington, Seattle, Washington  98195

Cancer pain has long been, and continues to be, one of
the most important pressing issues of modern society in general and the health care system of many countries throughout
the world.  This importance stems from two interrelated
facts:  (a) cancer afflicts millions of people throughout
the world annually; and (b) all too frequently the pain is
inadequately managed and consequently many patients spend
their last weeks and months, or even years of their lives
in great discomfort, suffering and disability which precludes a quality of life that is vital to these patients.
This paper includes a brief overview of:  a) prevalence of
pain in cancer patients; b) the physiologic, psychologic,
affective and sociologic effects of cancer pain; c) the
current status of its management and the reasons for deficiencies which exist in cancer pain therapy; and d) some
recommendations for future activities in order to improve
this serious health problem.

PREVALENCE

Because of lack of national epidemiologic studies, the
prevalence of pain associated with cancer throughout the
world cannot be defined.  However, one can gain some insight
by reviewing the incidence of cancer and cancer deaths and
from data derived from a number of local and regional surveys on the prevalence of pain among the general cancer
population and among those with various specific neoplasms.
Stjernswård (1981) basing on statistics for 1978, estimated
that its worldwide incidence (number of new cases) of cancer
is 8.7 million, the prevalence (new and old cases) is 37.1

million and 6.9 million people die from cancer each year
which represents 15% of all deaths throughout the world.
Moreover, in developed countries in Europe and North America and other parts of the world where major infectious
diseases and nutritional problems are no longer aiding
causes of deaths, cancer is responsible for 20% of the total deaths. For example, the American Cancer Society
(1981) estimates that in the United States, in 1981, there
were 815,000 new cases of cancer diagnosed and there were
420,000 deaths, which accounted for 21% of all deaths in
this country. Of these deaths, cancer of the lungs contributed 25%; colon/rectum 13%; of breast and leukemia/lymph-
omas each 9%; uterus/cervix, prostate, stomach/esophagus
each 5.2%; bladder/kidney and pancreas each 4.5%. Review
of data published by WHO reveals that age-adjusted death
rates per 100,000 population for selected cancer sites in
39 countries including all of the Western European countries, Canada, and most Central and South American countries, Australia, New Zealand, and Japan were similar to
those in the United States.

In view of the lack of epidemiologic data, on cancer
pain, it is reasonable to extrapolate from data acquired in
a number of surveys carried out in specific hospitals in
the United Kingdom, the U.S.A., Canada and Italy, these
provide some indication of the prevalence of cancer pain
in general, and the prevalence with specific types of
cancer. These are summarized in Table 1. The prevalence
of pain with different cancers is detailed elsewhere
(Bonica, 1978, 1979) and can be found in the report by
Foley (1979), Greenwald et al (1982), Pannuti and co-
workers (1979, 1980), Turnbull (1979), and Wilkes (1974).
Foley and her co-workers (1979) also reported that among
cancer patients who had pain in 78% the pain is due to
direct tumor involvement, in 19% it is a result of the
complication of anti-cancer therapy, and in 3% it is unrelated to the cancer of the therapy. Further analysis of
the data indicates that moderate to severe pain is experienced by about 40-45% of the patients when the lesion is
diagnosed, by about 35-40% of the patients with the intermediate stages of disease, and by 45-100% of the patients
with advanced cancer depending on the type and site of the
lesion. The data also suggests that the pain is severe or
very severe in an overall average of 60% of the patients
with advanced cancer. Extrapolation of these data and
those estimated by Stjernswärd (1981) suggest that world-

TABLE 1 CANCER STATISTICS: 1981 ESTIMATES (ACS)

| SITE | ESTIMATED NEW CASES DIAGNOSED | | ESTIMATED DEATHS | |
|---|---|---|---|---|
| | NUMBER | % OF TOTAL* | NUMBER | % OF TOTAL |
| 1. LUNG | 122,000 | 15.0 | 105,000 | 25.0 |
| 2. COLON/RECTUM | 120,000 | 14.7 | 56,000 | 13.0 |
| 3. BREAST | 111,000 | 13.6 | 37,000 | 8.8 |
| 4. UTERUS (OVARY, CERVIX,CORPUS) | 72,000 | 8.8 | 21,700 | 5.2 |
| 5. PROSTATE | 70,000 | 8.6 | 22,200 | 5.3 |
| 6. LEUKEMIAS AND LYMPHOMAS | 63,000 | 7.7 | 37,500 | 8.9 |
| 7. URINARY (BLADDER/KIDNEY) | 54,600 | 6.7 | 18,700 | 4.5 |
| 8. STOMACH/ESOPHAGUS | 32,700 | 4.0 | 22,000 | 5.2 |
| 9. ORAL CAVITY AND PHARYNX | 26,600 | 3.3 | 9,200 | 2.2 |
| 10. PANCREAS | 24,200 | 3.0 | 22,000 | 4.5 |
| 11. BONE/CONNEC. TISSUE | 20,900 | 2.6 | 10,000 | 2.4 |
| 12. LIVER/BILIARY | 13,000 | 1.6 | 9,400 | 2.3 |
| 13. CENTRAL NERVOUS SYSTEM | 12,100 | 1.5 | 10,200 | 2.4 |
| 14. LARYNX | 10,700 | 1.3 | 3,700 | 0.9 |
| 15. ALL OTHERS | 62,200 | 7.6 | 35,400 | 8.4 |
| TOTAL | 815,000 | 100.0 | 420,000 | 100.0 |

*Percent rounded to nearest decimal

wide, moderate to severe pain was experienced by 4 million patients with advanced cancer and died and by nearly 16 million cancer patients in the prevalence group.


EFFECTS OF CANCER PAIN

It is now well established that chronic persistant pain and suffering due to causes other than cancer produces a progressive physical deterioration due to disturbances in sleep and appetite and often excessive medication and undergo serious emotional, affective and behavioral changes including anxiety, depression, hypochondriasis, and an increased level of neuroticism (Pilowsky et al 1977, Sternbach 1974). There is also evidence that the physiologic and psychologic impact of cancer pain on the patient is greater than that of non-malignant chronic pain (Bond 1979, Bonica 1979). The physical deterioration is more severe because these patients have greater problems with sleep disturbance and with lack of appetite, nausea and vomiting.

Cancer patients also develop greater emotional reactions of anxiety, depression, hypochondriasis, somatic focussing and neuroticism to the pain when it develops than is found in patients with non-malignant chronic pain (Bond and Pearson 1969, Bond 1979, Woodforde and Fielding 1975). Woodforde and Fielding (1975) examined cancer patients with and without pain using the Cornell Medical Index and demonstrated that the former group was significantly more emotionally disturbed than the latter group and that they responded less well to treatment of their cancer and died sooner. The causes of emotional morbidity were depression, hypochondriasis and psychosomatic symptoms, which together with intractable pain represent symptomatology indicative of the state of helplessness or inability to cope with disease, damage to the body and the threat to life -- responses to having a progressive and potential fatal illness. Bond (1979) found that cancer patients with pain had raised levels of hypochondriasis and neuroticism, while pain-free cancer patients had low levels. He further noted that the scores of patients with high levels of emotionality fell after the pain was relieved by percutaneous cordotomy. This led Bond to conclude that personality factors are distorted by severe pain and that its relief results in restoration in the direction of normality.

The social effects of the uncontrolled cancer pain are equally devastating. Many patients develop interpersonal problems with members of their family, and the community. The fact that most patients with advanced cancer have to stop working poses not only an economic but also an emotional stress and a feeling of dependency and uselessness. The physical appearance and behavior produced by the patient's pain and suffering stresses the family emotionally which is, in turn, perceived by the patient and consequently aggravates the pain and suffering. Some patients with severe intractable pain become so discouraged and desperate as to contemplate suicide.


CURRENT STATUS OF CANCER PAIN CONTROL

Various sources in information suggest that like chronic pain in general, cancer pain all too frequently is improperly managed. A study carried out by Marks and Sachar (1973) of Montefiore Hospital in New York revealed that physicians prescribed amounts of narcotic analgesic for patients with moderate to severe pain due to cancer (and other medical disorders) which were about 50-65% of what had been established as effective doses of such drugs and that the nurses administered as little as 20-30% of the (inadequate) amount prescribed. For example, for patients with severe pain due to abdominal cancer, cancer of the pancreas and lymphosarcoma 50 mg of meperidine every four hours was prescribed and they received only 25-75 mg of the drug per day. Consequently, in most patients moderate to severe pain persisted after the narcotic therapy.

Parkes (1978) found that among the patients cared for in the hospital who had severe or very severe pain, it remained unrelieved during the terminal stage of the disease. Whereas in patients managed in their home, the incidence of unrelieved severe/very severe pain during the terminal phase increased nearly six-fold over that experienced during the period prior to the terminal phase of the disease. These figures suggest that pain control was inadequate in the hospital and even worse in the home. Aitken-Swan (1959) reported that of 52% of cancer patients who had significant pain over a continuous period of time, in 18% the pain was relieved "to a certain extent" and in 20% the "distressing pain" remained unrelieved. Hinton (1963) reported of 82 patients interviewed prior to dying

from cancer, 67% had pain and in 31% it remained unrelieved.
Other British clinicians who have reported unrelieved
cancer pain included Cartwright and associates (1973) and
Rees (1972) and this problem was the subject of an editorial comment by Cicely Saunders (1978). Turnbull (1979)
reported that at the end of palliative therapy pain was
present in 45% of the patients and two-thirds of the
patients died with unrelieved pain. In this epidemiologic
study by our group Greenward et al (1982) revealed that a
large percent of the patients receiving various forms of
anti-cancer therapy continued to have moderate to very
severe pain (Table 2).

REASONS FOR THERAPEUTIC DEFICIENCIES

In view of the great advances in biomedical scientific
knowledge and technology and especially the great amount
of interest in, and effort devoted to, cancer research and
therapy, why is cancer pain inadequately relieved? Serious
consideration of this important question by the author in
the course of the past quarter century has repeatedly
suggested that it is due to an inadequate appreciation or
outright neglect of the problem of pain (in contrast to the
problem of cancer) by oncologists, medical educators,
investigators, research institutions, and national and
international cancer agencies (Bonica 1953, 1978, 1982).
Consequently, there are great voids in our knowledge of
various clinically relevant aspects of cancer pain, and
whatever knowledge and therapeutic modalities that are
currently available often are improperly applied (Bonica
1979).

Lack of Knowledge

Great voids exist in our knowledge of the mechanisms
and physiopathology of acute and chronic pain in general
and cancer pain in particular. This is due to the fact
that until recently pain research was neglected by the
biomedical scientific community and only a few basic and
clinical scientists devoted efforts to this field (Bonica,
1978, 1982). Moreover, of those basic scientists who
studied pain, most did so in the isolation of the animal
laboratory and most were not concerned with pathologic
pain.

TABLE 2

PREVALENCE OF M/VS CANCER PAIN IN PATIENTS UNDER TREATMENT

(% OF PATIENTS INTERVIEWED)

| TYPE OF CANCER | TYPE OF THERAPY | | | | | | | |
|---|---|---|---|---|---|---|---|---|
| | SURGERY | | CHEMO-THERAPY | | RADIATION | | MULTIMODAL | |
| | 1 WK | 2 MOS | 1 WK | 2 MOS | 1 WK | 2 MOS | 1 WK | 2 MOS |
| LUNG | 49 | 85 | 50 | 60 | 50 | 50 | 54 | 70 |
| PANCREAS | 70 | 100 | -- | -- | -- | -- | 68 | 100 |
| PROSTATE | 37 | 57 | 21 | 50 | 65 | 75 | 31 | 75 |
| CERVIX | 23 | 70 | -- | -- | 34 | 60 | 30 | 30 |

These comments are especially true of cancer-related pain. To date there are no published reports of studies to the anatomic, physiologic, and biochemical substrates of cancer pain. Consequently we have no data on the basic mechanisms of the excruciating pain experienced by patients with cancer of the bone, pancreas and other types of advanced neoplastic processes. What are the biochemical events that produce the severe pain of mucositis? Why do some patients with various types of cancers have severe pain while others with the very same type of cancer and similar pathology do not have pain? Answers to these questions are not available.

A very important reason for the voids in our knowledge about pain in general and cancer pain in particular has been the lack of sufficient number of scientifically trained persons devoting their time to pain research. Related to this has been the meager amount of funds for research and training in this field. For example, in the United States over $2 billion will be spent this year for cancer research by the National Cancer Institute (NCI) and other federal, state, and municipal agencies, and by the American Cancer Society and other private agencies, private institutions, and the pharmaceutical industry. These funds will support the research of tens of thousands of scientists, physicians, and other health professionals who are investigating the cause, prevention, and treatment modalities of every form of cancer. However, until recently, research on cancer pain per se, which, from the viewpoint of the patient and his family is one of the most important aspects of this dreadful disease, was virtually non-existent. Analysis of a computer printout for the period from 1971 to 1975 revealed that NCI spent a total of nearly $2.5 billion to support its programs and of these only $560,000 were spent for cancer pain research. This total for the five year period represented 0.022% of the NCI budgets for those years (Bonica 1979). Since then, there has been a very modest progressive increase each year, with a total expenditure of $5,576,000 for the six-year period 1976-1981, representing about 0.1% of the total NCI budget for that period. For the coming fiscal year, $1.8 million, or 0.18% of the budget will be spent by NCI for cancer pain. While these trends are encouraging, they fall very far from the mark in relation to the importance of the problem. In view of the past neglect and the critical needs for research and research training in cancer pain, this area should be given special consideration, but NCI staff has made it clear that this will not be the case. It deserves emphasis that the situation is even worse in other affluent countries in Western Europe and other parts of the world, where virtually no funds are being spent for research on cancer pain.


Improper Application of Current Knowledge and Therapeutic Modalities

These are even more important reasons for inadequate cancer pain control, which in turn, are due to a number of interrelated factors: a) lack of organized teaching of medical students and physicians and other health professionals and the meager amount of published information about the proper symptomatic treatment of cancer pain. Review of the curricula of medical schools reveals that none teach students basis principles of the use of narcotics and other therapeutic modalities that effectively relieve cancer pain. Moreover, many physicians in residency training for specialization in surgical, medical and radiation oncology receive little or no teaching about the proper managment of cancer pain.

Inadequate or total lack of interest or concern about the problem of pain by oncologists is further attested by the fact that very little, if any, information about the proper management of the pain problem is found in the oncology literature, voluminous as it is. In the many textbooks on various aspects of cancer, a vast amount is written on the prevention, diagnosis and therapy of cancer, but only a few deal with the problem of controlling pain symptomatically, and they do it in a totally inadequate manner. For example, review of the ten important textbooks and monographs on the clinical management of cancer published in the United States reveals the startling fact that of a total of 9300 pages, only 18 pages are devoted to the symptomatic treatment of cancer pain (Ackerman and Del Regato 1970, American Cancer Society 1968, Becker 1975-1977, International Union Against Cancer 1978, Holland and Frei 1973, Horton and Hill 1977, Najerian and Delaney 1976, Raven 1977, Rubin and Bakemeier 1971). Moreover, review of the current literature reveals that of the thousands of articles written on some aspects of cancer each year, only a miniscule number, less than 0.1%, are concerned with pain therapy.

As the result of this lack of education of students and graduate physicians and other health professionals, the pain of cancer has been and continues to be treated in an empirical manner. Most practitioners rely on narcotic analgesics which, while they are very useful and have their definite role in the control of pain in cancer, many if not most, cancer patients with moderate to severe pain are given inadequate amounts because of insufficient knowledge of the pharmacology of these drugs. As part of the study previously mentioned, Marks and Sachar (1973) surveyed physicians in specialty training and found that most of them underestimated the effective dose range of narcotics, overestimated the duration of their action, and had an exaggerated opinion of the dangers of addiction. Apparently, this problem is widespread because many others have reported similar findings (Bond 1979, Saunders 1978, Twycross in press).

In some patients, even properly administered narcotics and other systemic drugs do not produce sufficient relief and other modalities need to be used alone or in combination with drugs. These include interruption of pain pathways chemically with nerve blocks or with neurosurgical operations, the use of neurostimulating techniques, hypnosis and other psychologic procedures. Unfortunately, for the aforementioned reasons, the role of these therapeutic modalities is not known by most practitioners and even many oncologists, and consequently, in patients who could be more effectively relieved by one of these procedures or a combination of therapies, they are not considered or, if they are considered, this is done too late. Moreover, in some of these patients the cancer pain problem is so complex that it requires the coordinated efforts of specialists from different disciplines working as a team.

FUTURE NEEDS AND GOALS

In order to rectify the current deficiencies, it is essential to mount and support a multi-pronged program consisting of greatly expanded pain research and research training, activation of a highly effective teaching program for students and practitioners, intensive educational campaign for the public, patients and families, and provision of a better source of information through the oncologic literature.

The urgent need for much greater research and research training on cancer-related pain cannot be overemphasized. Of course, the support for studies on the causes, prevention, and treatment of cancer must be sustained and expanded. However, until this dreadful disease can be effectively prevented, it is also essential to find better and more effective means to relieve cancer-related pain. Future research should include: a) comprehensive epidemiologic studies on the prevalence of pain with each type of tumor; b) study of the neurophysiologic, biochemical and pathophysiologic mechanisms of cancer pain; c) evaluation of the efficacy of methods currently available to relieve the cancer pain; and d) new therapeutic modalities.

Until we acquire new information, we should be able to effectively use the knowledge and therapeutic modalities currently available to do a much better job in relieving the suffering and pain of cancer. To achieve these goals, it is necessary to mount intensive educational and training programs for students of all the health professions, those in specialty training, and for practitioners which would include: a) knowledge of causes and pathophysiology of cancer pain; b) the efficacy, indications, limitations, and complications of current methods of pain relief; and c) specific guidelines for proper management of these patients. Moreover because cancer pain problems are often too complex for one health professional to manage, it is highly desirable to have multidisciplinary cancer pain diagnostic and therapy teams, especially in the larger comprehensive cancer centers. It is also important to develop active programs for the information and education of the public about cancer pain, in order to decrease or eliminate the unnecessary fear and apprehension the public has about this problem. All of these goals could best be achieved through the development of a broad-based multidisciplinary/interdisciplinary cancer pain program or center, which would be responsible to carry out the research, education, training and patient care. Such programs or centers should include critical masses of basic and clinical scientists and clinical oncologists who have special interest and expertise in cancer pain research and therapy.

Ackerman LV, Del Regato JAW (eds) (1970). "American Cancer Diagnosis, Treatment and Prognosis," 4th ed. St. Louis: Mosby, p 783.

Aitken-Swan J (1959). American Cancer Society: Nursing the late cancer patient at home. Practitioner 183:64.

American Cancer Society (1981). "Cancer Facts and Figures." New York: American Cancer Society.

American Cancer Society - Massachusetts Division (1968). "Cancer: A Manual for Practitioners." Boston: American Cancer Society, p 408.

Becker F (ed) (1975-1977). "Cancer: A Comprehensive Treatise." Vol 1-6. New York: Plennum Press, p 6v.

Bond MR (1979). Psychologic and emotional aspects of cancer pain. In Bonica JJ, Ventafridda V (eds): "Advances in Pain Research and Therapy, Vol 2," New York: Raven Press, p 81.

Bond MR, Pearson (1969). Psychologic aspects of pain in women with advanced cancer of the cervix. J Psychosom Res 13:13.

Bonica JJ (1953). "The Management of Pain." Philadelphia: Lea & Febiger.

Bonica JJ (1978). Cancer pain: A major national health problem. Cancer Nurs J 4:313.

Bonica JJ (1979). Cancer pain: Importance of the problem. In Bonica JJ, Ventafridda V (eds): "Advances in Pain Research and Therapy, Vol 2," New York: Raven Press, p 1.

Bonica JJ (1982). Management of cancer pain. Acta Anaesth Scand Suppl 74, 26:75.

Bonica JJ, Ventafridda V (eds) (1979). "Advances in Pain Research and Therapy, Vol 2, Proc of the International Symposium on Pain of Advanced Cancer." New York: Raven Press.

Cartwright A, Hockey L, Anderson ABM (eds) (1973). "Life Before Death." London: Routledge & Kegan Paul.

Foley KM (1979). Pain syndromes in patients with cancer. In Bonica JJ, Ventafridda V (eds): "Advances in Pain Research and Therapy, Vol 2," New York: Raven Press, p 59.

Greenwald H, Bonica JJ, Francis A, Bergner M (1982). Report on Epidemiology of Cancer Pain. Presented at the Meeting of the National Cancer Institute, 1982.

Hinton JM (1963). The physical and mental distress of the dying. Quarterly J Med MS 32:1.

Holland JF, Frei III E (eds) (1973). "Cancer Medicine." Philadelphia: Lea & Febiger.

Horton J, Hill GJ (eds) (1977). "Clinical Oncology." Philadelphia: Saunders.

International Union Against Cancer (1978). "Clinical
  Oncology: A Manual for Students and Doctors," 2nd ed.
  Berlin: Springer Verlag.
Marks RM, Sachar EJ (1973). Undertreatment of medical
  inpatients with narcotic analgesics. Ann Int Med 78:173.
Najerian JS, Delaney P (eds) (1976). "Advances in Cancer
  Surgery." New York: Stratton Intercontinental Medical
  Book Corp. p 608.
Pannuti E, Martoni A, Rossi AP, Piana E (1979). The role
  of endocrine therapy for relief of pain due to advanced
  cancer. In Bonica JJ, Ventafridda V (eds): "Advances
  in Pain Research and Therapy, Vol 2." New York: Raven
  Press, p 145.
Pannuti F, Rossi AP, Marraro D (1980). Natural history
  of cancer pain. In "Continuing Care of Terminal Pa-
  tients: Proc of the International Seminar on Continuing
  Care of Terminal Cancer Patients, Milan, October 19-20,
  1979." New York: Pergamon Press.
Parkes CM (1978). Home or hospital? Terminal care as seen
  by surviving spouse. J Roy Coll Gen Prac 28:19.
Pilowsky I, Chapman CR, Bonica JJ (1977). Pain, depression
  and illness behavior in a pain clinic population. Pain
  4:183.
Raven RW (ed) (1977). "Principles of Surgical Oncology."
  New York: Plennum.
Rees WK (1972). The distress of dying. Brit Med J
  2:105-108.
Rubin P, Bakemeier R (eds) (1971). "Clinical Oncology for
  Medical Students and Physicians. A Multidisciplinary
  Approach," 3rd ed. New York: American Cancer Society.
Saunders CM (1978). Editorial note to relief of pain. In
  Saunders CM (ed): "The Management of Terminal Disease."
  Chicago: Year Book Publishers, p 65.
Stjernswärd J (1981). Is cancer available? World Health,
  September/October, p 2.
Sternbach RH (1974) "Pain Patients, Traits and Treatments."
  New York: Academic Press.
Turnbull F (1979). The nature of pain that may accompany
  cancer of the lung. Pain 7:371-375.
Twycross RG (in press). Narcotic analgesics in clinical
  practice. In Bonica JJ, Lindblom U, Iggo A (eds):
  "Advances in Pain Research and Therapy, Vol 5,"
  New York: Raven Press.
Wilkes F (1974). Some problems in cancer management. Proc
  Roy Soc Med 67:23.
Woodforde JM, Fielding JR (1975). Pain and cancer. In

Weisenburg M (ed): "Pain, Clinical and Experimental Perspectives." St. Louis: Mosby, p 332.

**13th International Cancer Congress, Part D**
**Research and Treatment, pages 17–25**
© **1983 Alan R. Liss, Inc., 150 Fifth Avenue, New York, NY 10011**

MULTIMODAL APPROACH IN MANAGEMENT OF CANCER PAIN

Vittorio Ventafridda, M.D., Franco De Conno, M.D.
Marcello Tamburini and Enrico Pietrojusti, M.D.
Division of Pain Therapy,
Istituto Nazionale per lo Studio e la Cura dei
Tumori, Via Venezian 1 - 20133 Milan, Italy

INTRODUCTION

In approaching the treatment of cancer pain, it is necessary to always bear in mind two factors: I) the hormo-
chemo-radio sensitivity of pathological disease; II) the limits of treatments based on blocks of pain pathways. In effect, the latter involve, sooner or later, a reoccurrence of
the feeling of pain, due to the development of new pain pathways or to the manifestation of extremely painful dysesthesia complaints (Zimmermann 1979).

The first step to be taken is a correct assessment of
pain, carried out through a comparison of the medical indicators used for the detection of the noxiceptive focus (CT
scan, x-rays, scintigraphic studies, hormo-chemo-radio sensitivity, etc.) with the behavioural response indicators
(intensity and duration of pain, life activity, hours of
sleep, etc.). All these data should be collected and recorded onto appropriate history cards and compared during follow
up checks at least once a week.

The second step is to start treatment according to a
therapeutic strategy which should take into account the above
mentioned factors. This strategy is based on a continuous
control over pain, which is to be achieved by applying integrated methods of analgesic drugs, pain pathway blocks and
with continuing care. (Ventafridda 1981) (Fig. 1).

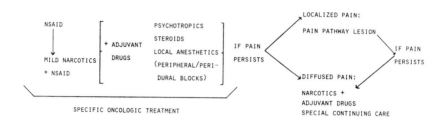

Fig. 1.  Therapeutic strategy in advanced cancer pain.

METHODOLOGY

The possibility of controlling pain through a multimodal approach has been verified in retrospect on 150 patients who underwent analgesic treatment for a minimum period of three months.

The subjects taken into consideration for the study were of both sexes, of an age range from 21 to 82 years, with severe pains due to an advanced stage of the disease, no longer responding to specific antitumoral treatments.

The parameters taken into consideration were the following:
- intensity and duration of pain expressed by means of an integrated score (IS) (Ventafridda 1981);
- primary pathology;
- number, sequence and duration in time of the analgesic treatment given.

The means used for keeping the pain under control were applied according to the sequence already defined in the therapeutic strategy.

The blocks of pain pathways or invasive techniques were:
1) thermorhizotomy of the Gasserian ganglion for cancer of the head and neck;
2) percutaneous chordotomy for pains in a half of the body from C7 to S5;
3) coeliac gangliolysis for abdominal pain of the coeliac

axis;
4) subarachnoidal chemical rhizotomy mostly used for peri-
neal pains;
5) chemical hypophysectomy for pains due to breast cancer;
6) peridural blocks with infusion of steroids in the lumbar
spaces.

The statistical evaluation of the results was made by
the Student's t test.

RESULTS
During a period of three months the 150 patients underwent a total of 1320 out-patient or home controls (means =
8.8 ± 0.25 S.E.) with a range of 5-22 controls.

Table 1 shows the frequency distribution of primary on-
cological pathology. A greater degree of incidence appears
in the pathology of lungs, of the breast and colon-rectum,
in a similar way to the incidence recorded epidemiologically.

TABLE 1. Frequency distribution of primary pathology
in 150 patients

|  | n. | % |
|---|---|---|
| COLON-RECTUM | 35 | 23.4 |
| BREAST | 28 | 18.7 |
| LUNG | 26 | 17.3 |
| HEAD AND NECK | 18 | 12.0 |
| GU FEMALE | 12 | 8.0 |
| GU MALE | 6 | 4.0 |
| SKIN | 6 | 4.0 |
| GASTRIC | 5 | 3.3 |
| OTHERS (HODGKIN'S, SARCOMA, SOFT-TISSUE, BONE, LYMPHOMA) | 14 | 9.3 |
|  | 150 | 100.0 |

Through the multimodal approach, the pain was kept under control in all 150 patients. As can be observed in Fig.
2, after 3 months, in spite of the evolution of the disease,
the pain was reduced to 1/5 of the initial value (To).

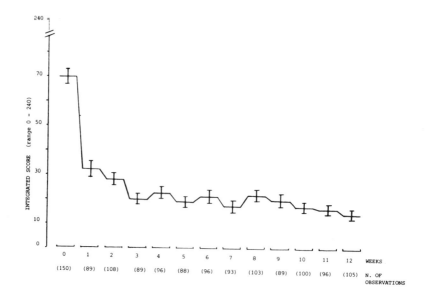

Fig. 2. Analgesic results obtained during the first three
months of treatment on 150 patients with advanced
cancer pain (mean ± S.E.)

Table 2 shows how most of the patients had required a
combined therapy. Of the 37 patients who, during the 12
weeks, underwent a single treatment, 13 (35%) were on narcotics, 19 (51%) on non-narcotic drugs, and only 5 (14%) were
submitted to invasive therapy. The sequence of the treatments, administered either one at a time or in association,
illustrated in Table 3, proves the importance of the approach
with analgesic drugs. The non-steroidal anti-inflammatory
drugs (NSAID), followed by narcotics and then by psychotropic drugs and steroidal anti-inflammatory drugs (SAID) represent, in that order, the methods most commonly used.
With regard to invasive techniques, we can observe, by looking at Figure 3 , that during the 12 weeks their effectiveness underwent a dramatic drop, probably due to the fact
that other noxiceptive foci developed as a consequence of
the dynamics of cancer.

TABLE 2. Distribution of frequency in the number of single and combined treatments carried out for a period of three months on 150 patients with advanced cancer pain.

| N° OF TREATMENTS SINGLE/COMBINED | N° OF PATIENTS | % |
|---|---|---|
| 1 | 37 | 24.7 |
| 2 | 52 | 34.6 |
| 3 | 36 | 24.0 |
| 4 | 16 | 10.7 |
| 5 OR MORE | 9 | 6.0 |
| | 150 | 100.0 |

VALUE OF MAXIMUM FREQUENCY N° 2 (MODE)
(AVERAGE) $\bar{x}$ = 2.4
(STANDARD DEVIATION) S.D. = 1.2
(STANDARD ERROR) S.E. = 0.1

TABLE 3. Sequence of single or combined analgesic treatments given to 150 patients.

| | THERAPY | 1° | 2° | 3° | 4° | 5° OR MORE | TOTAL N° | % |
|---|---|---|---|---|---|---|---|---|
| PHARMACOLOGIC | NSAID | 100 | 15 | 9 | 4 | 2 | 130 | 86.7 |
| | SAID | 23 | 6 | 2 | 2 | – | 33 | 22.0 |
| | MILD NARCOTICS | 59 | 9 | 5 | 3 | – | 76 | 50.7 |
| | NARCOTICS | 29 | 28 | 21 | 5 | 4 | 87 | 58.0 |
| | PSYCHOTROPIC DRUGS | 54 | 8 | 4 | 1 | – | 67 | 46.7 |
| INVASIVE | PERIDURALS | 15 | 7 | 3 | – | 1 | 26 | 17.3 |
| | COELIAC SYMPATHETIC | 10 | 6 | 3 | 2 | – | 21 | 14.0 |
| | GASSERIAN | 5 | 3 | 1 | – | 1 | 10 | 6.7 |
| | HYPOPHYSIS | 2 | 1 | – | – | – | 3 | 2.0 |
| | SUBARACHNOIDAL | 7 | 8 | 5 | – | 2 | 22 | 14.7 |
| | CHORDOTOMY | 14 | 16 | 3 | 3 | 1 | 37 | 24.7 |

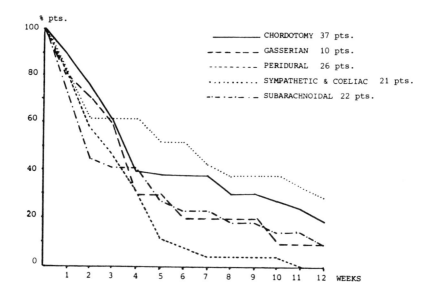

Fig. 3.  % of patients treated with invasive techniques who, during 12 weeks observation, did not require any other analgesic procedure.

Another point of interest is represented by the observation that 25% of the patients who underwent coeliac gangliolysis, after 12 weeks did not need further treatment. This percentage falls down to 22% for chordotomy and to 10% for thermorhizotomy (Gasser's) and chemical rhizotomy.

With regard to non-narcotic drugs, it was observed that, after 12 weeks, between 50% and 60% of the patients were still undergoing the treatment. (Fig. 4.)

Fig. 5 shows a comparison between those patients which had had the possibility of using the home care service and those patients who represented the balance of the group under observation. Starting from the 8th week, which coincides with a greater incidence of home care, a significant reduction of the pain was observed in comparison to patients who did not benefit from the home care service.

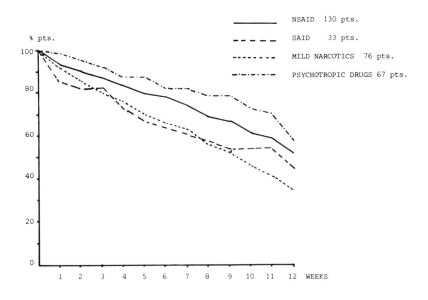

Fig. 4.  % of patients who, during 12 weeks observation,
continued the initial pharmacological treatment.

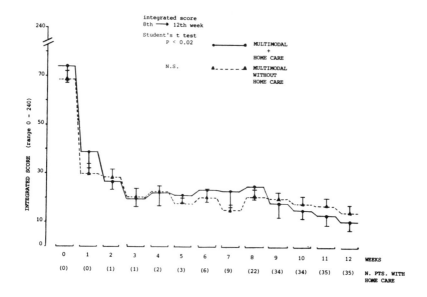

Fig. 5. Analgesic results obtained during the first three
months of treatment on 150 patients, of whom 35
were able to benefit from home care service (mean
± S.E.).

COMMENTS

The retrospective verification of the multimodal approach method, carried out according to a specific therapeutic strategy which takes into account an immediate at-
tack on pain as soon as it manifests itself again, proves
that this is the only possible method, in that it is capable of reaching 100% of the results. The analgesic drugs represent the main means, whereas the opium-based drugs, which
are used in the ratio of 2/3 during the subsequent treatments, represent the most important means after the non-steroidal anti-inflammatory drugs. The invasive techniques only
provide a respite to pain which lasts a few weeks and need
to be integrated with analgesic drugs at an earlier or later
stage. This implies that only rarely can a single technique
have a lasting effectiveness.

Lastly, home care for these patients who are almost always bedridden, brings about a marked contribution in reduceing pain.

In order to keep under control the pains of cancer patients, it is, therefore, necessary to follow an integrated methodology, as well as carrying out a continuous monitoring within the framework of a type of assistance which reaches the patients in their own homes.

ACKNOWLEDGEMENTS
The authors are grateful to the Floriani Foundation for assistance in preparation of the manuscript.

REFERENCES

Ventafridda V, De Conno F (1981). Strategia terapeutica nel dolore da cancro avanzato. Proceedings of Ottavo Corso di Aggiornamento in Oncologia Medica, Perugia. p 315.

Ventafridda V, De Conno F, Guarise G, Rigamonti G, Tamburini M, Gallico S (1981). A new method of pain quantification based on a weekly self-descriptive record of the intensity and duration of pain. In Bonica J.J. (ed): "Advances in Pain Research and Therapy Vol 5", New York: Raven Press, In press.

Zimmermann M (1979). Peripheral and central nervous mechanisms of nociception, pain, and pain therapy: facts and hypotheses. In Bonica JJ, Liebeskind JC, Albe-Fessard DG (eds):"Advances in Pain Research and Therapy Vol 3", New York: Raven Press, p 3.

**13th International Cancer Congress, Part D
Research and Treatment, pages 27–32**
© **1983 Alan R. Liss, Inc., 150 Fifth Avenue, New York, NY 10011**

SURGICAL APPROACHES TO PAIN CONTROL

Hubert L. Rosomoff, M.D., D. med.Sc.

Department of Neurological Surgery
University of Miami, School of Medicine
Miami, Florida U.S.A.

The management of pain falls into two broad categories of approach. The first is non-invasive, and the second is in the purview of the neurosurgeon with the utilization of invasive techniques (Rosomoff, 1974).

Among the non-invasive techniques are 1) psychotropic anti-depressant drugs, 2) trans-cutaneous neural stimulation, and the not totally non-invasive techniques of 3) percutaneous neural stimulation, and 4) nerve blocks, then 5) behavioral modification of aversive affect or maladaptive pain behavior.

The invasive techniques include 1) chemical and surgical rhizotomy, 2) stimulator implants, 3) percutaneous chordotomy, nerve coagulation, 4) thalamic ablation or stimulation, periaqueductal gray stimulation, 5) psycho-surgery, and 6) hypophysectomy.

Chemical rhizotomy has been performed utilizing either absolute alcohol or varying concentrations of phenol in glycerol or pantopaque. These techniques have limited application in that the necrotizing substance must be applied to the sensory roots so as to not produce an associated significant neurologic deficit. This almost entirely limits the use of these substances to the thoracic area of the spine or to isolated cranial nerves.

Approximately 77% of those individuals in whom the chemical rhizotomy can be accomplished will receive satisfactory relief of pain. More often than not, the period of pain relief is short, ranging from six weeks to

six months, but there has been an occasional exception for
as long as four years. One limiting factor, when applied
to the patient with cancer, is an inability of the agent
to penetrate the nerve root, if it is encased in tumor.

Complication rates are low, primarily bladder or
muscle weakness. Of course, with pain ablation, numbness
or dysesthesia must be an acceptable consequence.

Surgical rhizotomy, or root section, has primary
application to the cranial nerves where an autonomous dermatomal supply is seen. The trigeminal nerve is the most
common candidate and rhizotomy can be accomplished by either
open surgery or thermal coagulation. Thermal coagulation
is the present treatment of choice, and it is accomplished
by a percutaneous insertion of the needle into the area of
the Gasserian ganglion by way of the foramen ovale. Once
the needle has been placed, there is the alternative of
using a necrotizing agent like alcohol or phenol, hot water
or glycerol, or the radiofrequency current.

Unfortunately, the result is not always as salutary as
desired in that there may be distressing side effects in the
form of dysesthesiae and complicating cranial nerve palsies.
When posterior roots of nerves in the thoracic area are to
be cut, in order to be effective, it is necessary not only
to section the immediate root giving rise to pain, but at
least two or three above and below that level. This is a
major operation for which the indication is relatively rare.

Another form of peripheral nerve ablation is
neurectomy. This also has limited application, for the
same reason. It is primarily applied to peripheral portions
of the cranial nerves and, again, the duration of relief is
short-lived, ranging from five months to three years.

The procedure of greatest use is percutaneous
chordotomy. This procedure is applicable to pain originating
anywhere from below the level of the mandible, whether the
pain be unilateral or bilateral in origin. Among a series
of 1300 chordotomies in some 800 patients, there have been
468 cancer patients who have undergone chordotomy for pain
(Rosomoff, 1969).

The most prevalent site of malignancy was pain from
cancer of the lung, followed by colon and rectum. The GI

tract, female genital tract, and breast were the next most common etiologies. Almost all forms of cancer have had chordotomy for relief of pain.

The most common location of pain has been in the back and lower extremities, followed by the abdomen, thorax, and neck and upper extremities.

Unilateral chordotomies were more common than bilateral, despite the presence of pain in the abdominal viscera which commonly is thought to require a bilateral procedure. When the pain is on one side of the abdomen, a unilateral procedure does suffice. Approximately 14% of the chordotomies had to be repeated, when the original procedure was found to be ineffective or there was a failure to hold the chordotomy level. This was usually a problem with technique, which was easily corrected, when the repeat procedure was accomplished.

In order to afford maximum protection, high levels of analgesia were purposefully sought, since it is necessary to allow for a fall in analgesic level of somewhere between four and eight dermatomal segments, or else the fall of analgesia may come within the area of the painful stimulation.

It was found that the chordotomy levels, by and large, were maintained at follow-up examination; in fact, some were even higher. It was true that some did slip, as would have been anticipated, and there were some in which the levels disappeared completely or became spotty in nature. If pain was still present or returned, it was necessary to repeat the chordotomy in order to regain the pain-free state.

Permanent complications were infrequent, although there was a temporary incidence of paresis in 4% of the patients. If the patient lived sufficiently long, the weakness improved or disappeared. In fact, the weakness would have disappeared in all, had the survival time been long enough to effect rehabilitation. Ataxia was a more common phenomenon, because it is necessary to trespass the ventral spinocerebellar tract in order to reach the pain fibers. Surprisingly, urinary retention was not common. This makes percutaneous chordotomy much more desirable than open surgical chordotomy, where the incidence of paresis, urinary bladder, and bowel complications is extremely high. With the necessity for high levels of analgesia, particularly with

bilateral lesions in the upper thorax or brachial plexus,
the risk of respiratory complications in the form of sleep-
induced apnea was found. This was seen particularly where
there was major impairment of pulmonary function from
disease. The 4% incidence of this complication is still
acceptable, since sleep-induced apnea is most often self-
limiting, if the patient can be supported during the period
of recovery. Spontaneous ventilation will return, with a
pain-free existence.

The very nature of the cancer problem precludes long-
term follow-up. The majority of patients died within the
first year following the procedure, and most did not survive
beyond the second year.

Initial success for the procedure was high, some 94%.
This did tend to fall off with time, but at the end of the
first year there was still an 80% effective level of relief.
This certainly proved to be a major contribution to a
happier existence with the elimination of pain and its
associated dependence on narcotics.

Another form of pain tract ablation is section of the
descending tract for pain subserving the cranial nerves.
This requires exposure of the brain stem, and it is
applicable to head and neck pain deriving from cancer of
that area. It is possible to selectively ablate areas served
by the trigeminal or other cranial nerves; the procedure
can be most effective.

Unfortunately, the ability to display the anatomy in
true life is not as easy as in the anatomical charts. The
major complication in this procedure is the inadvertent
section or occlusion of brain stem vessels which can give
rise to ischemia of that area and ensuing neurologic
deficits.

As we move up the brain stem, stimulation of the periaqueductal gray area by an implanted electrode has been
utilized with cancer patients. This is an attempt to
stimulate the release of endogenous opioids. The number of
patients so treated has been too small for statistical
analysis. It is presently an investigational technique
with some promise (Richardson, 1979).

Thalamotomy for pain relief is another procedure with

limited application. This is another form of stereotactic
surgery with insertion of electrode into the thalamus and
the receptive areas for pain fibers. Generally, a
bilateral thalamotomy is necessary in order to produce
effective relief and this may become a problem when a
bilateral procedure produces hypokinesia or paucity of movement
and flatness of affect. It has not proved to be long-lasting
in its effectiveness, but it is another alternative for pain
relief (Sano, 1979).

The psychosurgical approach, or leukotomy, removes the
suffering from the pain and suffering cycle. Individuals
who have undergone leukotomy do not complain of pain,
although they will indicate pain is present when asked
directly. It is the interpretive mechanism that has been
destroyed. The patient may appreciate the reception of
pain, but it has no meaning and is not distressing. This,
too, is a procedure of very limited application and short-
lived expectation. This was once used extensively for
carcinoma of the lung with brachial infiltration. It was a
reasonably successful procedure for periods as long as
three months, but thereafter was doomed to fail.

The last surgical approach to be discussed is that of
hypophysectomy. Originally, the procedure was proposed for
endocrine dependent cancers like breast and prostate. This
was accomplished by craniotomy and the results varied from
series to series. It was estimated that some 50% of
individuals were placed into remission by this technique.

More recently, chemical hypophysectomy has been
popularized by Moricca, 1974. It is claimed that pain
relief can be achieved for all forms of cancer, whether or
not the tissue be endocrine-dependent. The procedure is
accomplished by insertion of needles through the nasopharynx
and base of the skull into the pituitary gland where alcohol
is injected. Some 40% or more have good pain relief after
pituitary alcohol injection (Miles, 1979). They may become endocrine-dependent because of pituitary ablation and,
of course, this is a drawback to the procedure.

The complication rate is low; the most important ones
being that of CSF rhinorrhea and cranial nerve palsies.

SUMMARY AND CONCLUSIONS: The neurosurgeon has many
approaches to pain control, depending on the location of the

cancer and its tissue characteristics. By far, the most common procedure to be employed is percutaneous chordotomy, which is relatively risk-free and easy for the patient to undergo. It is most important to recognize that pain relief should be effected early in the course of the disease before the ravages of drug addiction and the complications of directed therapy like radiation or chemotherapy have taken their toll. Inanition, under these circumstances, may well be the result of treatment and drugs, rather than the disease itself. We have often seen patients, once given pain relief, make sudden weight gains and go on to a comfortable existence for a surprisingly long period of time thereafter. It is urged that pain relief be considered early, as a major contribution to enhanced quality of living and longevity of survival.

Miles, J (1979) Chemical Hypophysectomy in Bonica, JJ Ventafridda, V (ed): Advances in Pain Research and Therapy Vol 2 Raven Press New York p 373.

Moricca (1974) Chemical Hypophysectomy for Cancer Pain in Bonica, JJ (ed): Advances in Neurology Vol 4 Raven Press New York p 707.

Richardson, DE (1979) Central Gray Stimulation for Control of Cancer Pain in Bonica, JJ Ventafridda, V (ed): Advances in Pain Research and Therapy Vol 2 Raven Press New York p 487.

Rosomoff, HL (1969) Neurosurgical Control of Pain Ann Rev Med 20:189.

Rosomoff, HL (1974) Percutaneous Radiofrequency Cervical Cordotomy for Intractable Pain in Bonica, JJ (ed): Advances in Neurology Vol 4 Raven Press New York p 683.

Sano, K (1979) Sterotaxic Thalamolaminotomy and Posteromedial Hypothalamotomy for Relief of Intractable Pain in Bonica, JJ Ventafridda, V (ed): Advance in Pain Research and Therapy Vol 2 Raven Press New York p 475.

13th International Cancer Congress, Part D
Research and Treatment, pages 33–53
© 1983 Alan R. Liss, Inc., 150 Fifth Avenue, New York, NY 10011

CANCER PAIN: EVALUATION OF ELECTROMYOGRAPHIC AND
ELECTRODERMAL FEEDBACK

Sophia S. Fotopoulos, Mary R. Cook,
Charles Graham, Harvey Cohen, Mary Gerkovich,
Susan S. Bond, and Theodore Knapp

Midwest Research Institute

Pain is highly prevalent in patients with metastatic
or recurrent cancer and in certain tumor types such as primary bone tumor or carcinoma of the cervix (Bonica, 1980;
Foley, 1979). Cancer pain is a complex neuropsychophysio-
logic phenomenon which incorporates physical sensations,
underlying biochemical and physiological mechanisms, and
affective and cognitive factors. These components interact
and determine the totality of pain sensation and perception
(Graham, Bond, Gerkovich and Cook, 1980; Crue and Pinsky,
1981). When perpetuated, pain causes progressive psychophysiological deterioration which contributes to the overall
energy depletion and severe debilitation of the patient.
As Bonica's (1980) review aptly points out, there are many
facets of somatogenic and psychogenic cancer pain, including:
emotional, behavioral, social and physiological, as well as
pain induced by the oncologic process itself, e.g., infiltration of nerve roots by the tumor.

Physiological mechanisms underlying the neuropsychophys-
iological aspects of pain are still being delineated. Stem-
ming from the current rudimentary knowledge of neurochemistry/
physiology, theories such as central versus peripheral, and
pain as sensation versus perception, etc., are still being
argued (Crue, 1981). The spinocervical tract, neospinal
tract and possibly the postsynaptic elements in the dorsal
column seem to influence the sensory-discriminative aspects
of pain (Melzack and Dennis, 1980). Affective and emotional
components of pain are reflections of the limbic system and
brainstem reticular formation which are influenced by the
spinoreticular and paleo-spinothalamic parts of the

anterolateral somatosensory pathway (Melzack, 1968). Receptors play an increasingly important role in understanding underlying mechanisms and in establishing treatment regimes for patients with cancer pain. Pain perception thresholds and pain tolerance thresholds are decreased in patients with chronic pain, which may be due to the depletion of endorphins found in these people compared to healthy normals (Almay et al., 1978).

Affective, sensory and perceptual components of pain can all be modulated by cognitive functions of identification, evaluation and selective input which are neurally transmitted rapidly to the cortex. Explicitly, the dorsal column and dorsolateral projection pathways play an important role in carrying information about the pain stimulus to the cortex, thus activating central control processes (Melzack and Dennis, 1980).

Cognitive functions appear to alter either pain perception or the pain threshold as exemplified by men who feel no pain after a serious wound, but feel considerable pain with a venipuncture (Beecher, 1959), the placebo response, and pain relief through suggestion (Orne, 1980). Electrophysiological and certain behavioral techniques are recent developments in pain treatment which aim at activating the putative endogenous pain-inhibitory mechanisms in the brain and spinal cord. Electrical stimulation (peripheral, spinal cord and deep brain) are used to ameliorate pain syndromes (Bonica, 1980); e.g., spinal axis stimulation (Campbell, 1981; Krainick et al., 1980; Lang et al., 1981; Shimoji et al., 1982; Speigel, 1982). In some cases, intracranial stimulation has been introduced to provide central control over pain mechanisms (e.g., Richardson and Akil, 1977; Thoden et al., 1979). While the precise mechanisms of action are under current debate, it is acknowledged that changes in the electrical responses of the central and peripheral nervous systems can result in reduction of perceived pain (e.g., Abols and Basbaum, 1981).

Chronic pain associated with cancer is a particularly important issue both for clinicians and research scientists (Bonica, 1980; Foley, 1981). Concurrent with the work of others in the area of cancer pain management (e.g., Levenson, 1981; McKegney et al., 1981), our laboratory has evaluated the efficacy of using certain electrophysiological and behavioral techniques in alleviating pain in cancer patients

(Fotopoulos et al., 1979; Graham et al., 1980; Fotopoulos et al., 1981). Electrophysiological monitoring and control of physiological processes through biofeedback techniques have been reviewed (e.g., Rees, 1981; Turk et al., 1981). Behavioral techniques such as hypnosis have also been used in pain management (Isele, 1982; Orne, 1980; Bonica, 1980), and recently have been applied to control of cancer pain (Barber, 1978; Barber, 1980; Orne, 1976; Sacerdote, 1970; Hilgard, 1975). However, few controlled studies on the effects of hypnosis on cancer pain (Noyes, 1981) have been reported. Minimal numbers of subjects (Bonica, 1980), lack of appropriate measures and methods of pain alleviation, and changes in the course of the disease or its treatment have hampered research in the area.

The present study utilized an A-B-A design, with subjects as their own controls, in evaluating skin conductance level (SCL) and electromyographic (EMG) feedback and hypnosis as possible techniques for controlling cancer pain. Half the subjects were assigned to a long baseline prior to treatment (5 weeks) and half to a long baseline after treatment (5 weeks). The experimental design is summarized in Table 1.

## EXPERIMENTAL METHODS AND PROCEDURES

The following measures were included: (a) extensive pre- and post-treatment physiologic and psychologic assessments; (b) multiple measures of physiological activation during biofeedback sessions; (c) assessment of pain parameters in the laboratory and at home; and (d) evaluation of the relationship between therapeutic success and the degree of physiologic control achieved.

The overall experimental program called for separate evaluation of the use of biofeedback or self-hypnosis in the treatment of cancer pain. Participation in the program was voluntary. Criteria for participation included: medical diagnosis involving carcinoma; current medical treatment specifically for pain; and ambulatory condition. When subjects completed the pretreatment assessment procedures described below, they were assigned on a pseudo-random basis to receive either biofeedback or self-hypnosis. Material presented in this article focuses on those subjects who were assigned to the EMG/SCL biofeedback experimental condition.

## T A B L E   1

### E X P E R I M E N T A L   D E S I G N

| CODE | NO. OF DAYS | SHORT BASELINE GROUP | LONG BASELINE GROUP |
|---|---|---|---|
| 10 | 14 | Day of Intake to Day of Hypnosis Evaluation | Day of Intake to Day of Hypnosis Evaluation |
| 20 | 35 | Day of Hypnosis Evaluation through Last Day of Treatment | Day of Hypnosis Evaluation through Day of Last Weekly Review (20) |
| 30 | 14 | Day after Last Treatment through Day of 2nd Weekly Review (Includes 2nd administration of psychological tests and interview) | Day after Last Weekly Review through Day of 2nd Weekly Review (30) (Includes psychological tests and interview) |
| 40 | 35 | Day after 2nd Weekly Review (30) through Day of Last Weekly Review (40) | Day after 2nd Weekly Review (30) through Last Day of Treatment |
| 50 | 14 | Day after Last Weekly Review (40) through Day of 2nd Weekly Review (50) (Includes psychological tests and interview) | Day after Last Treatment through Day of 2nd Weekly Review (Includes psychological tests and interview) |

SCL was selected as a physiological feedback parameter because it is a direct measure of sympathetic nervous system (SNS) activity. EMG feedback was chosen in an attempt to control or decrease skeletomuscular activity resulting in a general physiological state of low autonomic activation with a concomitant subjective state of comfort. Experimentation evaluating 4-8 Hz electroencephalographic (EEG) plus EMG feedback and results of a psychophysiologic battery were previously reported (Fotopoulos et al., 1979).

## Pretreatment Measures

Pretreatment psychologic and demographic measures were taken. The initial interview included a short sociodemographic inventory (age, sex, race, ethnic origin, and background) and a detailed pain history. In the second assessment session, a psychologic test battery was administered which consisted of: Eysenck Personality Inventory (EPI), Repression-Sensitization Scale (RS), Ego-strength (ES), Locus of Control (LOC), and the McGill Pain Questionnaire (MPQ). As a final pretreatment measure, all subjects were individually administered a standardized hypnotic susceptibility scale (Stanford Scale of Hypnotic Susceptibility, Form C: Weitzenhoffer and Hilgard, 1962).

## Subjects

The subject population, pseudorandomly assigned to the EMG/SCL biofeedback condition, consisted of eight females and four males between the ages of 41 and 62 with a $\bar{x}$ age of 52.3 years. The most common diagnoses were carcinoma of the breast and lung (see Table 2). Subjects had been in pain an average of 12.1 months and were using both narcotics ($\bar{x}$ = 10.04 mg morphine equivalent per day) and nonnarcotic analgesics ($\bar{x}$ = 1,204 mg aspirin equivalent per day).

## Biofeedback Procedures

The study protocol consisted of 11 biofeedback treatment sessions to be administered over a 5-week period; during the first week, three sessions were scheduled, with two sessions a week scheduled for each of the remaining 4 weeks.

T A B L E   2

PRE-TREATMENT  CHARACTERISTICS  OF  SUBJECTS'
SOCIODEMOGRAPHIC  AND  MEDICAL  DATA

| Subject | Age | Sex | Race | Marital Status | Hollingshead Index | Months Since Diagnosis | Months of Reported Pain | Diagnosis |
|---|---|---|---|---|---|---|---|---|
| 21 | 51 | M | C | M | 32 | 12 | 4 | Malignant Melanoma |
| 25 | 53 | M | C | M | 35 | 11 | 12 | Adenocarcinoma, Lung |
| 27 | 48 | F | C | M | 53 | 35 | 5 | Adenocarcinoma, Vagina |
| 28 | 47 | F | 0 | M | 66 | 38 | 32 | Metastatic carcinoma |
| 29 | 57 | F | C | D | 50 | 49 | 5 | Metastatic carcinoma |
| 30 | 62 | M | N | W | 16 | 26 | 26 | Squamous cell carcinoma |
| 31 | 53 | M | N | S | 19 | 103 | 8 | Metastatic adenocarcinoma |
| 32 | 41 | F | C | M | 66 | 9 | 3 | Adenocarcinoma |
| 34 | 60 | F | C | D | 42 | 32 | 9 | Leiomyosarcoma |
| 35 | 58 | F | C | M | 32 | 32 | 1 | Uterine carcinoma |
| 36 | 47 | F | C | M | 38 | 23 | 23 | Adenocarcinoma |
| 37 | 51 | F | C | M | 42 | 49 | 17 | Adenocarcinoma |

Prior to each biofeedback session, the subject rated his/her pain, using a 100-point analog scale. Measures of weight, oral temperature, blood pressure, pulse, and respiration rate were obtained. Electrodes were then attached to standard recording sites over the frontalis to monitor EMG activity and to the second and fourth fingers of the nondominant hand to measure SCL (see Table 3). The session protocol is shown in Table 4. Three 2-min physiologic baselines were obtained: sitting quietly with eyes open; then eyes closed; followed by a volitional control period during which the subject was asked to relax (e.g., decrease muscle firing) as much as possible without feedback. Then a 15-min biofeedback period ensued, during which the subject heard a tone whose pitch was proportional to the degree of muscle firing in the frontalis muscle. The lower the tone, the lower the muscle activity. The subject was instructed to let the tone go lower and lower. An operant conditioning shaping procedure was used to reinforce reduction of muscle potentials. Specified levels of EMG activity at or below baseline EMG activity were established as thresholds. Each subject was required to produce EMG activity below this specified microvolt threshold 50% of the time in order to obtain (hear) the feedback tone. Based on this criterion, and the subject's physiological (EMG) changes, the threshold was changed at 1-min intervals. A generalization of training technique was also instituted, consisting of a standard deep breathing respiratory maneuver paired with biofeedback during each session. Following the EMG biofeedback, there was a 15-min SCL feedback period. Again, according to the subject's session baseline, SCL activity thresholds were set where the subject would receive a biofeedback tone which decreased in pitch with decreasing SCL. At the end of each session EMG and SCL measurement were repeated under baseline eyes closed, eyes open, and volitional control conditions. Transducers were then removed from the subjects, and they were asked to rate their pain again on the pain rating scale, as well as their success in controlling the feedback tone.


Apparatus

EMG signals from bipolar biopotential electrodes were amplified by an Autogen Model 1500 and quantified with a voltage-to-frequency converter and counter system, Model 910, ANL 600, made by Med Associates. Skin conductance was measured by the constant voltage method using a 9844 coupler in a Beckman RM Dynagraph recorder.

TABLE 3

P H Y S I O L O G I C   M E A S U R E S

| MEASURE | RECORDING SITE | PURPOSE |
|---|---|---|
| ELECTROMYOGRAPH (EMG) | FRONTALIS | EVALUATION OF PATTERNS OF SKELETAL MUSCLE RESPONSE |
| SKIN CONDUCTANCE LEVEL (SCL) | 2ND & 4TH FINGERS OF NONDOMINANT HAND | EVALUATE AUTONOMIC BASE LEVEL RESPONSIBILITY |
| TEMPERATURE (TEMP) | ORAL | EVALUATE METABOLIC AND HOMEOSTATIC LABILITY |
| BLOOD PRESSURE (BP) | NONDOMINANT ARM | CARDIOVASCULAR MONITORING |
| RESPIRATION (R) | HALFWAY BETWEEN UMBILICUS AND XYPHOID PROCESS | EVALUATE RELATIONSHIP BETWEEN RESPIRATORY AND AUTONOMIC CHANGES |

## T A B L E   4

### E X P E R I M E N T A L   B I O F E E D B A C K
### S E S S I O N S

PRE & POST SESSION:

    PAIN RATING
    ORAL TEMPERATURE
    BLOOD PRESSURE
    PULSE RATE
    RESPIRATION RATE

SESSION:

    BASELINES:

| | |
|---|---|
| UNINSTRUCTED SITTING | 2 MIN |
| INSTRUCTED EYES OPEN | 2 MIN |
| INSTRUCTED EYES CLOSED | 2 MIN |
| INSTRUCTED VOLITIONAL CONTROL | 2 MIN |

    TREATMENT:

| | |
|---|---|
| EMG FEEDBACK | 15 MIN |
| SCL FEEDBACK | 15 MIN |

    BASELINES:

| | |
|---|---|
| INSTRUCTED EYES OPEN | 2 MIN |
| INSTRUCTED EYES CLOSED | 2 MIN |
| INSTRUCTED VOLITIONAL CONTROL | 2 MIN |
| UNINSTRUCTED SITTING | 2 MIN |

RESULTS

Pretreatment Characteristics of Subjects

Table 2 summarized major sociodemographic and medical information about the subjects; Table 5 presents psychological test data, subjective pain ratings, and analgesic medication usage during the baseline period. Correlational analysis indicated that females reported less pain than males, and had lower average intake of narcotic analgesics. Subjects with higher educational levels reported less pain. It is of particular interest that while scores on the "chance" sub-scale of the Locus of Control Scale were positively correlated with subjective pain ratings, no such relationship was seen for the "internal" sub-scale. Repression-sensitization (RS) scores predicted non-narcotic analgesic use, with the greater the sensitization the more non-narcotic use; but RS was not related to subjective pain reports. Brief Symptom Index scores (GT, GSI, PSDI, SOM)* were positively correlated with subjective pain, but were unrelated to analgesic drug use. To further investigate this correlational result, t-tests were conducted between "high" and "low" pain patients (median split on baseline home pain ratings). The results are shown graphically in Figure 1.

Table 6 shows the effects of biofeedback on pain ratings and medication usage. Note that complete data are available on only five of the twelve subjects; six subjects died or became too ill to complete the protocol, and one moved away from the area. Significant pain relief in the laboratory was shown by three of the six subjects on whom sufficient data were available for analysis. Two of five subjects showed pain relief on a daily basis outside the laboratory, and three of five reduced their usage of analgesic medications. These data suggest that subjects 25 and 37 obtained good clinical pain reduction. Subject 21 had increased pain over the course of the treatment period, and subjects 29 and 32 remained relatively constant.

---

*  GT = Grand Total; GSI = General Severity Index; PSDI = Positive Symptom Distress Index; SOM = Somatization.

T A B L E   5

### Pre-Treatment Characteristics of Subjects'
### Psychological Test and Pain Data

| Instrument | Mean | S.D. | Range |
|---|---|---|---|
| State Trait Anxiety Inventory | | | |
|    Form 1 | 47.8 | 11.4 | 30 - 64 |
|    Form 2 | 50.2 | 9.1 | 33 - 60 |
| Repression - Sensitization Scale | 14.2 | 4.1 | 8 - 21 |
| Brief Symptom Index | 51.2 | 20.1 | 14 - 99 |
| Self-Esteem | 2.4 | 1.3 | 1 - 4 |
| Locus of Control | | | |
|    Internal | 13.7 | 5.0 | 5 - 21 |
|    Powerful Others | -9.3 | 10.9 | -24 - 9 |
|    Chance | -6.6 | 10.4 | -24 - 13 |
| Ego Strength | 33.2 | 7.7 | 23 - 46 |
| Hopelessness | 5.4 | 2.6 | 1 - 9 |
| Pain Rating (0 - 100) | | | |
|    Laboratory | 33.7 | 28.3 | 0 - 95 |
|    Home | 39.9 | 20.9 | 9 - 82 |
|    Physicians' Ratings | 49.9 | 25.5 | 10 - 90 |
| Medications | | | |
|    Morphine Equivalents | 10.1 | 21.4 | 0 - 80 mg |
|    Aspirin Equivalents | 2232 | 1737 | 0 - 4825 mg |

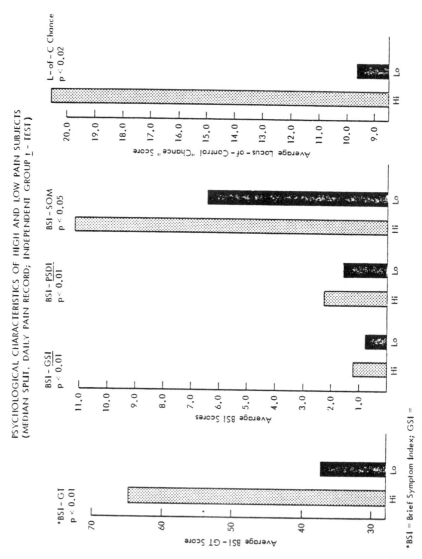

FIGURE 1

PSYCHOLOGICAL CHARACTERISTICS OF HIGH AND LOW PAIN SUBJECTS
(MEDIAN SPLIT, DAILY PAIN RECORD; INDEPENDENT GROUP $t$ - TEST)

*BSI = Brief Symptom Index; GSI =

T A B L E   6

EFFECTS  OF  TREATMENT  ON  SUBJECTIVE  PAIN  RATINGS
AND  ANALGESIC  DRUG  USE

| | Primary Site (Effects of BF Session) | | | Average Pain (Home Ratings) | | | Medication Use: MG Equivalent | | | | | |
|---|---|---|---|---|---|---|---|---|---|---|---|---|
| | | | | | | | Narcotic | | | Non-Narcotic | | |
| S | $\bar{X}$ Pre | $\bar{X}$ Post | p< | $\bar{X}$ Pre TX | $\bar{X}$ Post TX | p< | $\bar{X}$ Pre TX | $\bar{X}$ Post TX | p< | $\bar{X}$ Pre TX | $\bar{X}$ Post TX | p< |
| 21 | 27.7 | 28.2 | NS | 29.3 | 36.7 | NS | .1 | 0 | NS | 3140 | 10621 | .001 |
| 25 | 30.5 | 22.3 | .05 | 25.0 | 15.7 | .01 | 19.2 | 17.6 | .01 | 3853 | 3510 | .005 |
| 29 | 1.4 | .9 | NS | 3.8 | 3.3 | NS | | NA | | 279 | 0 | .05 |
| 32 | 30.9 | 23.6 | .10 | 50.3 | 50.0 | NS | .4 | 2.8 | NS | 1057 | 578 | .05 |
| 37 | 2.4 | .5 | .002 | 13.8 | 7.1 | .005 | | NA | | 3394 | 2879 | .05 |
| 27 | 27.5 | 15.8 | .05 | SUBJECT DIED BEFORE COMPLETING TREATMENT | | | | | | | | |

30  UNABLE TO COMPLETE PROGRAM

31  DIED AFTER FIRST BF SESSION

34  NEUROSURGERY PRIOR TO COMPLETION OF BASELINE PERIOD

35  UNABLE TO COMPLETE PROGRAM: DAILY RADIO THERAPY REQUIRED

36  UNABLE TO COMPLETE PROGRAM: TERMINAL HOSPITALIZATION AFTER BF SESSION 6

28  UNABLE TO COMPLETE PROGRAM: SUBJECT MOVED FROM AREA BEFORE COMPLETING BASELINE PERIOD

Table 7 presents data from the McGill Pain Questionnaire administered before and after treatment. Again, subjects 25 and 37 showed marked reduction in pain, subject 21 reported increased pain, and subjects 29 and 32 did not change.

Physiological learning data were examined to determine whether there was a relationship between learned control of EMG and SCL and clinical outcome. The learning criteria employed and the results are summarized in Table 8. Subjects 25 and 37, who reported the greatest pain relief, did not show the greatest physiological learning. Subject 25 appeared to learn control of SCL, but not of EMG, while subject 37 did not meet criterion on either system. Subject 21, whose pain ratings and medication usage increased during the treatment period, met learning criteria for SCL, but not for EMG. No relationship is, therefore, apparent between physiological learning and pain alleviation.

## DISCUSSION

These results clearly indicate the need for further work in the area using a different experimental paradigm. A double-blind crossover design is essential to determine actual learning of the biofeedback technique. As stated previously, the physiologic variables chosen for conditioning should be closely linked to the disease processes. Death and debilitation caused by the carcinomas and diverse treatment regimes are major problems in implementing research in the cancer pain area. In lieu of placebo groups, we chose an experimental paradigm which had long (5 week) pretreatment baselines. Since our patients were terminal and their prognosis poor, this lengthly baseline was a mistake. Many of the patients died or were incapacitated by the time they entered the treatment part of the study. Although in the past, placebos have not been considered appropriate in dying patient populations, that approach, in conjunction with a crossover, needs to be considered. It would also be advantageous to have a large number of subjects diagnosed at the same stage, with the same disease, in order to be able to choose the appropriate physiological feedback parameter. In addition, differences in baseline physiology could dictate the type of feedback to be utilized or explain subjects' ability to learn control over certain physiologic functions.

TABLE 7

## McGILL PAIN QUESTIONNAIRE DATA

| | SENSORY | | AFFECTIVE | | EVALUATIVE | | PRESENT PAIN INTENSITY | |
|---|---|---|---|---|---|---|---|---|
| | PRE | POST | PRE | POST | PRE | POST | PRE | POST |
| 21 | 10.0 | 15.0 | 2.5 | 7.0 | 2.0 | 3.0 | 2.0 | 2.0 |
| 25 | 21.5 | 10.5 | 6.5 | 2.5 | 4.0 | 3.5 | 3.0 | 2.0 |
| 29 | 3.0 | 3.0 | 0 | 0 | 0 | 1.0 | 0 | 0 |
| 32 | 22.5 | 26.5 | 0 | 0 | 1.5 | 2.0 | 2.5 | 2.5 |
| 37 | 31.5 | 20.5 | 5.5 | 2.0 | 2.5 | 2.0 | 1.5 | 1.0 |

TABLE 8

SUMMARY OF PHYSIOLOGICAL LEARNING DATA

| CRITERION | S: | 21 | | 25 | | 27 | | 29 | | 32 | | 37 | |
|---|---|---|---|---|---|---|---|---|---|---|---|---|---|
| | | EMG | SCL | EMG | SCL | EMG | SCL | EMG | SCL | EMG | SCL | EMG | SCL |
| **WITHIN SESSIONS** | | | | | | | | | | | | | |
| BASELINE: PRE > POST | | NO | YES | NO | .10 | YES | NO | NO | YES | NO | YES | .10 | YES |
| VOLITIONAL CONTROL: PRE > POST | | NO | YES | NO | NO | .10 | NO | NO | YES | YES | NO | NO | NO |
| LEVELS DURING FB < DURING BASELINE | | YES | YES | YES | YES | YES | NO | YES | YES | YES | YES | NO | YES |
| ORDERLY DECREASE OF LEVEL | | NO | YES | NO | YES | NO | YES | NO | YES | YES | NO | NO | NO |
| SPECIFICITY (LEVEL OF FB VARIABLE LOWER THAN LEVEL OF NON-FB VARIABLE) | | YES | YES | NO | .10 | NO | NO | NO | YES | YES | NO | NO | NO |
| **ACROSS SESSIONS** | | | | | | | | | | | | | |
| ORDERLY DECREASE OF LEVEL | | YES | YES | YES | YES | NO | NO | YES | YES | NO | NO | NO | YES |
| MEETS 60% OF LEARNING CRITERIA? | | NO | YES | NO | YES | NO | NO | NO | YES | YES | NO | NO | NO |

YES = P < .05
NO = P > .10
.10 = TREND

Theoretically, and on the basis of our previous experience with cancer patients and stress alleviation in other populations, we expected that decreasing SNS and/or skeletal muscle activity would result in decreased pain. Because of the minimal physiological learning observed in the present study, this question remains unanswered. However, in addition to a possible placebo effect, there are several other issues which need to be addressed. These are: appropriateness of the physiologic feedback parameters; and appropriateness of the experimental procedures.

The low level of learning observed suggests that the biofeedback parameters chosen were not right or the specific manner in which the study was implemented was not appropriate. Using the frontalis as the site for monitoring and controlling EMG activity was probably an error. Electrode placement at the major site of pain, at the innervation of a major muscle group near the pain site, or at a muscular site where the patient "feels" the most stress appear to be appropriate sites for EMG feedback. Although we used this approach in our original study of cancer pain and found no differences related to electrode placement, the issue should be examined again using a different operant or classical/operant procedure. Skin conductance activity was learned in some subjects and shows some promise for use in future work. Electrode placement appears to be appropriate although conductance levels from other parts of the body (e.g., abdominal), or near the major pain site, etc., should be evaluated.

Reduction of autonomic activity is theoretically sound in attempting to alleviate pain. The specific biofeedback method(s) for controlling or decreasing pain have not as yet been determined. For example, the most appropriate shaping procedures and reinforcement schedules for controlling EMG and SCL are still unknown and need to be studied in a controlled manner. The current study used a fixed interval and fixed ratio schedule for EMG; in this instance a fixed ratio alone linked to physiological threshold changes might have been more effective in obtaining learning. In addition, the SCL feedback was implemented using high versus low tones to indicate changes in SCL. A better procedure would include periods of no sound when subject's SCL went above baseline level or out of the established threshold range established through the session.

Appropriate feedback parameters based on the disease process and conditioning procedures (shaping, schedules of reinforcement, etc.), be they operant, classical, or combinations, need to be delineated. In addition, bootstrapping techniques such as electrical stimulation, pharmacology plus biofeedback need to be considered.

Many of us have stated the difficulties in performing studies in patients suffering with chronic pain. The disease process itself, which is often unpredictable and progressive, makes the control of these types of studies extremely difficult. Changes in metabolic functioning, ANS and CNS, and medical regime changes, related to various aspects of the disease, cause changes in the motivation, participation ability, pre-post comparisons, and generalization of treatment techniques and effects. Since the patients' health is always foremost, we cannot change chemotherapy or other medications in order to gain more experimental control. However, such factors can be taken into account when designing experimental studies for the treatment for cancer-related pain.

As indicated in our previous studies (Fotopoulos et al., 1979), the efficacy of using biofeedback techniques should continue to be evaluated. Factors of note which need to be considered when discussing the current study are numerous. For example, the cancer pain patients who participated in this study were referred only after other sources of pain relief were exhausted and had proved unsuccessful and biofeedback was presented as the "last resort." In addition, patients had been taking considerable pain medication (narcotic and nonnarcotic) for a period of more than 10 months in which they were in pain. As previously indicated, the choice of feedback parameters, autonomic, CNS, or a combination, is yet to be determined, as is the effectiveness of this technique(s) in controlling cancer pain in patients, when used earlier in the patients' pain/disease process.

Taking into consideration the aforementioned factors, a series of experiments needs to be designed and systematically implemented in order to determine the types of feedback and/or combined techniques which would be effective in alleviating cancer pain and its concomitant deleterious effects. In addition, the efficacy of using these techniques versus state-of-the-art pharmacological regimens needs to be determined.

There is one critical point of which we can not lose sight--the needs of the cancer patient. The success of any treatment method must be based not only on the validity of the research techniques but, as importantly, on the timeliness and effectiveness of the treatment in mitigating the symptoms to the utmost benefit of the patient.

# REFERENCES

Abols IA, Basbaum AI (1981). Afferent connections of the rostral medulla of the cat: A neural substrate for midbrain-medullary interactions in the modulation of pain. J Compar Neurol 201:285.

Almay BGL, Johansson F, von Knorring L, Terenius L, Wahlstrom LA (1978). Endorphins in chronic pain 1. Differences in CSF endorphin levels between organic and psychogenic pain syndrome. Pain 5:153.

Barber J (1978). Hypnosis as a psychological technique in the management of cancer pain. Cancer Nursing 1:361.

Barber J, Gitelson J (1980). Cancer pain: Psychological management using hypnosis. CA-A Cancer J Clin 30:131.

Beecher HK (1959). "Measurement of Subjective Responses." New York: Oxford University Press.

Bonica JJ (1980). Cancer pain. Res Publ - Assoc Res Nervous and Mental Diseases 58:335.

Campbell JN (1981). Examination of possible mechanisms by which stimulation of the spinal cord in man relieves pain. Appl Neurophys 44:181.

Crue BL, Pinsky JJ (1980). Chronic pain syndrome four aspects of the problem: New hope pain center and pain research foundation. Natl Inst Drug Abuse Res Monog Series 36:137.

Foley KM (1979). Pain syndromes in patients with cancer. In Bonica JJ, Ventafridda V (eds.): "Advances in Pain Research and Therapy," New York: Raven Press.

Foley KM (1979). The management of pain of malignant origin. In Tyler HR, Dawson DM (eds.): "Current Neurology Vol II," Boston: Haughton, Mifflin, p 279.

Foley KM (1980). Current issues in the management of cancer pain: Memorial Sloan-Kettering Cancer Center. NIDA Res Monog Ser 36:169.

Fotopoulos SS, Graham C, Cook MR (1979). Psychophysiological control of cancer pain. In Bonica JJ, Ventafridda V (eds.), "Advances in Pain Research and Therapy Vol 2," New York: Raven Press.

Fotopoulos SS, Knapp TM, Bond SB, Gerkovich MM, Cook MR, Graham C (1981). Evaluation of EEG, EMG and SCL feedback for cancer pain alleviation. Biol Psychol.

Graham C, Bond SS, Gerkovich MM, Cook MR (1980). Use of the McGill Pain Questionnaire in the assessment of cancer pain: Replicability and consistency. Pain 8:377.

Hilgard ER (1975). The alleviation of pain by hypnosis. Pain 1:213.

Isele FW (1982). Biofeedback and hypnosis in the management of pain. NY State J Med 82:38.

Krainick J, Thoden U, Riechert T (1980). Pain reduction in amputees by long-term spinal cord stimulation: Long-term follow-up study over 5 years. J Neurosurg 52:346.

Levenson BS (1981). A multidimensional approach to the treatment of pain in the oncology patient. Frontiers Rad Ther Oncol 15:138.

Long DM, Erickson D, Campbell J, North R (1981). Electrical stimulation of the spinal cord and peripheral nerves for pain control: A 10-year experience. Appl Neurophys 44:207.

McKegney FP, Bailey LR, Yates JW (1981). Prediction and management of pain in patients with advanced cancer. Gen Hosp Psychiat 3:95.

Melzack R, Dennis SG (1980). Neurophysiological foundations of pain. In Sternback RA (ed.), "The Psychology of Pain," New York: Raven Press, p 1.

Melzack R, Casey KL (1968). In Kenshalo D (ed.), "The Skin Senses," Springfield: Thomas.

Myers SJ, Janal MN, Pai LT, Clark WC (1982). A model of clinical pain: Technique for evaluation of analgesic agents. Am J Phys Med 61:1.

Noyes R Jr (1981). Treatment of cancer pain. Psychosom Med 43:57.

Orne MT (1974). Pain suppression by hypnosis and related phenomena. In Bonica JJ (ed.), "Advances in Neurology," New York: Raven Press, p 563.

Orne MT (1976). Mechanisms of hypnotic pain control. In Bonica JJ, Albe-Fessard D (eds.), "Advances in Pain Research and Therapy Vol 1," New York: Raven Press, p 717.

Orne MT (1980). Hypnotic control of pain: Toward a clarification of the different psychological processes involved. Res Publ - Assoc Res Nervous and Mental Diseases 58:155.

Rees L (1981). Biofeedback. J Irish Med Assoc Suppl 72:19.

Richardson DE, Akil H (1977). Pain reduction by electrical brain stimulation in man. J Neurosurg 47:178.

Richardson RR, Meyer PR, Cerullo LK (1980). Neurostimulation in the modulation of intractable paraplegic and traumatic neuroma pains. Pain 8:75.

Sacerdote P (1970). Theory and practice of pain control in malignancy and other protracted or recurring painful illness. Int J Clin Exp Hypn 18:160.

Shimoji K, Shimizu H, Maruyama Y, Matsuki M, Kuribayashi H, Fujioka H (1982). Dorsal column stimulation in man: Facilitation of primary afferent depolarization. Anesth Analg 61:410.

Spiegel EA (1982). Relief of pain and spasticity by posterior column stimulation. Arch Neurol 39:184.

Thoden U, Doerr M, Dieckmann G, Krainick JU (1979). Medial thalamic permanent electrodes for pain control in man: An electrophysiological and clinical study. Electroenceph Clin Neurophys 47:582.

Turk DC, Meichenbaum DH, Berman WH (1981). Application of biofeedback for the regulation of pain: A critical review. Psych Bull 86:1322.

Weitzenhoffer AM, Hilgard ER (1962). "Stanford Hypnotic Susceptibility Scale, Form C." Palo Alto, California: Consulting Psychological Press.

CONGRESS SYMPOSIA

LIVER AND PANCREATIC NEOPLASIA Johannessen, J.V.,
Norway, Chairman; Weinhouse, S., USA, Co-Chairman;
Opera House

Early Detection - A Component of Prevention Strategy
of Liver Cancer. *Tsung-tang, S., and Xing-yao, H.,
Beiking, People's Republic of China.

Morphologic Expression of Neoplasia in Human and
Experimental Liver Tumors. *Lapis, K., Budapest,
Hungary.

Hepatitis B Virus and the Pathogenesis and Prevention of
Prevention of Cancer of the Liver. *Blumberg, B. S.,
Philadelphia, PA USA.

Biochemical Phenotype in Human and Animal Liver
Tumors. *Prajda, N., Budapest, Hungary.

Surgical Treatment of Human Liver Neoplasia.
*Fortner, J. G., New York, NY USA. (By Title Only)

Carcinoma of the Pancreas: Progress or Stalemate?
Hutchinson Jr., William B. and Wagner, Donald E.,
Seattle, WA USA.

Please note: Papers that are listed as "By Title
Only" were presented at the 13th International
Cancer Congress, but are not included in these
volumes.

13th International Cancer Congress, Part D
Research and Treatment, pages 57–66
© 1983 Alan R. Liss, Inc., 150 Fifth Avenue, New York, NY 10011

EARLY DETECTION –A COMPONENT OF PREVENTION
STRATEGY OF LIVER CANCER

Sun Tsung-tang, M.D.      Huang Xing-yao

Chief Dept of Immunol     Chief Surgeon
Cancer Institute CAMS      Cancer Institute
Beijing, China            Qidong, China

Liver cell cancer, arising from the hepatic parenchymal cells, constitutes more than 90% of human primary liver malignancies. Crude estimation indicated that more than 200,000 people died of this cancer each year in the world. It is a global health problem especially when its closely associated chronic liver disease is also taken into consideration (Sun in press). It appears to be certain that the basic approach which might lead to the ultimate control of liver cancer could only be offered by primary prevention, the prospect of which seems to be optimistic in the light of recent advances in this field. However, it needs a long time. Millions of people will die from this cancer before primary prevention starts to show its significant effect. Therefore, secondary prevention including early detection and successful treatment of liver cancer at its most curable stage of development should still be explored and be considered as an important component of control strategy on liver cancer. Serum AFP had been demonstrated to be a good marker of liver cell cancer (Abelev 1971), and its application in early detection had yielded encouraging results (Sun, Chu 1981; Chu 1981). In the present paper, the long term survival data and the biological basis of early detection of liver cancer will be summerized. In addition, the prospect and limitation of early detection approach will also be discussed on the basis of field trials.

EARLY DETECTION LEADS TO SIGNIFICANT INCREASE OF
6 YEAR SURVIVAL RATE

The real possibility of early detection of
liver cancer was demonstrated by the mass screening
conducted in Qidong and Shanghai areas of China
since 1974 (Sun, Tang, Chu 1981). The follow-up data
of one of the first series of patients detected and
treated during 1974-1975 in the high incidence Qidong
field was summerized in Table 1. The sero-positive

Table 1. 6 year survival rate of liver
cancer patients following AFP survey

| Patient group | I | II | III |
|---|---|---|---|
| AFP (ng/ml) | ≤1,000 | >1,000 | ≤1,000 |
| Treatment | surgery | surgery | medicine |
| 6 yr survival | 13/33(39%) | 4/64(6.3%) | 0/12(0%) |

individuals detected in screening were followed.
Those showing rising pattern of serum AFP were advi-
sed to accept surgical treatment. Patients with very
high level of AFP and in advanced stage were not
included. 12 patients of Group III who were found
early but refused to accept surgery after repeated
advises were treated by ordinary chemotherapy. They
all died of liver cancer development within 3 years.
In Group I, 33 patients treated by surgery before
their serum AFP had exceeded 1,000 ng/ml, 13 of them
(39%) had their tumor found and resected. They all
survive over 6 years after treatment and are still
healthy except one who had recurrence of hepatic
tumor in the sixth year. Since these patients were
detected from the general population without selection, their survival data will indicate the potential value of early detection of liver cancer in
areas of high incidence where the positivity rate
of AFP generally exceeds 80%. Several points pertinent to early detection merit further emphasis.

1. Gradually rising concentrations of serum AFP in
2 or more months over 400 ng/ml with an average
doubling time of 30-45 days is a reliable indication
of the presence of an expanding population of liver
cancer cells (Ji, Sun et al, 1979).

2. Early surgical treatment is the deciding factor
effecting the survival rate. Although the 6 year

survival rate of the group operated at AFP level around 1,000 ng/ml is significantly higher than other groups as well as the previous records, however, this empirically chosen operation moment was already too late for many cases in the same group due to the difference in AFP secretion capacity of the individual tumors.

3. Rapid fall of serum AFP after surgery to normal or to low fluctuating levels for more than 1 year is a good prognostic sign. Among the 13 patients surviving over 6 years after treatment, all had their post-operative AFP concentration maintained at low levels for more than 18 months.

4. Spatial identification of liver cancer at its earliest possible stages indicated by AFP serology is the critical procedure to stabilize and to further improve the results of early detection.

Liver cancer is a relatively fast growing malignancy. Estimation based on the doubling time of serum AFP indicated that the natural course of liver cancer developing through 30 doublings to become clinically evident will require about 3 years. Survival over 6 years after resection of the tumors could be considered to be cured of the original cancer. Recurrence later may more likely be the occurence de novo rather than the relapse of the first tumor. The relatively high long term survival rate of the consecutive series following early detection of an otherwise fatal disease gives encouragement to explore further the full potential of such an approach.

BIOLOGICAL BASIS OF EARLY DETECTION OF LIVER CANCER

The conventional concept on the growth of liver cancer is that multiple cancer nodules develop in various parts of hepatic tissue simultaneously as a result of multifocal origin of the malignant change. This concept was based on the observations made in clinical and autopsy cases. This issue is important for better understanding of the natural history of liver cancer development (Sun 1983), and also for rational approach to early detection. Surgical and pathological analysis on early liver cancers offered unique opportunities to re-examine this important issue.

Table 2. Surgico-pathological data showing localized growth of early liver cancer

| Patient name | Tumors found | Liver retained | Patient status |
|---|---|---|---|
| Chen W. | 6 cm. R.Ant. | 80% | 8 yr DFS* |
| Sung | 1.5cm. R.Post. | 95% | 8 yr DFS |
| Chen C. | 1.4cm. L.L. | 85% | 8 yr DFS |
| Mao | 2.5cm. L.M. | 80% | 8 yr DFS |
| Zeh | 2.3x2. L.L. | 80% | 7 yr DFS |
| Sze | 1.7cm. L. | 65% | 7 yr DFS |
| Chang Z. | 11 cm. R. | 60% | 7 yr DFS |
| Lu | 2 cm. L.L. | 80% | relapse in 6th yr |
| Chang Y. | 3 x 2. R. | 50% | 7 yr DFS |
| Chen L. | 18 cm. R. | 55% | 7 yr DFS |
| Wang | 2.5cm. R.Ant. | 90% | 7 yr DFS |
| Hou | 4 cm. L. | 65% | 7 yr DFS |
| Chen T. | 12 cm. R. | 55% | 7 yr DFS |
| King | 5 cm. L.M. | 85% | 7 yr DFS |
| Chen S. | 1.2x2. R.Post. | 80% | 6 yr DFS |

DFS*   Disease free survival

In second column, tumor size (its largest diameter), number of nodules (x 2 means two nodules) and its location (L. for left lobe; R. for right lobe) were given.

Exploratory laparotomies on patients detected early demonstrated that in contrast to situations seen in late cases, usually single or two nodules in close vicinity were found in such patients. Table 2 showed the surgico-pathological data of 15 patients, including the 13 from Group I of Table 1. These data showed that cancer might occur in any location within the hepatic mass, but the tumors in each case were confined in the limited resected part. Since majority of the hepatic tissues were conserved after the operation, new liver cancer might quickly develop from the major background if the tumor was multifocal in origin and thus occurred randomly in space within the liver. However, limited resection results in long term survival of the patients. Obviously, liver cancer at its early stages of development detectable by AFP serology still remain in majority of cases in localized state, being surgically resectable whenever identified spatially. The localized growth is probably of unifocal origin (Sun, Chu 1981). Multiple nodules occuring in vicinity is more likely the result of local spread, since it is frequent to observe several small satelite foci of tumor cells growing close-by the major cancer nodule. In addition to the 40% 6 year survivals of the Group I following limited resection, there were several cases found to have solitary tumors which were unresectable either due to its unfavorable locations or to the poor liver background. Taking together, they constituted more than 50% of the series of 33 patients. In the remaining part, there were either extensive growth of tumor or failures to locate the cancer in the depth of right lobes. They all died of advanced liver cancer within 3 years of follow-up. Although the growth behaviors of liver cancers in these patients could not be definitely assessed, evidences in favor of their multifocal origins were also lacking. Therefore, localized growth, probably as a result of the development of a single focus of cancer cells, appears to be the common biological behavior of human liver cell cancer at early stages. Widespread distribution of cancer nodules throughout the liver mass were late manifestations of the cancer growth, and did not constitute the proof of its multifocal origins. The concept of unifocal origin of hepatic cancer is also consistent with the estimation of the probability of concomitant occurrence of two or more tumors in the same individual. Liver cancer generally arises on the background of chronic liver disease having conspicuous liver cell hyperplasia (Sun et al 1979). The liver cancer incidence among individuals having such precancerous lesions was exceedingly high, reaching 3 to 6% per annum (Sun, Chu 1981; Chu 1981). The probability of two independent foci occuring simultaneously or overlappingly in the 3 year growth period will be well below 5%. The probability of more than 2 foci to grow in the same period is virtually negligible. Therefore, multifocal origin of liver cell cancer, if happened, would be a rare clinical phenomenon.

Liver cancer occurs in younger age groups in areas of prevalence where AFP positivity rate is also high. The capacity of such tumor cells to secret significant amount of AFP into the general circulation enables its detection much earlier than itself becoming clinically evident. Analysis of cell density and cell population data of early liver cancers indicated that the maximum population while still remaining in the localized state were in the range of $1.4 \times 10^8$ to over $10^9$ cells, depending on the biological behaviors of individual tumors (Sun in press). They should pass at least 27 doublings to reach this stage above which metastasis will occur in high likelihood. Since the 'borderline' level of serum AFP is around 1,000 ng/ml and sensitive immunoassays can detect it down to 20 ng/ml, which is close to its physiological levels, AFP serology permits earlier detection at 6 doublings ahead. Hence, the earliest liver cancer detectable by AFP screenings will be at 21 doublings. The six doublings, which extend about 6 months, offer the precious time period for early detection and curative treatment. As a conclusion, the unifocal origin, localized growth behavior at early stages and the relatively high capacity of AFP secretion forms the biological basis of possible early detection of human liver cell cancer in areas of high prevalence.

## SPATIAL IDENTIFICATION OF EARLY LIVER CANCER

The chief difficulties encountered so far in the early detection of liver cancer arose as the result of wide difference in AFP secretion capacity of individual tumors. On the basis of previous experience, 1,000 ng/ml was empirically selected as the demarcation line to urge prompt surgical intervention. However, many tumors already grew to the extent beyond resection, whereas some with high secretion capacity remained in small size and hid in the deep mass of the right lobe. Early liver cancer may be soft enough to escape even careful bimanual palpation. Thirdly, the extent of cirrhosis also limited the surgical approach. Only in cases of local resection of very small tumors, indications for

surgical treatment might be extended to. These 3
situations constituted the major causes of failure
in around 50% of the consecutive cases in Group I
mentioned previously where surgical intervention had
been adopted.Identification and spatial localization
of small liver cancers, if successfully solved, might
provide the common solution to the problems thus encountered. Hepatic angiography had been tried with
some success (Okuda, Nakashima 1979; Tang Zhaoyou
1980). However, non-traumatic approach, such as CT
and/or B-scan ultrasonography might be more desirable since they permit repeated examinations in
correlation with AFP dynamics. Analysis of the morphological characteristics of early liver cancers
indicated that their size, contour and possible difference in consistency might fascilitate such an
approach (Sun, Chu 1981). Preliminary study on 8
patients found in subclinical stages by serum AFP
measurements showed close correlation between AFP
dynamics, CT findings and subsequent clinico-pathological observations in each case(Huang Xing-yao et
al, 1982). Thus, in 3 patients having stabilized
serum AFP exceeding 2,000 ng/ml, CT scans revealed
large space occupying lesions in all cases. They
died within 6 months after being detected. 2 of them
got  pathological confirmation during surgery.  In
another 4 patients having rising pattern of serum
AFP approaching the level of 1,000 ng/ml, CT scans
demonstrated translucent areas of less absorbancy
having diameters from 2 to 5 cm  with regular  ·

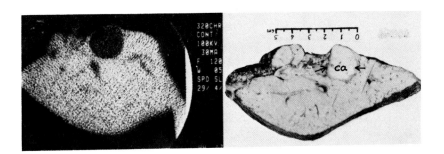

Fig. 1. CT scan and pathological picture of liver
cancer at early stage. CT scan of resected left lobe
showed well circumscribed area of reduced absorbancy
which correlated well with the morbid anatomy of
the tumor both in size and in location (right).

contour. Surgery was done in 3 of them, and the presence and location of liver cancers were confirmed in 2 patients. The resection of the localized tumor was followed by restoration of serum AFP to normal. CT scans showed clearer image of the tumor in the surgical specimen immersed in L-15 solution (Fig.1. left), and the reduced absorbancy of early cancers was partly related to the high lipid content as shown in Sudan stained histological sections. In one case, liver cancer could not be identified during surgery and in another, operation was postponed due to the acute epidsode of hepatitis. They died of advanced liver cancer 6 months later, having clinical signs consistent with location of tumors in right lobe as indicated by the CT scans. The 8th patient had a fluctuating type of serum AFP, with negative CT findings. He recovered from chronic hepatitis in the 2 years follow-up. The close correlation found in this small but varied group between AFP, CT and clinico-pathological observations will encourage further trials on a larger series detected early through AFP serology. However, surgical identification of small tumors even on the basis of positive CT indication still remains to be the issue to be solved. Besides, the large cost and additional risks associated with repeated examinations also poses limitation to the use of CT for this purpose.

B-scan ultrasonography might be an attractive approach for spatial identification of early liver cancers, but its potential in this area remains to be explored. Preliminary study on subclinical liver cancer patients showed some promise, but the contrast between tumor and adjacent tissue appeared to be less sharp than in case of CT scan (Huang et al, in preparation). The possible value of ultrasonography guided needle biopsy in identifying small cancers during operations also needs to be clarified.

LIMITATIONS AND PROSPECT OF EARLY DETECTION

Early detection of liver cancer so far presented is based on the use of AFP marker. Obviously, it is not applicable to AFP negative or weakly positive tumors. The percentage of such tumors may account for 20 to 50% of all liver cancer cases in some areas.

Therefore, efforts to seek for new markers should be stressed to expand the spectrum of early detection of liver cancers. Among the AFP positive members, the percentage of patients having multi-focal growth chiefly as a result of early intra-hepatic spread actually set the limit for the detectability of AFP positive cancers at the early stages resectable by surgical approach. The background liver disease also set limit to surgical indications among those who might suffer from severe hepatic decompensation following conventional operations. Obviously, if the identification and localization of small liver tumors could not be solved by the presently available technology, early detection of liver cancer will still remain in the stage of clinical investigations.

In spite of the limitations mentioned above, the prospect of early detection of liver cancer still appears to be optimistic. It is fortunate that AFP positivity rate is usually high in areas of prevalence where early detection should be expected. On the basis of field trials so far, it is rational to predict that majority of liver cancer could be found at the early resectable stages by means of AFP serology. The key link to push forward the early detection of liver cancer to its full potential is the solution of spatial identification of cancer sufficiently early to fascilitate prompt local excision. This will lead to the significant increase of survival probability among those detected through sero-surveys in areas of very high incidence and also among those people having chronic liver disease regularly monitored by liver function tests, including the serum AFP assay. Early detection will then become an important component of secondary prevention which might bring immediate benefit to patients of this otherwise fatal disease.

## REFERENCES

Abelev GI (1971). Alpha-fetoprotein in ontogenesis and its association with malignant tumors. Advances Cancer Res 14:295.
Chu Yuan-yun (1981). AFP sero-survey and early diagnosis of liver cell cancer in the Qidong field. Chin J Oncology 3:35. (in Chinese)

Huang X, Su X, Yu H, Chang Q, Sun T (1982). Preliminary study on CT localization of subclinical liver cell cancer. Kiangsu Med 8:42.

Huang X, Wang M, Chang Q, Chu S (1983). Ultrasonographic identification of early liver cancers. submitted for publication. (in Chinese)

Ji Zhen, Sun T, Wang L, Ding G, Chu P, Li F (1979). Characteristics of AFP serology in early liver ca & high risk group. Chin J Oncol 1:96. (in Chinese)

Okuda K, Nakashima T (1979). Hepatocellular carcinoma: A review of the recent studies and developments. In Popper H, Schaffner F (eds): "Progress in liver diseases" vol.V, New York: Grunne & Stratton, p.639.

Sun T, Wang N, Xia Q, Wang L, Zhang Y (1979): Pathological and serological investigation on early primary hepatocellular carcinoma and its liver disease background. Chin J Oncol 1:13. (in Chinese)

Sun T, Chu Y (1981). Early diagnosis of liver cancer and its preceding stage through AFP serology. In Burchenal JH, Oettgen HF (eds): "Cancer" vol.1, New York: Grunne & Stratton, p.651.

Sun T, Tang Z, Chu Y (1981). Epidemiology, early diagnosis and treatment of liver cell cancer. In DeCosse JJ & Sherlock P (eds): "Gastrointestinal cancer 1", Hague:Martisnus Nijhoff, p.387.

Sun T (1983). Studies on human liver carcinogenesis. In Harris CC, Autrup HN (eds): "Human carcinogenesis", New York: Academic Press, in press.

Sun T (in press). Prevention strategy of liver cancer. In WHO publication on Cancer Prevention Strategies.

Tang Z (1980). Screening and early treatment of primary liver cancer - with special reference to the eastern part of China. Annals Acad Med Singapore 9:234.

13th International Cancer Congress, Part D
Research and Treatment, pages 67-76
© 1983 Alan R. Liss, Inc., 150 Fifth Avenue, New York, NY 10011

MORPHOLOGIC EXPRESSION OF NEOPLASIA IN HUMAN AND
EXPERIMENTAL LIVER TUMORS

Károly Lapis, M.D.

Director, I. Institute of Pathology
and Experimental Cancer Research
Semmelweis Medical University
Budapest 1085, Hungary

There is an increasing interest in primary hepatocellular carcinoma /PHC/, first of all because
of the close association observed between hepatitis
B virus infection and liver cancer and because of
the trend of increasing incidence all over the world
/Popper 1978/. Clinically human liver cancer seems
to exist in two forms: one is characteristic for
the low, the other for the high incidence areas.

Macroscopically both types may be massive, nodular and diffuse in appearance /Edmondson 1958/.
Histologically highly, moderately differentiated,
undifferentiated, mixed and rare forms can be distinguished /Edmondson 1958; Lapis, Johannessen
1979/, each of which appears in various patterns
like trabecular, tubular, solid, sclerosing, clear
cell or hypernephroid, pleomorphic and spindle cell
form.

The degree of cytologic differentiation varies
considerably, in the judgement of which electronmicroscopy is particularly useful. Even in the differentiated form there is a decrease in the number
of bile canaliculi and their structure is also altered. Frequently in the undifferentiated form the
liver cell origin of the tumor can be proved only
by electronmicroscopy, revealing abortive bile canaliculi among the anaplastic tumor cells /Lapis,
Johannessen 1979/. Electronmicroscopy is also reliable in clarifying the nature of the frequent nuc-

lear and cytoplasmic inclusions, a special type of
which is the surface component of the hepatitis B
virus /HBsAg/. HBsAg containing orcein positive
ground glass hepatocytes have been frequently demonstrated also in tumorous livers, particularly in
the non-tumorous part of the liver. In certain cases
orcein positive materials were found also in some
of the liver cancer cells and the presence of HBsAg
could be demonstrated by electronmicroscopy as well.

While the morphologic aspects of fully developed liver cancer are known in detail, rather few
established knowledge is available concerning the
precancerous lesion in the human liver.

In most regions 80% of liver cancer occur in
cirrhotic liver. In a broader sense, the cirrhosis
itself, particularly the hyperplastic regenerative
nodules associated with it, could be regarded as a
precancerous condition, just as the nodular regenerative hyperplasia in the absence of fibrosis
/Qizilbash, Castelli 1980/, the partial nodular
transformation of the liver /Sherlock et al. 1966/,
and the hepatocellular adenomatosis. Liver cell
dysplasia /Anthony 1976/ has also been proven to be
a premalignant lesion. The focal nodular hyperplasia and the adenoma showing increasing incidence
with the wide-spread use of oral anticoncipients
should also be considered as possible premalignant
lesions /Christopherson, Mays 1979/.

In spite of these numerous potentially precancerous lesions the early events of hepatocarcinogenesis in human beings are not yet known.

Hepatocarcinogenesis has been, however, extensively studied in animal experiments /Williams 1980;
Bannasch et al. 1982/ and proved to be a multistep
process /Farber 1982/. In most of the various model
systems /Becker 1981; Emmelot, Scherer 1980; Peraino
et al. 1973; Pitot, Sirica 1980; Solt, Farber 1976/
used for such studies carcinogens as initiators and
promoters were applied in combination. We have also
carried out hepatocarcinogenesis experiments using
several model systems.

Independently of the model system used the basic alterations induced are similar, the time of appearance of which, however, varies according to treatment schedule. The first morphologically observable alterations are the foci of altered liver cells, which lesions are smaller than the size of a lobule, they do not compress the adjacent liver tissue and the architectural pattern is only slightly altered. They can be most easily revealed by their glycogen storage. Four distinctive types of foci: the clear cell, eosinophilic, basophilic and mixed cell foci have been described, recognizable by changes in staining characteristics, cell size and glycogen storage. Foci are followed by appearance of hyperplastic and neoplastic nodules, being larger lesions than the area of several lobules, roughly round, sometimes observable by the naked eye /Pitot, Sirica 1980/ and they disrupt and compress the surrounding liver parenchyma /Williams 1980/. Both altered foci and neoplastic nodules have several common properties, distinguishing their composing cell population from the surrounding hepatocytes.

At ultrastructural level cells of clear cell and eosinophilic foci are characterized by large fields of accumulated glycogen granules, storage of lipid droplets, decreased amount of parallel-arrayed rough endoplasmic reticulum /Bannasch et al. 1982; Williams 1980/, pronounced proliferation of smooth endoplasmic reticulum with fingerprint formation. The basophilic cell type is characterized by increased amount of polyribosomes accompanied by loss of cytoplasmic glycogen.

Both altered foci and neoplastic nodules can be recognized most reliably by the number of their functional abnormalities which can be revealed by special histochemical techniques. The loss, decrease, or increase of activity of a branch of enzymes were found to be characteristic for these early lesions /Pitot, Sirica 1980/, out of which the loss of glycose-6-Pase and membrane-bound canalicular ATPase and the increase of $\gamma$-glutamyl-transpeptidase /GGT/ are the most striking and constant. Slight variations may exist in enzymatic pattern between foci, but each focus displays a rather uniform profile of histochemical abnormalities /Ogawa et al. 1980/.

Concerning the coincidence of the various enzymatically altered foci we have found by morphometric methods that at least in the case of the three enzymes studied /GGT, G-6-P, ATP/ the proportion of the enzymatically altered areas was almost the same.

The neoplastic nodules may be more heterogeneous in enzymatic pattern; persistent and remodeling types have been distinguished /Enomoto et al. 1981/. While the persistent type remains uniform like the foci, the remodeling type shows irregular patchy staining for some marker enzymes.

Analysing separately the isolated nodules, biochemically the most striking alteration observed was the high GGT activity. There were nodules in which practically no G-6-Pase could be detected, while in others only its modest decrease was observable. In a large majority of the nodules the amount of cytochrome P450 is extremely low. This might be the basis of increased resistence of the cells composing the foci and the nodules against the cytotoxic effect of the carcinogen applied.

Out of the other distinctive biologic features of these lesions the most constant is the loss of concentration ability for iron of the tumor cells /Williams 1980/. Recently we have studied the alteration of fibronectin production in injured livers among others during hepatocarcinogenesis /Szendrői et al. 1982/. In normal liver small amount of fibronectin can be found along the sinusoids. In the neoplastic nodules, its amount is remarkably increased, the distribution changed and even more interesting is that the altered hepatocytes composing the nodules seem to produce fibronectin as demonstrable by immunfluorescence technique.

The fully developed chemically induced liver cancer usually has the same histologic types as human hepatocellular carcinomas.

The progress for development of carcinomas from foci or nodules is poorly understood. Over 90% of foci disappeared if exposure to carcinogen or promoter was terminated. This phenomenon is called phenotypic reversion. Some foci, however, may possess a more stable alteration in phenotype providing them an independent growth ability /Williams 1980/.

Views are more differing concerning the nature and possible further development of the nodules. By some authors they are considered hyperplastic and not neoplastic in nature, as their persistence and continued proliferation frequently proved to be environment dependent and reversible /Farber 1982/. On the other hand, two international workshops /National Academy of Sciences 1980; Squire, Lewitt 1975/ took the definitive standpoint that these nodules do progress and "the use of the term "hyperplastic nodule" as a synonym for neoplastic nodule is to be discouraged" /National Academy of Sciences 1980/. There are differences even in the views of those who consider the nodules neoplastic. Some authors regard them as the main link between altered foci and carcinomas, others - although pronouncing their neoplastic nature - consider them to be of end stage benign neoplasias, that is to say as adenomas, pointing out that no conversion or only occasional progression to carcinoma was observed /Williams 1980/. Remodeling /Farber 1982/ or even regression of nodules by extensive cystic degeneration /Williams 1980/ was also reported. The main reason for these strikingly differing views may be the heterogeneity of the induced nodules and of the individual tumors for the marker enzymes. So far there is no known single phenotype specific for both early lesions and carcinomas. Thus in hepatocarcinogenesis, the delineation of the progenitor cells of carcinomas is a problem still to be solved. The possible ways for development of chemically induced hepatocellular carcinomas are shown on the Figure. The majority of the altered foci do regress and/or may become the source of latent initiated cells, while some may persist. Out of the heterogeneous population of altered foci, however, in some - particularly in the basophilic type - a direct conversion to carcinoma may occur, while others may progress into neoplastic nodules. Carcinomas may also develop from neoplastic nodules and the possibility that they arise from latent initiated cells can not be excluded either.

HYPOTHETIC WAYS OF NEOPLASTIC DEVELOPMENT DURING CHEMICAL HEPATOCARCINOGENESIS

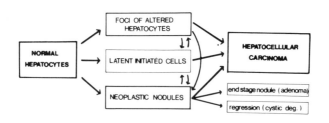

Contrary to the numerous model systems of chemical carcinogenesis there is only one or few animal models of viral hepatocarcinogenesis /Beard et al. 1975; Snyder et al. 1982/. In 1975 Beard and his co-workers /Beard et al. 1975/ described liver tumors induced by MC-29, myelocytomatosis virus in chickens from which I succeeded /Lapis et al. 1975/ to establish a virus-derived transplantable hepatoma line. We carried out hepatocarcinogenesis experiments with the same virus in turkeys, too /Schaff et al. 1978/.

In the turkey chicks infected by i.v. administration of $5 \times 10^5$ virus particles at the age of one day, liver tumors developed in strikingly short period, within 12-14 days. Up to the 8th day following infection no morphologic, cytologic or cytochemical alterations were seen. Afterwards, however, in extremely rapid manner, randomly dispersed foci of transformed hepatocytes appeared all over the liver. These foci, however, in contrast to the foci described in connection with chemical hepatocarcinogenesis were strictly speaking real neoplastic lesions, irreversible and progressive in nature. The main features of the composing transformed hepatocytes were the enlarged nuclei

containing extremely hypertrophic nucleoli, giving
the nuclei of owl-eye appearance. At the beginning
the transformed cells were lying in the frame of
the trabecules without obvious disruption of the
liver architecture. Later on, growing in number,
they formed foci of various shapes and sizes,
standing out from the background by their pronounced basophilia. Their size was rapidly growing
and at the end of experiments larger proportion of
liver tissue was replaced diffusely by such transformed neoplastic cell population.

At ultrastructural level the cells composing
the tumors showed various degrees of similarities
to hepatocytes. Bile canaliculi formed by tumor
cells, connected by desmosome type cell junctions,
were regularly seen in the tumorous foci. One of
the main characteristics of this tumor is the continuous virus production. Large amount of virus
particles can be observed in the intercellular
space, some in intracellular vacuoles and the budding process can also be observed regularly on the
surface of the tumor cells.

During viral hepatocarcinogenesis the loss of
G-6-Pase and ATPase activity could be demonstrated,
but we did not succeed to demonstrate increased
GGT activity by histochemical methods. Biochemically, however, in the liver of the newly hatched
turkey-chicks there was a substantially high level
of GGTase, decreasing very much on the second day
after infection. Later, however, a continuous increase was observed.

The most striking difference between chemical
and viral carcinogenesis was seen in the latency
period. It seems that one can not speak of a multistep process in the case of viral induced tumor
formation, in the sense used in connection with
chemical carcinogenesis. Another difference was
the absence of glycogen storage in the virus transformed hepatocytes. On the other hand, the trend of
the changes of enzyme activities proved to be similar in certain respects.

Changes in enzyme activity were also reported

in human hepatocellular carcinomas /Gerber, Thung
1980/. They appeared in various combination indicating a significant heterogeneity in enzyme phenotype of fully developed tumors similar to that seen
in chemically induced carcinomas. Concerning the
preneoplastic lesions of human liver tumors, studies
on the enzyme pattern were only sporadically carried
out. Recently /Thung, Gerber 1981/, increase in
GGTase, loss of G-6-Pase and canalicular ATPase
was demonstrated in a case of nodular "regenerative"
hyperplasia of the liver, while a human adenoma
studied exhibited ATPase and G-6-Pase, but no
GGTase activity.

We have studied three cases of focal nodular
hyperplasia /FNH/ by both histochemical and biochemical methods. The GGTase activity was highly
increased, just as in the case of the previously
mentioned nodular regenerative hyperplasia, in
contrast to the adenoma. No loss of G-6-Pase activity, however, the loss of ATPase activity was
detected /Schaff et al. 1982/. According to presently available data, even more pronounced heterogeneity seems to exist in the human preneoplastic
and neoplastic hepatic lesions than in those seen
in experimental models.

The precise delineation of the process of hepatocarcinogenesis is still ahead us. To achieve
this, much more studies on the supposed human preneoplastic lesions are needed, while in experimentation more attention should be paid to models of
viral hepatocarcinogenesis and the process of neoplasia formation should be studied in animals with
cirrhotic liver, too.

Anthony PP /1976/. The background to liver cell
    cancer. In Cameron HM, Linsell DA, Warwick GP
    /eds/: "Liver Cell Cancer", Amsterdam: Elsevier,
    p. 93.
Bannasch P, Moore MA, Klimek F, Zerban H /1982/.
    Biological markers of preneoplastic foci and neo-
    plastic nodules in rodent liver. Toxicol Pathol
    /under publication/.
Beard JW, Hillman EA, Beard D, Lapis K, Heine U
    /1975/. Neoplastic response of the avian liver to

host infection with strain MC 29 leukosis virus. Cancer Res 35:1603.

Becker FF /1981/. Recent concepts of initiation and promotion in carcinogenesis. Amer J Pathol 105:3.

Christopherson WM, May ET /1979/. Relation of steroids to liver oncogenesis. J Toxicol Environ Health 5:207.

Edmondson HA /1958/. "Tumors of the Liver and Intrahepatic Bile Ducts". Atlas of Tumor Pathology. Sect. 7. Fasc. 25. Washington: Armed Forces Institute of Pathology.

Emmelot P, Scherer E /1980/. The first relevant cell stage in rat liver carcinogenesis: A quantitative approach. Biochem Biophys Acta 605:247.

Enomoto K, Ying TS, Griffin MJ, Farber E /1981/. Immunohistochemical study of epoxide hydrolase during experimental liver carcinogenesis. Cancer Res 41:3281.

Farber E /1982/. Chemical carcinogenesis. A biologic perspective. Amer J Pathol 106:271.

Gerber MA, Thung SN /1980/. Enzyme patterns in human hepatocellular carcinoma. Amer J Pathol 98:395.

Lapis K, Beard D, Beard JW /1975/. Transplantation of hepatomas induced in the avian liver by MC29 leukosis virus. Cancer Res 35:132.

Lapis K, Johannessen JV /1979/. Pathology of primary liver cancer. J Toxicol Environ Health 5:315.

National Academy of Sciences /1980/. Histologic typing of liver tumors of the rat. J Natl Cancer Inst 64:179.

Ogawa K, Solt DB, Farber E /1980/. Phenotypic diversity as an early property of putative preneoplastic hepatocyte populations in liver carcinogenesis. Cancer Res 40:725.

Peraino C, Fry RJM, Staffeldt E, Kisieleski WE /1973/. Effects of varying the exposure to phenobarbital on its enhancement of 2-acetylaminofluorene-induced hepatic tumorigenesis in the rat. Cancer Res 33:2701.

Pitot HC, Sirica AE /1980/. The stages of initiation and promotion in hepatocarcinogenesis. Biochem Biophys Acta 605:191.

Popper H /1978/. Introduction: the increasing
importance of liver tumors. In Remmer H, Bolt HM,
Bannasch P, Popper H /eds/: "Primary Liver Tumors",
Lancaster: MTP Press, p 3.

Qizilbash AH, Castelli M /1980/. Nodular regenerative hyperplasia of the liver: diagnosis by
liver biopsy. CMA Journal 122:1151.

Schaff Zs, Lapis K, Széchény A, Feller J /1982/.
Enzyme histochemical phenotypes in focal nodular
hyperplasia of the liver. In preparation.

Schaff Zs, Tálas M, Stőger I, Lapis K, Földes I
/1978/. Neoplastic response of turkey liver to
MC29 leukosis virus. Acta Morphol Acad Sci Hung
26:325.

Sherlock S, Feldman CA, Moran B, Scheuer PJ /1966/.
Partial nodular transformation of the liver with
portal hypertension. Amer J Med 40:195.

Snyder RL, Tyler G, Summers J /1982/. Animal model
of human disease: Chronic hepatitis and hepatocellular carcinoma associated with woodchuck
hepatitis virus. Amer J Pathol 107:422.

Solt DB, Farber E /1976/. A new principle for the
analysis of chemical carcinogenesis. Nature
263:701.

Squire RA, Lewitt MH /1975/. Report of a workshop
on classification of specific hepatocellular
lesions in rats. Cancer Res 25:3214.

Szendrői M, Lapis K, Schaff Zs /1982/. Changes in
fibronectin production and distribution in the
liver during hepatocarcinogenesis. In preparation.

Thung SN, Gerber MA /1981/. Enzyme pattern and
marker antigens in nodular "regenerative"
hyperplasia of the liver. Cancer 47:1796.

Williams GM /1980/. The pathogenesis of rat liver
cancer caused by chemical carcinogens. Biochem
Biophys Acta 605:167.

13th International Cancer Congress, Part D
Research and Treatment, pages 77-78
© 1983 Alan R. Liss, Inc., 150 Fifth Avenue, New York, NY 10011

# HEPATITIS B VIRUS AND THE PATHOGENESIS AND PREVENTION OF CANCER OF THE LIVER

Baruch S. Blumberg, M.D., Ph.D.

Institute for Cancer Research
Fox Chase Cancer Center
Philadelphia, PA    19111

There is now a substantial body of evidence that persistent infection with the hepatitis B virus (HBV) is required for the development of primary cancer of the liver (primary hepatocellular carcinoma, PHC), one of the most common cancers in the world. The evidence includes the following. Essentially all patients with PHC have been infected with HBV. The DNA of HBV is found integrated in the liver cells of a very large percentage of patients with PHC. In areas where there is a high frequency of infection with HBV (i.e., Asia, Africa), males who are carriers of HBV (that is, persistently infected but not apparently ill) have more than a 350 greater risk of developing PHC than controls. Woodchucks infected with a virus very similar to the human hepatitis B virus also show integration of viral DNA, high risk of PHC in viral carriers and other phenomena similar to that seen in humans with PHC. This plus other related findings are sufficient to warrant the development of primary prevention programs, and such programs are now starting in areas where HBV infection is common.

We have developed a vaccine prepared from the peripheral blood of carriers of the virus containing only the coat protein. This is now available in the USA and abroad, and field trials have shown it to be effective in preventing infection with HBV. By the use of this vaccine and other public health measures, we believe that it will, in due course, be possible to prevent primary cancer of the liver.

This line of investigation has, along with other scientific studies, encouraged the search for additional virus-cancer relations in humans which may also be preventable.

We have developed a model to explain certain clinical epidemiologic, pathologic and molecular characteristics of the HBV-PHC relation. These include: 1) the long period (incubation time) between infection and onset of clinical cancer (20-25 years), 2) the absence or low concentration of whole virus and its antigens in transformed cells. Whole virus present in the non-transformed cells immediately surrounding the tumor, 3) the association of HBV with chronic liver disease in addition to PHC, 4) PHC usually produces fetal proteins of which alpha fetoprotein is the best studied example, 5) there is a higher frequency of PHC in males than females, 6) the presence of integrated HBV-DNA in the liver cells of patients with PHC as well as patients with chronic liver disease and chronic carriers.

The model postulates the existence of two kinds of liver cells. S cells are susceptible to productive infection with HBV, while R cells are resistant to such infection, although HBV-DNA can integrate into the DNA of R cells. The S cells are derived from mature differentiated cells. These rarely divide, but when they do they produce only S cells. The R cells derive from undifferentiated or partially differentiated cells. When they divide, which they can do readily, they can produce R cells only, S cells only or both R and S cells.

The productive infection of S cells by HBV leads to their eventual death. The death of S cells stimulates the division of R cells. When this division becomes uncontrolled, a clinically perceptible cancer can develop.

This model focuses attention both on the transformed and non-transformed infected cells and has interesting implications for diagnosis, secondary prevention and treatment of PHC.

**13th International Cancer Congress, Part D**
**Research and Treatment, pages 79–88**
© **1983 Alan R. Liss, Inc., 150 Fifth Avenue, New York, NY 10011**

BIOCHEMICAL PHENOTYPE IN HUMAN AND ANIMAL LIVER TUMORS

Noemi Prajda, Ph.D.

National Institute of Oncology

Budapest, Hungary

The purpose of this paper is to discuss the strategy of liver cancer cells as expressed in the biochemical phenotype, focusing on the following questions: 1. Is the biochemical pattern of imbalance in liver cancer ordered or diverse and random? 2. Is the pattern characteristic to neoplasia? 3. Does the biochemical pattern in liver cancer reflect the impact of various carcinogenic agents or is it independent from the etiology? 4. Is the pattern species-specific? 5. Is the pattern in experimental models applicable to human hepatocellular carcinoma? 6. Is the biochemical phenotype of experimental and human hepatomas relevant to the design of clinical chemotherapy?

HISTORICAL DEVELOPMENT OF APPROACHES TO THE BIOCHEMISTRY OF LIVER TUMORS

Numerous ideas have been introduced some of which were surveyed by Potter 1982. The most frequently cited are shown in table 1. I will approach the biochemical phenotype of liver cancer with the application of the molecular correlation concept, a useful experimental and conceptual tool in analyzing the biochemical phenotype in model systems and in primary human neoplasms (Weber 1963).

BIOLOGICAL MODEL SYSTEMS

In the biochemical characterization of liver cancer, biological models were used (Morris 1978). Much of the framework of our understanding of the biochemical phenotype of liver tumors was achieved through examination of chemically-induced, transplantable hepatomas in rat (Morris, Wagner 1968, Weber 1977).

| CONCEPTS | PROPOSAL |
| --- | --- |
| Warburg theory (1935) | Respiratory defect followed by increased glycolysis |
| Convergence hypothesis Greenstein (1943) | Tendency to converge to a similar biochemical phenotype |
| Deletion hypothesis Miller and Miller (1943) Potter (1953) | "Loss of proteins" "Loss of enzymes related to catabolic cellular functions" |
| Minimal deviation concept Potter (1960) | Essential changes for cancer status |
| Altered feedback hypothesis Monod, Jacob, Pitot, Potter (1965) | Does not imply presence or absence of somatic mutation |
| Molecular correlation concept Weber (1963, 1977) | Ordered pattern of opposing key enzymes and pathways Reprogramming of gene expression |

Table 1. Historical development of biochemical approaches to cancer.

The phenotypic alterations in hepatomas were analyzed in several main areas (Morris, Criss 1978).

From the wealth of information this paper will focus on metabolic regulation and enzymology. In the hepatoma spectrum an ordered pattern of metabolism was detected in transformation- and progression-linked alterations (Weber 1977). There was an increased capacity for glucose catabolism, glycolysis and an increased capacity for biosynthesis of purines and pyrimidines. There was a decreased potential for glucose synthesis, gluconeogenesis, and for the catabolism of purines and pyrimidines.

From my own work, I cite an example of reciprocal regulation of the behavior of activities of opposing key enzymes
of purine metabolism. The activity of amidophosphoribosyltransferase, the rate-limiting enzyme of IMP synthesis,
increased and that of the rate-limiting catabolic enzyme,
xanthine oxidase, decreased in all the examined hepatomas.
Since these changes occurred even in the slowest growing,
most liver-like hepatomas and there was no progressive enzymic change, these alterations are transformation-linked
(Prajda et al 1975, 1976). Immunological studies showed
that the increased amidotransferase activity was due to an
increased amount of enzyme (Tsuda et al 1979). This observation supports the idea that the enzymatic changes are due
to a reprogramming of gene expression in cancer cells.

PHENOTYPES OF CHEMICALLY- AND VIRAL-INDUCED HEPATOMAS

Lapis and his associates provided a useful virus-
induced, transplantable hepatoma model in the chicken,
(Lapis, Beard 1975) which answered the question whether the
biochemical phenotypes of viral-induced and chemically-
induced hepatomas are similar and whether species difference
is reflected in the tumor biochemical phenotype.

Lapis and associates reported an increased amount of
DNA and decreased concentrations of RNA, protein and phos-
pholipids in the virus-induced hepatomas (Kovalszky et al
1976) which are similar to those found in chemically-induced
hepatomas (Weber 1957, Lea et al 1966). The increased DNA
content may be accounted for by the increased activity of
DNA polymerase. This key enzyme increased 10-fold in viral-
induced hepatomas as reported by Lapis (Lapis 1980) which
agrees with the findings in chemically-induced liver tumors
(Ove et al 1969, Chiu et al 1978).

An important aspect of the biochemical phenotype in
hepatomas is the decrease and loss of responsiveness to reg-
ulatory mechanisms, including endocrine controls (Weber 1958,
Feigelson, DeLap 1978, Weinhouse 1978, Baumann, Held 1981).
The loss of responsiveness to hormonal stimulation was first
reported by Weber. The Novikoff hepatoma failed to respond
to glucocorticoid injection, which in normal liver induced
an increase of glucose-6-phosphatase activity. A similar
failure of enzyme induction by steroid hormones was observed
in the MC-29 virus-induced chicken liver (table 2). There

was a decreased binding of the hormone to the receptors which may explain the decreased response to hydrocortisone of glucose-6-phosphatase and aryl hydrocarbon-hydroxylase (Kovalszky et al 1976). The binding capacity of the cytosolic receptors to steroids was the same in liver and tumor, but the rate of interaction between DNA and the steroid in the hepatoma was only one-half of that of the liver.

| TISSUE | ENZYME INDUCTION % of control | | BINDING OF ($^3$H) HYDROCORTISONE to cytosol receptor | | to DNA | |
|---|---|---|---|---|---|---|
| | AHH | G-6-Pase | % of control | | % of control | |
| Liver | 260 | 210 (200) | 100 | (100) | 100 | (100) |
| Hepatoma | 100 | 100 (100) | 93 | (102) | 51 | (98) |

Values in parentheses refer to chemically-induced rat hepatomas. AHH = aryl hydrocarbon hydroxylase; G-6-Pase = glucose-6-phosphatase. (Kovalszky et al., 1976).

Table 2. Enzyme induction and receptor binding in hydrocortisone treated chicken liver and hepatoma MC-29.

ENZYMIC PHENOTYPES OF RAPIDLY GROWING HEPATOMAS IN CHICKEN AND RAT

The applicability of the biochemical phenotype of the chemically-induced hepatomas was tested in the MC-29 virus-induced tumor by several groups of Hungarian investigators (Elek et al 1979, Jeney et al 1979, Prajda et al 1979).

Comparing the enzymic phenotypes of virally- and chemically-induced rapidly growing hepatomas (table 3), we observed that in both tumors the glycolytic capacity was increased, as reflected in the elevated activities of the key enzymes, hexokinase and pyruvate kinase. The activity of the key gluconeogenic enzyme, glucose 6-phosphatase, decreased. The activity of glucose 6-phosphate dehydrogenase, increased in all the examined chemically-induced hepatomas, was also elevated in the avian hepatoma (Kovalszky 1976). The activity of amidophosphoribosyltransferase increased whereas that of xanthine oxidase decreased. In thymidine metabolism,

there was an increase in the activity of the synthetic enzyme, thymidine kinase, which should provide a stepped-up
capacity for pyrimidine production.  These investigations
suggest that the enzymic phenotype is independent from both
the carcinogenic agent and the species.

| ENZYMES | SPECIFIC ACTIVITY:  % OF NORMAL LIVER | |
| --- | --- | --- |
| | Chicken hepatoma MC-29 Virus-induced | Rat hepatoma 3924A Chemically-induced |
| Glycolytic | | |
| Hexokinase | 303 | 500 |
| Pyruvate kinase | 13,519 | 499 |
| Gluconeogenic | | |
| Glucose-6-Pase | 6 | < 1 |
| Pentose phosphate | | |
| Glucose-6-P DH | 593 | 751 |
| Pyrimidine synthesis | | |
| Thymidine kinase | 1,361 | 1,114 |
| Uridine kinase | 428 | 238 |
| Purine synthesis | | |
| Amidotransferase | 135 | 196 |
| Purine catabolism | | |
| Xanthine oxidase | 31 | 10 |

All differences are statistically significant ($p < 0.05$).
Prajda et al. (1979).

Table 3.  Comparison of enzymic phenotypes of rapidly
growing hepatomas in chicken and rat.

COMPARISON OF ENZYMIC PHENOTYPES OF ADULT AND DIFFERENTIATING
LIVER AND OF HEPATOMA MC-29 IN CHICKEN

The marked changes in the virus-induced tumor in activities of key enzymes were either not observed or found only
in a minor extent in the differentiating chicken liver (Fig.
1).  A clear-cut difference was observed in xanthine oxidase
activity which in the hepatoma decreased to 31%, whereas it

increased to 154% in the 2-week-old liver as compared to the
values in normal adult chicken liver. Thus the enzymic
phenotype of the hepatoma is different from that of the differentiating liver. Most biochemical alterations reported
were in amount or activity of enzymes and in activity of
metabolic pathways.

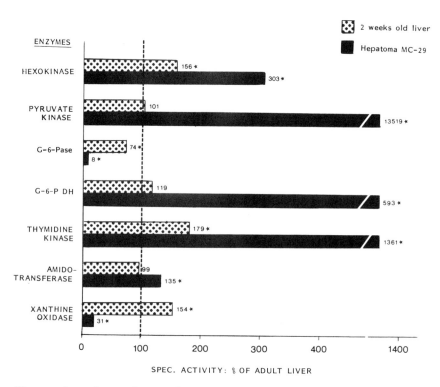

Figure 1.  Comparison of enzymic phenotypes of adult and
differentiating liver and in hepatoma MC-29 in chicken.

However, changes in the isozyme pattern may be considered as
qualitative changes in phenotype.  Important advances in this
field have been made by Weinhouse and his associates and
various investigators (Ono, Weinhouse 1972, Hatayama, Sato
1980, Dunaway 1981) in chemically-induced tumors, and Lapis
and associates (Lapis 1980) in Hungary, studying behavior of
ornithine transaminase in virus-induced hepatoma.  The interesting results of Weinhouse (Weinhouse 1976) illustrate the
isozyme shift.  The liver-type pyruvate kinase present in

normal liver and very slowly growing, well differentiated hepatoma was replaced in the more rapidly growing and less differentiated hepatomas and particularly in the poorly differentiated tumors by non-liver type isozyme.

## TRANSFORMATION-LINKED DELETION OF CHOLESTEROL FEEDBACK IN HEPATOMAS

A neoplastic transformation-linked alteration was shown (Siperstein 1971) to occur in all hepatomas examined in rat and mouse and also in human. When cholesterol was administered in the diet (table 4) in the normal liver the synthesis of cholesterol was markedly decreased due to feedback inhibition of the activity of the key enzyme, hydroxymethylglutaryl Coenzyme A reductase. When hepatoma-bearing rats were fed cholesterol there was no inhibition in cholesterol synthesis in the hepatoma because of the absence of this feedback in the tumor. Since this occurred even in the slowest growing hepatomas, this is a transformation-linked alteration in the phenotype of liver cancer.

| TISSUES | TREATMENT | HMG-CoA REDUCTASE* |
|---------|-----------|--------------------|
| Liver | - | 100 |
| Liver | 5% cholesterol | 1 |
| Hepatoma | - | 100 |
| Hepatoma | 5% cholesterol | 99 |

*Hydroxymethylglutaryl Coenzyme A reductase Siperstein et al. (1971).

Table 4. Feedback control of HMG-CoA reductase in normal liver and hepatoma 3924A.

## SPECIFICITY OF ALTERATIONS TO NEOPLASIA

Detailed evidence has been presented that although some alterations in enzymic activities overlapped with those in normal, fetal, developing or regenerating liver the overall phenotype of biochemical imbalance in the hepatomas was characteristic to neoplasia and could be distinguished from all other patterns (Siperstein 1966, Weber 1977).

COMPARISON OF BIOCHEMICAL PHENOTYPES OF HUMAN AND RAT HEPATOMAS

The phenotype (table 5) shows that biochemical alterations in the human hepatoma are similar to those in rat for key enzymes (Weber 1975), abnormal glycoproteins, glycosyltransferase (Waxman 1980) and phosphoprotein kinase (Chiu 1978). Thus, the biochemical phenotype of liver cancer is independent both from the carcinogen and from the species. Thus, the chemically and virally-induced, transplantable hepatomas are useful models for primary human hepatomas.

| Metabolic Pathways | Enzymes[a] | % of Normal Liver | |
|---|---|---|---|
| | | Human hepatoma | Rat hepatoma[b] |
| Glycolysis | Pyruvate kinase | 389 | 200 |
| Gluconeogenesis | Glucose 6-phosphatase | 38 | 27 |
| | Fruct-1,6-diphosphatase | 41 | 34 |
| Pentose phosphate | | | |
| Oxidative pathway | Glucose 6-P DH | 1,159 | 1,862 |
| | 6-Phosphogluconate DH | 204 | 468 |
| Non-oxidative pathway | Transaldolase | 187 | 284 |
| | Transketolase | 164 | 167 |
| Purine synthesis | PRPP amidotransferase | 331 | 218 |
| DNA | TdR to DNA | 100 | 291 |
| | TdR to $CO_2$ | 76 | 52 |
| RNA | UDP kinase | 299 | 244 |

[a]Activities were calculated in $\mu mol/hr/cell \times 10^{-7}$ and expressed as % of normal liver values. [b]Slowly growing hepatomas 9618A and 66.

Table 5. Comparison of enzymic phenotype of human and rat hepatomas.

CLINICAL RELEVANCE OF ALTERED ENZYME ACTIVITY IN HUMAN HEPATOMAS

The transformation- and progression-linked alterations are markers of malignancy and of degrees of malignancy, respectively. These phenotypic alterations assist in clinical diagnosis and grading of tumor malignancy. The activities of key enzymes in tumors and in host tissues are the targets of drugs and are responsible for the side effects. Thus, the biochemical phenotype is relevant to the design of clinical selective chemotherapy and the toxicity that occurs in treatment.

Baumann H, Held WA (1981). Biosynthesis and hormone regulated expression of secretory glycoproteins in rat liver and hepatoma cells. J Biol Chem 256:10145.

Chiu F, Hnilica LS, Belanger L, Morris HP (1978). Nuclear macromolecular changes in hepatomas. Adv Exp Med Biol 92: 181.

Dunaway G (1981). Phosphofructokinase isozymes in Morris hepatomas. Arch Biochem Biophys 212:1.

Elek G, Lapis K, Foldes I (1979). Comparative study of tumor-specific transplantation antigens of MC-29 chicken hepatoma and Rous sarcoma virus-induced sarcomas in mice. In "Liver carcinogenesis" ed. Lapis K, Johanessen FV Washington Hemisphere Publ. Corp. 359.

Feigelson P, DeLap LW (1978). Control of specific m-RNA species in liver and hepatoma. Adv Exp Med Biol 92:307.

Hatayama T, Sato K (1980). Changes in the glycogen phosphorylase isozyme pattern of AH130 during cell growth. Gann 71:875.

Jeney A, Kovalszky I, Gyapay G, Lapis K, Suba ZS (1979). Chromatin alterations and gene function disorder in MC-29 virus-derived hepatoma. J Toxicol Environ Health 5:509.

Kovalszky I, Jeney A, Asbot R, Lapis K (1976). Biochemistry and enzyme inducibility in MC-29 virus-induced transplantable avian hepatoma. Cancer Res 36:2140.

Lapis K (1980). Biological characterisation of virus-induced hepatoma. Orvostudomany 31:277.

Lapis K, Beard D, Beard TW (1975). Transplantation of hepatomas induced in the avian liver by MC-29 leukosis virus. Cancer Res 35:132.

Lea MA, Morris HP, Weber G (1966). Comparative biochemistry of hepatomas VI. Thymidine incorporation into DNA as a measure of hepatoma growth rate. Cancer Res 26:465.

Morris HP, Wagner BP (1968). Induction and transplantation of rat hepatomas with different growth rates (including "minimal deviation" hepatomas). Methods Cancer Res 4:125.

Morris HP, Criss WE (1978). Morris hepatomas. Adv Exp Med
    Biol Vol 92 New York Plenum Press.
Ono T, Weinhouse S (1972). Isozymes and enzyme regulation
    in cancer. Gann Mono Univ Tokyo Press, Tokyo 13.
Pitot H, Cho YS (1965). Control mechanism in the normal and
    neoplastic cell. Progr Exp Tumor Res 7:158.
Potter R (1982). Biochemistry of cancer. In Holland TF,
    Frei E "Cancer Medicine" p. 133.
Prajda N, Katunuma N, Morris HP, Weber G (1975). Imbalance
    of purine metabolism in hepatomas of different growth rates
    as expressed in behavior of glutamine PRPP amidotransferase
    (EC 2.4.2.14). Cancer Res 35:3061.
Prajda N, Morris HP, Weber G (1976). Imbalance of purine
    metabolism in hepatomas of different growth rates as
    expressed in behavior of xanthine oxidase (EC 1.2.3.2).
    Cancer Res 36:4639.
Prajda N, Eckhardt S, Suba ZS, Lapis K (1979). Biochemical
    behavior of MC-29 virus-induced transplantable chicken
    hepatoma. J Toxicol Environ Health 5:503.
Siperstein WD, Fagan VM, Morris HP (1966). Further studies
    on the deletion of the cholesterol feedback system in
    hepatomas. Cancer Res 26:7.
Tsuda M, Katunuma N, Morris HP, Weber G (1979). Purification,
    properties and immunotitration of hepatoma glutamine phos-
    phoribosylpyrophosphate amidotransferase (amidophosphoribo-
    syl transferase, EC 2.4.2.14). Cancer Res 39:305.
Waxman S, Liu C, Schmied R (1980). Abnormal glycoproteins
    and glycosyltransferases in human hepatoma. Ann NY Acad
    Sci 394:411.
Weber G, Cantero A (1957). Phospholipid content in Novikoff
    hepatoma, regenerating liver and in liver of fed and fasted
    normal rats. Exper Cell Res 13:125.
Weber G, Cantero A (1958). Glucose-6-phosphate utilization
    in hepatoma regenerating and new born rat liver and in the
    liver of fed and fasted rats. Cancer Res 17:995.
Weber G (1963). Behavior and regulation of enzyme systems in
    normal liver and in hepatomas of different growth rates.
    Adv Enzyme Regul 1:321.
Weber G, Prajda N, Williams JC (1976). Molecular basis of
    malignancy. In: Biological characterisation of human
    tumors. ed.: Davis M, Maltoni C Excerpta Med Amsterdam.
Weber G (1977). Enzymology of cancer cells I, II. New Engl
    J Med 296: 486 and 541.

ACKNOWLEDGEMENT: The authors work was supported, in part,
by USPH Grant CA-13526.

**13th International Cancer Congress, Part D**
**Research and Treatment, pages 89–95**
© **1983 Alan R. Liss, Inc., 150 Fifth Avenue, New York, NY 10011**

CARCINOMA OF THE PANCREAS: PROGRESS OR STALEMATE?

William B. Hutchinson, Jr., M.D., F.A.C.S., and
Donald E. Wagner, M.D., F.A.C.S.
Fred Hutchinson Cancer Research Center
Seattle, Washington  98104

Historically, carcinoma of the pancreas has been one
of the most difficult diseases to diagnose and treat.
Whipple, in the 1930's, designed an operation for treatment
of this disease which gave hope to the surgeon and the
patient alike.  Since that time, much has been done, but
little progress has been made in the areas of effective
early diagnosis and treatment.  Epidemiologic investigators
today allude to the steady increase in the incidence of
pancreatic cancer in the United States and other industrialized nations (American Cancer Society: Cancer Facts and
Figures, 1981).  They also refer to diagnostic criteria to
determine which patients would benefit from a radical pan-
createctomy. However, biologically and anatomically, cancer
of the pancreas is not well suited to curative surgical
extirpation.  Since there is an increase in incidence of
carcinoma of the pancreas and an apparent stalemate in
early diagnosis and treatment, a careful review of our current methods of detection, our approach to treatment, and
an attempt to understand the natural course of the disease
seems indicated.

When a single test or procedure for work-up of a
suspected lesion does not exist, we usually rely on multiple
inferior studies.  The diagnosis of the patient with suspected carcinoma of the pancreas is no exception and
includes ultrasonography, computerized tomography, radionuclide scanning, endoscopic retrograde cholangiography,
duodenal drainage studies, cytology, selective arteriography,
carcinoembryonic antigen assay and pancreatic oncofetal
antigen assay.  These tests vary in accuracy from 86% using

successful ERCP cytology and drainage studies in combination
to less than 20% for other procedures (Pollock, Taylor 1981).
The accuracy of radiologic studies vary greatly depending on
the radiologist and the equipment available to him. Positron-
Omission computerized tomography of the pancreas has been
reported as offering a new diagnostic imaging technique and
is superior to earlier scanners because it allows imaging
of the biologic activity of the pancreas. This would help
us diagnose as well as follow progression of the disease
when one is undergoing treatment. Nuclear Magnetic Reson-
ance is a new diagnostic device which may offer hope for
earlier detection of cancer of the pancreas. Carcinoembryonic antigen, and other tumor antigens, would be
particularly helpful in detecting early stages of carcinoma
of the pancreas and recurrences, if such assays were found
to be more consistent and specific for disease growth. Pancreatic oncofetal antigen is another tumor marker which is
being investigated for future use, but to date significant
data is not available for evaluation in clinical practice.

Ultrasonography, CAT scanning, and arteriography each
provide indirect information about the pancreas but technical problems often make interpretation difficult. However,
it has been hoped that combinations of these studies would
lead to earlier diagnosis and selection of patients for
radical surgical procedures.

The data for carcinoma of the pancreas were analyzed
at St. John's Hospital and Health Center. Two time periods
were selected: 1960-1969 and 1973-1982. Data from inter-
vening years was not used because of insufficient follow-up
during those years. There were 78 patients in the period
between 1960-1969 and there were 112 patients in the period
from 1973-1982. (Fig. 1). In analyzing these groups,
attempts were made to separate them into different categories
to see if perhaps one surgically treated group or non-
surgically treated group did any differently than the rest.
Some interesting data did become apparent.

First, the surgically treated patients, as opposed to
those non-surgically treated, appeared to survive longer.
(Fig. 2). However, after 12 months the curves come together
and bear no significant differences. Second, those surgically explored in our series with a clinical diagnosis of
carcinoma of the pancreas, but who did not have a patho-
logically proven CA. of the pancreas, seemed to survive much

Figure 1
## CARCINOMA OF THE PANCREAS
### SAINT JOHN'S HOSPITAL AND HEALTH CENTER

AGE - SEX DISTRIBUTION - - COMPARISON OF TIME PERIODS 1973-81 AND 1960-69

| Age Group | 1973-81[*] | | | | 1960-69 | | | |
|---|---|---|---|---|---|---|---|---|
| | M | F | Tot | % | M | F | Tot | % |
| Under 45 | 1 | 1 | 2 | 2 | 2 | 0 | 2 | 2 |
| 45 - 54 | 4 | 5 | 9 | 8 | 7 | 4 | 11 | 14 |
| 55 - 64 | 14 | 14 | 28 | 25 | 20 | 12 | 32 | 41 |
| 65 - 74 | 22 | 21 | 43 | 38 | 7 | 10 | 17 | 22 |
| 75 & over | 7 | 23 | 30 | 27 | 6 | 10 | 16 | 21 |
| TOTAL | 48 | 64 | 112 | 100 | 42 | 36 | 78 | 100 |

*1981 Data Incomplete; Tumor Registry, 10-1-81 AA/VC.

the same as those with histologic proof of diagnosis. (Fig. 3). Third, when we analyzed the diagnostic cases of carcinoma of the pancreas as to stage, all seemed to do very poorly by 24 months with a 10% survival rate. (Fig. 4). Fourth, 94% of the tumors were adenocarcinomas. All ampullary distal bile duct and duodenal carcinomas were excluded from our series. The age, sex, methods of achieving diagnosis, and surgical bypass as well as resections, are no different in this series than the statistics from the Surveillance Epidemiologic End Results data ( Cancer Incidence and Mortality in the United States, SEER, 1978).

Summary

Has treatment for cancer of the pancreas progressed or has a stalemate been reached? This is a difficult question to answer. Cancer of the pancreas has several unique features. First, it has been an extremely difficult tumor to study because of its anatomic location and our present invasive and non-invasive studies have failed to provide for truly early detection of this disease when cure may be possible. Second, assuming that we are able to diagnose early, radical surgical resection (our best treatment to date) still carries a substantial morbidity and mortality.

The direction certainly has to be in early detection and screening in the asymptomatic patient. To date all of our therapy is directed to the patient who already has

Figure 2. Carcinoma of the Pancreas — Saint John's Hospital and Health Center: Observed Survival for Surgically Treated Cases and Those Not Surgically Treated*, Cases Diagnosed 1973–1981**

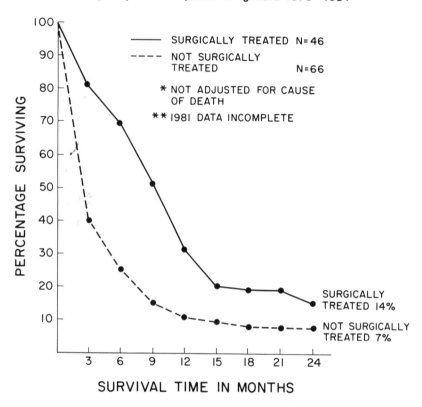

*Tumor Registry, 10-1-81 AA*

Figure 3. Carcinoma of the Pancreas — Saint John's Hospital and Health Center: Observed Survival for Clinically Diagnosed Cases and Total Cases*, Cases Diagnosed 1973—1981**

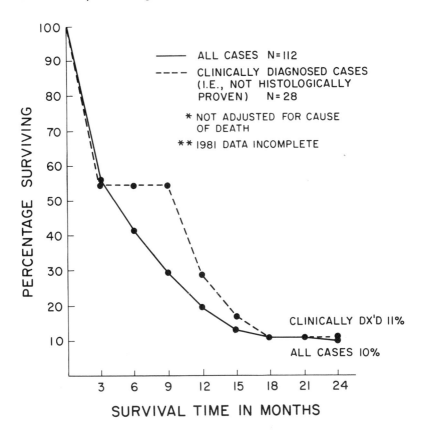

*Tumor Registry, 10-1-81 AA*

Figure 4. Carcinoma of the Pancreas — Saint John's Hospital and Health Center: Comparison of Observed Survival*, Cases Diagnosed 1973–81** and 1960–69

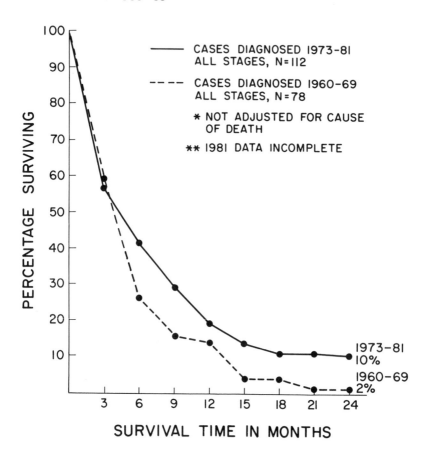

symptoms. Diagnosis prior to this stage of the disease is imperative. This would entail the use of biological and serum antibody-type screening procedures with specific tumor markers and better epidemiologic studies to identify risk factors which would aid in screening procedures. It is apparent that present day techniques in the diagnosis and treatment of pancreatic cancer are inadequate and that new directions are needed before any significant improvement in survival rates are realized.

Bibliography

Cancer Facts and Figures, 1981. New York, American Cancer Society, Inc. 1980.

Cancer Incidence and Mortality in the United States, SEER 1973-1976. Bethesda, MD, US Dept. of Health, Education, and Welfare, NIH Publication No. 78-1837, 1978.

Pollock, D, Taylor KJW: Ultrasound scanning in patients with clinical suspicion of pancreatic cancer: a retrospective study. Cancer 47:1662-1665, 1981.

CONGRESS SYMPOSIA

THE PATHOLOGY OF INCIPIENT NEOPLASIA Sugano, H.,
Japan, Chairman; Koss, L., USA, Co-Chairman;
Playhouse

Intraepithelial Stage of Squamous Cell Carcinoma
of the Uterine Cervix: A Multifactorial Dynamic
Process. *Rilke, R., Milan, Italy.

Microcarcinoma of the Stomach Measuring Less Than
5 mm in the Largest Diameter and Its Histogenesis.
*Nakamura, K. and Sugano, H., Tokyo, Japan.

Early Development in the Progression of Lung Cancer:
Squamous Cell Carcinoma. *Frost, J. K.,
Erozan, Y. S., Gupta, P. K., Eggleston, J. C.,
Ball, W. C., Jr., Levin, M. L., Tockman, M. S.
and Pressman, N. J., Baltimore, MD USA. (By Title
Only)

Morphologic Aspects of the Genesis of Colo-Rectal
Carcinoma and Its Relationship to Adenoma.
*Enterline, H. T., Philadelphia, PA USA.

Incipient Neoplasia of the Urinary Bladder.
*Friedell, G. H., Worcester, MA USA. (By Title
Only)

Please note: Papers that are listed as "By Title
Only" were presented at the 13th International
Cancer Congress, but are not included in these
volumes.

**13th International Cancer Congress, Part D**
**Research and Treatment, pages 99–105**
© **1983 Alan R. Liss, Inc., 150 Fifth Avenue, New York, NY 10011**

INTRAEPITHELIAL STAGE OF SQUAMOUS CELL CARCINOMA OF THE
UTERINE CERVIX: A MULTIFACTORIAL DYNAMIC PROCESS

Franco Rilke, M.D.

Division of Pathology
Istituto Nazionale Tumori
Milano, Italy 20133

Squamous cell carcinoma of the uterine cervix is preceded in most cases by a preinvasive stage that encompasses
a spectrum of lesions that include dysplasia and carcinoma
in situ and are also defined by comprehensive terms such as
cervical intraepithelial neoplasia (CIN) (Koss, 1979;
Richart, 1967) or precancerous epithelial atypia. Less
commonly, the invasive cancer arises de novo or following a
short preinvasive stage (Ashley, 1966; Hakama, Penttinen,
1981; Laskey et al., 1976), especially in young women
(Macgregor, 1982). Risk factors of cervical neoplasia are
numerous (Kessler, 1981) and mainly related to age, race,
and sexual habits. In spite of its limitations, cytology
is suitable in most cases for the detection of cells that
derive from all grades of CIN and is also useful to monitor
the progression or regression of the lesions. The progression rate is higher in the more severe grades of CIN and
may be influenced by external factors (Stern, 1977).

A variety of causative factors have been taken into
consideration in the etiology of CIN and, hence, of invasive
cervical cancer, ranging from in utero exposure to diethyl-
stilbestrol (Herbst et al., 1971) to several infectious and
non-infectious agents. In keeping with the opinion shared
by many investigators that squamous cell carcinoma of the
uterine cervix behaves as a venereal disease (Kessler, 1976),
herpes simplex virus type 2 (HSV-2) (Naib et al., 1966, 1969;
Rawls et al., 1968), which is one of the major sexually
transmitted infectious agents worldwide, has been shown to
act either as an initiator or a promotor of the neoplastic
event, possibly in association with other viruses or

carcinogens (Fenoglio, 1982).

The strong evidence supporting a role for HSV-2 in squamous cell carcinoma of the cervix has never pointed to the existence of a special subgroup of this tumor particularly related to the virus. Even though it has never been stated that squamous cell carcinoma of the cervix is always etiologically related to HSV-2, there seems to be no morphological difference between those cases in which RNA complementary to HSV-2 DNA could be found by the in situ cytological hybridization method in cells derived from CIN (McDougall et al., 1980) and those in which it could not. The results reported by various groups (Dreesman et al., 1980; McDougall et al., 1981) of localizing HSV-2 antigens were essentially in line with those obtained with in situ hybridization.

The recent interest in the causative role of one or possibly more members (Gissman et al., 1982; zur Hausen et al., 1981) of the human papilloma virus (HPV) group in condylomata of the uterine cervix was stimulated by the ultrastructural identification of typical papilloma virus particles in about 50% of the cells of those lesions (Della Torre et al., 1978; Laverty et al., 1978; Morin, Meisels, 1980) and by the demonstration of papilloma viral antigens also in about 50% of mild dysplasias (Shah et al., 1980) and condylomas (Ferenczy, 1981; Meisels et al., 1981; Morin et al., 1981; Woodruff et al., 1980). Cervical HPV-related lesions are characterized at a light microscopic level by cellular changes such as koilocytosis (Koss, Durfee, 1956) and dyskeratosis. Similarly to HSV-2, cervical condylomata are venereally transmitted and are commonly associated with CIN. This association may be visualized either by the contiguity of the two or by the presence of the same cellular lesions that characterize cervical condylomata in the upper layers of CIN (Pilotti et al., 1981).

We correlated the cytologic findings of an unselected series of consecutive CVE smears obtained from 202 women aged between 17 and 66 years and containing koilocytotic cells or cells deriving from CIN with koilocytotic changes, or both, with the histology of the cervical biopsies and found that 136 had condylomata only (67%) and 66 had CIN either associated with condylomata (19%) or with koilocytosis (14%). These data confirmed the overall experience that cervical condylomata are at least twice as prevalent as

CIN and that the majority of the cases diagnosed as mild dysplasia are, in fact, HPV-related cervical lesions (Meisels et al., 1977).

In another study (Pilotti et al., 1982) designed primarily to verify the histologic diagnoses of CIN made a decade earlier, after the recognition of the HPV-induced changes in cervical epithelium and contestually to correlate the histologic findings with the prior cytology, all the cytologic and histologic material pertaining to patients who had undergone cervical conization for advanced CIN was reviewed. The revision of the histology of the biopsies and cones showed in 56% the association of CIN with viral cytopathic effects (VCE) attributable to HPV and in 93% of these the coexistence of a flat condyloma. The comparison of the two groups of CIN, with and without VCE, showed that in the first the association had favored in 20% of the cases the histologic overestimation of the severity of the lesion. Of the patients with CIN III, 46% showed additional changes due to VCE. The mean age of the patients with CIN and VCE was 39.8 years and that of the patients with CIN was 48.6 ($P < 0.001$). The exocervix was significantly more often involved by CIN with VCE than by CIN alone ($P < 0.00001$). Cytologic sensitivity for VCE in cervical smears was high (95%) in the cases of CIN II and somewhat lower (81%) in those with CIN III. Cytologic follow-up studies revealed in both groups the same percentage of residual disease and, preliminarily, a trend to a better control of CIN with VCE. New disease also involving the vagina developed only in the group of patients with CIN without VCE. Cytologic follow-up showed the persistence of VCE in 17% of the patients treated surgically for CIN and VCE.

The availability of an antiserum (kindly supplied by Dr. Keerti V. Shah) prepared by immunization of a rabbit with disrupted virions from a pool of plantar warts (Jenson et al., 1980) enabled us to perform on the majority of the cases an immunohistochemical staining by use of an avidin-biotin-peroxidase complex (Vectastain ABC Kit, Vector Laboratories, Burlingame, Ca.) as developed by Hsu et al. (1981). The antiserum stained discrete nuclei of the most superficial and intermediate layers of the epithelium in 30% of the cases with CIN associated with VCE, whereas all cases of CIN alone tested were negative. The proportion of positivity varied greatly from case to case and from area to area. In some cases, a few nuclei only were positive. No difference was otherwise noted between positive and negative koilocytotic lesions. The discrepancy between the percentage of cases of CIN with light microscopic evidence of HPV-induced changes and positively reacting cases for papilloma virus antigens has already been reported (Kurman et al., 1982) and, in part, correlated with the intraepithelial extent of koilocytotic cells (Ferenczy, 1981). In a few cases of CIN II, ultra-structural studies showed a rather small size of the peri-nuclear halo, the very irregular nuclear contour due to deep involding of the membrane, the coarse clumps of chromatin, and the intranuclear presence of viral particles identical to those already described (Della Torre et al., 1978).

Utilizing a different approach to the problem of whether CIN with VCE is an entity or not, the outcome of several cases originally diagnosed cytologically as having CIN I or II with cytologic evidence of persistence or progression of the disease and followed for at least 24 months without any surgical interference is currently under investigation. Three main groups of patients were identified. The first group consisted of cases originally diagnosed as CIN I that were in part (70%) rediagnosed cytologically as condylomata. The majority of the condylomata progressed to CIN II or III within 40 months and all showed CIN with VCE at histology. The cases of reconfirmed CIN I progressed to CIN III within 32 months. These data show that a) 70% of CIN I diagnosed about a decade ago are nowadays recognizable as condylomata, b) a number of cases of condylomata of the cervix may pro-gress to advanced CIN, and c) the progression may be com-pleted within a time lapse similar to that of true CIN I.

In the second group of patients originally diagnosed cytologically as having CIN II, 60% were rediagnosed as CIN II with VCE and 40% as CIN II. The progression rate to CIN III and invasive carcinoma was similar in the two subsets of patients. The third group consisted of those cases, originally diagnosed as CIN II, whose smears revealed at revision the presence of a few small immature cells, possibly related to subcylindrical cell anaplasia (Christopherson, 1977; Spriggs, Boddington, 1980). Overall, 67% of the cases showed cytological evidence of HPV-infection, whose persis-tence was confirmed histologically years later in over 85%. Progression to more advanced lesions was shown by 78% of the cases in the HPV-infected subgroup as well as in the VCE-negative group.

In conclusion, advanced cervical intraepithelial

neoplasia associated with HPV-induced cellular lesions and/or flat condylomata appears to be a distinct variant among the precursors of squamous cell carcinoma of the uterine cervix because it is not uncommon, it displays a peculiar morphology, it has a special topographic extension, and it is diagnosed in patients who are younger than those with CIN alone.

REFERENCES

Ashley DJB (1966). Evidence for the existence of two forms of cervical carcinoma. J Obstet Gynaecol Br Commonw 73:382.
Christopherson WM (1977). Dysplasia, carcinoma in situ, and microinvasive carcinoma of the uterine cervix. Hum Pathol 8:489.
Della Torre G, Pilotti S, De Palo G, Rilke F (1978). Viral particles in cervical condylomatous lesions. Tumori 64:549.
Dreesman GR, Burek J, Adam E, Kaufman RH, Melnick JL, Powell KI, Purifoy DJM (1980). Expression of herpesvirus-induced antigens in human cervical cancer. Nature 283:591.
Fenoglio CM, Galloway DA, Crum CP, Levine RU, Richart RM, McDougall JK (1982). Herpes simplex virus and cervical neoplasia. In Fenoglio CM, Wolff M (eds): "Progress in Surgical Pathology," vol. 4, New York: Masson, p 45.
Ferenczy A, Braun L, Shah KV (1981). Human papillomavirus (HPV) in condylomatous lesions of cervix. A comparative ultrastructural and immunohistochemical study. Am J Surg Pathol 5:661.
Gissmann L, de Villiers E-M, zur Hausen H (1982). Analysis of human genital warts (condylomata acuminata) and other genital tumors for human papillomavirus type 6 DNA. Int J Cancer 29:143.
Hakama M, Penttinen J (1981). Epidemiological evidence for two components of cervical cancer. Br J Obstet Gynaecol 88:209.
Herbst AL, Ulfelder H, Poskanzer DC (1971). Adenocarcinoma of the vagina: Association of maternal stilbestrol therapy with tumor appearance in young women. N Engl J Med 284:878.
Hsu S-M, Raine L, Fanger H (1981). Use of avidin-biotin-peroxidase complex (ABC) in immunoperoxidase techniques: A comparison between ABC and unlabeled antibody (PAP) procedures. J Histochem Cytochem 29:577.
Jenson AB, Rosenthal JD, Olson C, Pass F, Lancaster WD, Shah K (1980). Immunologic relatedness of papillomaviruses from different species. J Natl Cancer Inst 64:495.

Kessler II (1976). Human cervical cancer as a venereal disease. Cancer Res 36:783.

Kessler II (1981). Etiological concepts in cervical carcinogenesis. Gynecol Oncol 12:S7.

Koss LG (1979). "Diagnostic Cytology and Its Histopathologic Bases." Philadelphia: Lippincott, p 292.

Koss LG, Durfee GR (1956). Unusual patterns of squamous epithelium of the uterine cervix. Cytologic and pathologic study of koilocytotic atypia. Ann N Y Acad Sci 63:1245.

Kurman RJ, Lancaster WD, Jenson AB (1982). Frequency and distribution of papillomavirus antigens in cervical dysplasia and carcinoma in situ (abstract). Lab Invest 46:46A.

Laskey PW, Meigs JW, Flannery JT (1976). Uterine cervical carcinoma in Connecticut, 1935 — 1973: Evidence for two classes of invasive disease. J Natl Cancer Inst 57:1037.

Laverty CR, Russell P, Hills E, Booth N (1978). The significance of noncondylomatous wart virus infection of the cervical transformation zone. A review with discussion of two illustrative cases. Acta Cytol 22:195.

Macgregor JE (1982). Rapid onset cancer of the cervix. Br Med J 284:441.

McDougall JK, Galloway DA, Crum C, Levine R, Richart R, Fenoglio CM (1981). Detection of nucleic acid sequences in cervical tumors. Gynecol Oncol 12:S42.

McDougall JK, Galloway DA, Fenoglio CM (1980). Cervical carcinoma: Detection of herpes simplex virus RNA in cells undergoing neoplastic change. Int J Cancer 25:1.

Meisels A, Fortin R, Roy M (1977). Condylomatous lesions of the cervix. II. Cytologic, colposcopic and histopathologic study. Acta Cytol 21:379.

Meisels A, Roy M, Fortier M, Morin C, Casas-Cordero M, Shah, KV, Turgeon H (1981). Human papillomavirus infection of the cervix. The atypical condyloma. Acta Cytol 25:7.

Morin C, Braun L, Casas-Cordero M, Shah KV, Roy M, Fortier M, Meisels A (1981). Confirmation of the papillomavirus etiology of condylomatous cervix lesions by the peroxidase-antiperoxidase technique. J Natl Cancer Inst 66:831.

Morin C, Meisels A (1980). Human papilloma virus infection of the uterine cervix (letter to the Editor). Acta Cytol 24:82.

Naib ZM, Nahmias AJ, Josey WE (1966). Cytology and histopathology of cervical herpes simplex infection. Cancer 19:1026.

Naib ZM, Nahmias AJ, Josey WE, et al. (1969). Genital herpetic infection: Association with cervical dysplasia and carcinoma. Cancer 23:940.

Pilotti S, Rilke F, De Palo G, Della Torre G, Alasio L (1981). Condylomata of the uterine cervix and koilocytosis of cervical intraepithelial neoplasia. J Clin Pathol 34:532.

Pilotti S, Rilke F, Alasio L, Fontanelli R (1982). Histologic evidence for an association of cervical intraepithelial neoplasia with human papilloma virus infection. Diagn Gynecol Obstet (in press).

Rawls WE, Laurel D, Melnick JL, et al. (1968). A search for viruses in smegma, premalignant and early malignant cervical tissues: The isolation of herpesviruses with distinct antigenic properties. Am J Epidemiol 87:647.

Richart RM (1967). Natural history of cervical intraepithelial neoplasia. Clin Obstet Gynecol 10:748.

Shah KH, Lewis MG, Jenson AB, Kurman RJ, Lancaster WD (1980). Papillomavirus and cervical dysplasia (letter to Editor). Lancet 2:1190.

Spriggs AI, Boddington MM (1980). Progression and regression of cervical lesions. Review of smears from women followed without initial biopsy or treatment. J Clin Pathol 33:517.

Stern E (1977). Steroid contraceptive use and cervical dysplasia. Science 196:1460.

Woodruff JD, Braun L, Cavalieri R, Gupta P, Pass F, Shah KV (1980). Immunologic identification of papillomavirus antigen in condyloma tissues from the female genital tract. Obstet Gynecol 56:727.

zur Hausen H, de Villiers E-M, Gissmann L (1981). Papillomavirus infections and human genital cancer. Gynecol Oncol 12:S124.

13th International Cancer Congress, Part D
Research and Treatment, pages 107–116
© 1983 Alan R. Liss, Inc., 150 Fifth Avenue, New York, NY 10011

MICROCARCINOMA OF THE STOMACH MEASURING LESS THAN 5 mm IN
THE LARGEST DIAMETER AND ITS HISTOGENESIS

Kyoichi Nakamura, M.D., D.M.Sc.* **
and Haruo Sugano, M.D., D.M.Sc.**
Department of Pathology, Tsukuba University, Ibaraki 305*,
and Cancer Institute, Tokyo 170**, Japan

Carcinomas arising from metaplastic epithelium of the
intestinal type have been reported by Järvi, Lauren(1951),
Mulligan, Rember(1954), Morson(1955), Lauren(1965), and
Ming, Goldman, Freiman(1967). These studies concern the
histogenesis of several cases of small or large carcinomas.

Microcarcinoma of the stomach, defined as carcinoma
measuring less than 5 mm in the largest diameter, is very
suitable for analysing histogenesis because it may be assumed
that the histological aspects of both the microcarcinomas
and of the adjacent mucosa are at the incipient phase of
cancer development. We have studied the histogenesis of
gastric carcinoma by histologically analysing microcarcinomas
(Nakamura, Sugano, Takagi 1968). The conclusion was that
undifferentiated carcinoma (gastric type) in which cancer
cells do not form tubuli, arises from the ordinary mucosa of
the stomach, while differentiated carcinoma (intestinal type)
in which cancer cells do form tubuli, arises from metaplastic
mucosa of the intestinal type. The purpose of this paper is
to summarize the histogenesis of gastric carcinomas studied
histologically by using 145 microcarcinomas of the stomach.

The stomachs resected for small or early carcinoma,
ulcer, or polyp were examined by systematical mapping of all
resected stomachs, as shown in Fig. 1. One hundred thirty-
four microcarcinomas were histologically discovered in this
way. Only 11 patients were diagnosed preoperatively as
having microcarcinomas (Figs. 1 and 2). Tissue paraffin
blocks including the microcarcinoma were serially cut from

the original face or from the opposite face, and all slides were stained with hematoxylin and eosin, periodic acid-Schiff, or alcian blue.

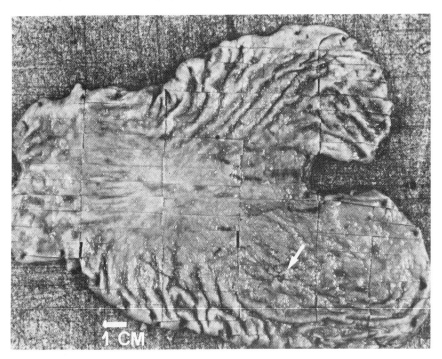

Fig. 1  A resected stomach removed for a microcarcinoma pre-operatively diagnosed (46 year-old man). This photograph shows method of examination by systematical mapping of the resected stomach. The microcarcinoma shows macroscopically a depression with slightly elevated contour (arrow).

The 145 microcarcinomas tended to be localized in the antrum along the lesser curvature (Table 1). The tendency is similar to the localization of advanced carcinoma infiltrating the proper muscle and serosa.

Macroscopic findings of the microcarcinomas were examined retrospectively in enlarged photographs of resected stomachs (Table 2). Eleven foci (7.6%) were recognized as minute depressed lesions and 31 foci (21.4%) as depressed lesions with slightly elevated contour (Fig. 1). One hundred and two foci of the microcarcinomas (70.3%) could

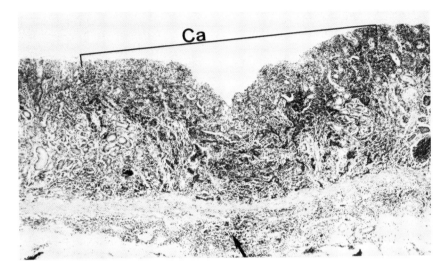

Fig. 2  A cut-surface of the microcarcinoma in Fig. 1.  The microcarcinoma measures approximately 3 mm in the largest diameter.  Small cancer cells show trabecular arrangement and invade microscopically the submucosa (arrow).  The surface of the microcarcinoma is slightly depressed.

|  | Antrum | Middle | Corpus | Total |
|---|---|---|---|---|
| Anterior wall | 16 | 9 | 8 | 33 foci |
| Lesser curvature site | 31 | 23 | 8 | 62 |
| Posterior wall | 22 | 8 | 9 | 39 |
| Greater curvature site | 6 | 4 | 1 | 11 |
| Total | 75 | 44 | 26 | 145 foci |

Table 1  Localization of microcarcinoma

| Macroscopic appearance | Histologically discovered | Preoperatively diagnosed | Total |
|---|---|---|---|
| Obscure | 102 | 0 | 102 foci |
| Depressed(IIc) | 5 | 6 | 11 |
| Protruded(IIa) | 0 | 1 | 1 |
| IIc+IIa* | 27 | 4 | 31 |
| Total | 134 | 11 | 145 foci |

*Depressed lesion with slightly elevated contour

Table 2  Macroscopic appearance of microcarcinoma

not be macroscopically recognized as a minute lesion.

One hundred forty out of the 145 microcarcinomas (97%) were found in mucosa essentially within normal limits or in atrophic mucosa. Three foci (2%) were associated with ulcer or ulcer-scar, and two (1%) extended into a slightly elevated lesion of benign atypical epithelium meauring about 4 cm in the largest diameter. The majority of the microcarcinomas were situated at the mucosa essentially within normal limits or at the atrophic mucosa independent of the localized benign lesions of the stomach.

Histological patterns of the microcarcinomas are generally uniform and simple. The microcarcinomas were classified into two types: i.e. whether the cancer cells form tubuli or not. Tubular adenocarcinomas whose cuboidal to cylindrical cells form tubular structures are defined as

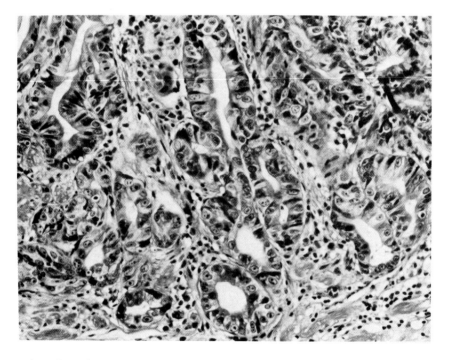

Fig. 3 High-power view of microcarcinoma in Fig. 7. Showing tubular adenocarcinoma (Differentiated carcinoma).

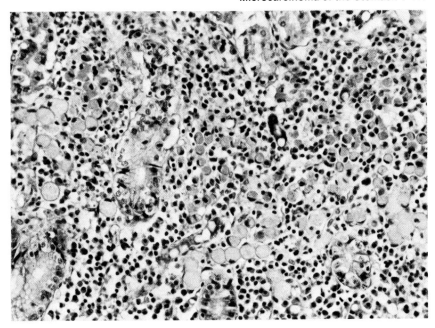

Fig. 4 High-power view of microcarcinoma in Fig. 8 showing mucocellular adenocarcinoma (Undifferentiated carcinoma).

differentiated carcinoma (Fig. 3). Mucocellular (Fig. 4) and anaplastic (Fig. 2) adenocarcinomas, whose small cells are individually spread and/or show trabecular arrangement and do not form tubuli, are defined as undifferentiated carcinomas. At the level of light-microscopy, cells of the differentiated carcinoma have a striated border (Fig. 5) and their cytoplasms are generally not stained with PAS and Alcian blue. Similar characteristics are noted in the metaplastic epithelial cell. In contrast, cells of undifferentiated carcinoma do not have a striated border. The mucus is positive for PAS and negative for Alcian blue stain and this is demonstrated to a greater or lesser degree in the cytoplasm (Fig. 6). These characteristics are similar to the surface mucous cells of the ordinary mucosa and the pyloric gland cells.

Table 3 shows the relation between histological type of the 140 microcarcinomas and the nature of the mucosae neighboring them. There is a tendency for tubular adenocarcinomas belonging to the differentiated carcinoma to be

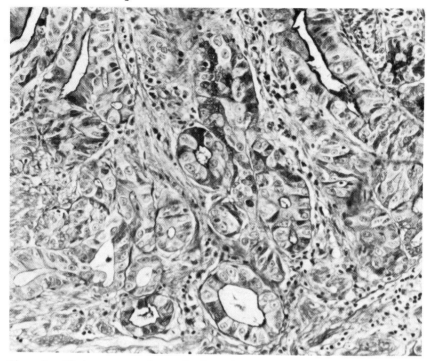

Fig. 5  High-power view of the microcarcinoma of Fig. 3
stained with PAS.  Cancer cells have striated border at the
free surface of tubuli.

surrounded by metaplastic mucosa of intestinal type (Fig. 7).
Mucocellular and anaplastic adenocarcinomas belonging to the

| Grade of intestinal metaplasia | Histological type | |
|---|---|---|
| | Differentiated | Undifferentiated |
| Prominent | 97 | 0 foci |
| Focal | 22 | 4 |
| None | 1 | 16* |
| Total | 120 | 20 foci |

* Four out of 16 foci: carcinomas completely surrounded by
  the fundic gland mucosa.
$X_0^2$ (1, 0.01) = 6.635, $X^2$ = 28.6 (Yates correction)

Table 3  Histological type of microcarcinoma situated at the
normal or atrophic mucosa and grade of intestinal metaplasia
at the mucosa surrounding it.

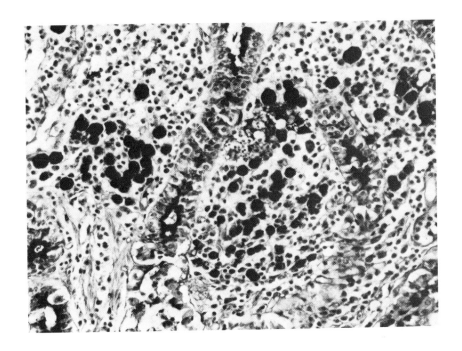

Fig. 6 High-power view of the microcarcinoma of Fig. 4
stained with PAS. Cancer cells and the mucous cells of the
foveolar epithelium are deeply stained with PAS.

undifferentiated carcinoma are surrounded by the ordinary
mucosa of the stomach consisting of the pyloric or fundic
gland mucosa without intestinal metaplasia (Figs. 2 and 8).
Application of the chi-square test between those two categories yields a significant difference (P is less than 0.01).

It may be considered that the microcarcinoma and its
neighboring mucosa may retain conditions conducive to the
development of cancer. The majority of the microcarcinomas
are situated within the boundary of normal or atrophic
mucosa, independent of ulcer and polyp. Furthermore, there
is a tendency for the tubular or well differentiated
microcarcinoma to be found in or near the mucosal layer
manifesting intestinal metaplasia. The undifferentiated
microcarcinomas are situated in the normal pyloric or
fundus mucosa and the individual tumor cells have the
morphological features of normal mucous cells. Based on

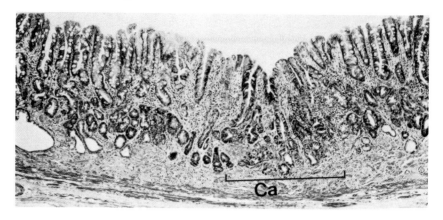

Fig. 7   A cut-surface of the microcarcinoma of Figs. 3 and 5, measuring about 1 mm in the largest diameter and situated at atrophic mucosa consisting completely of metaplastic epithelium of intestinal type.

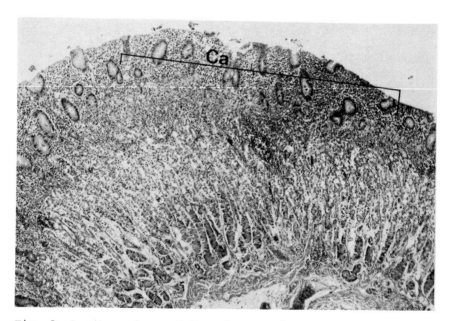

Fig. 8   A cut surface of the microcarcinoma of Figs. 4 and 6, measuring about 2 mm in the largest diameter and situated at the fundic gland mucosa, essentially within normal limits. Cancer cells invade diffusely the propria mucosae at the neck portion of the fundic gland.

those findings, a hypothesis of histogenesis of the gastric carcinoma may be drawn as follows: the differentiated carcinoma arises from metaplastic epithelium of intestinal type, while the undifferentiated carcinoma arises from the ordinary mucosa of the stomach, independently of the localized benign lesions.

Cells of the microcarcinomas belonging to the undifferentiated carcinoma are generally limited to the superficial half of the ordinary mucosa (Fig. 8), while tubuli of the microcarcinomas belonging to the differentiated carcinoma occupy the entire mucosa consisting of metaplastic epithelium from the mucosal surface adjacent to the muscularis mucosae (Fig. 7). Those findings may support the hypothesis of histogenesis because the mitotic zone of the pyloric and fundic glands for cell renewal is present at the neck portion, while the mitotic zone of intestinalized gland of the stomach occurs at the bottom. Cancer cells occur at the mitotic zone.

Järvi and his co-workers have studied extensively the histogenesis of gastric carcinoma since 1953. From the viewpoints of growing mode, individual cell structure, and mucin histochemistry, Lauren(1965) has reported that the gastric carcinoma is classified into two groups, diffuse carcinoma and intestinal-type carcinoma. The undifferentiated and differentiated carcinomas almost correspond to diffuse and intestinal-type carcinomas classified by Lauren, and to infiltrative and expanding carcinomas classified by Ming(1977). They have observed that the intestinal-type carcinoma arises from metaplastic epithelium of intestinal-type and that diffuse carcinoma also can arise from this. Morson(1955) has stated that 30% of all gastric carcinomas might arise from metaplastic epithelium of the intestinal type. No one suggests that mucocellular and anaplastic adenocarcinomas arise from the ordinary mucosa of the stomach. Nagayo (1975) has reported a study of the microcarcinomas, and observed that there is a relationship between the histological type of the microcarcinoma and the nature of the mucosa neighboring it. Johansen(1981) has reported that 17 early carcinomas out of 27 diffuse carcinomas had originated from a mucosa virtually depleted of intestinal metaplastic epithelium.

Järvi, O., Lauren, P.(1951). On the role of heterotopias
    of the intestinal epithelium in the pathogenesis of
    gastric cancer. Acta pathol. microbiol. scand. 29:26.
Johansen, A.(1981). "Early Gastric Cancer. A contribution
    to the pathology and to gastric cancer histogenesis."
    Copenhagen: Bispebjerg Hospital, P 194.
Lauren, P.(1965). The two histological main types of
    gastric carcinoma. An attempt at a histo-clinical
    classification. Acta pathol. microbiol. scand. 64:31.
Mulligan, R. M., Rember, R. R.(1954). Histogenesis and
    biologic behavior of gastric carcinoma. Study of one
    hundred thirty-eight cases. Arch. Path. 58:1
Morson, B. C.(1955). Carcinoma arising from areas of
    intestinal metaplasia in the gastric mucosa. Br. J.
    Cancer 9:377.
Ming, Si-C., Goldman, H., Freiman, D. G.(1967). Intestinal
    metaplasia and histogenesis of carcinoma in human
    stomach. Cancer 20:1418.
Ming, Si-C.(1977). Gastric carcinoma - a pathological
    classification. Cancer 39:2475.
Nakamura, K., Sugano, H., Takagi, K.(1968). Carcinoma of
    the stomach in incipient phase: Its histogenesis and
    histological appearances. Gann 59:251.
Nagayo, T.(1975). Microscopical cancer of the stomach.
    A study on histogenesis of gastric carcinoma. Int. J.
    Cancer 16:52.

**13th International Cancer Congress, Part D**
**Research and Treatment, pages 117–127**
© **1983 Alan R. Liss, Inc., 150 Fifth Avenue, New York, NY 10011**

MORPHOLOGIC ASPECTS OF THE GENESIS OF COLO-RECTAL CARCINOMA
AND ITS RELATIONSHIP TO ADENOMA

Horatio T. Enterline, M.D.

Professor of Pathology and Laboratory Medicine
University of Pennsylvania School of Medicine
Philadelphia, Pennsylvania 19104

Epidemiologic and experimental studies indicate that
the basic pathogenesis of colo-rectal carcinoma is due to an
endogenous diet related carcinogen activated through the action of various microflora and present in the colonic lumen
(Correa 1978, Hill 1975, Reddy 1974). The effect of such
carcinogens in experimental models is modified by the species
and genetic strain of the animals used. The precise dietary
and microfloral factors involved are not agreed upon (Graham
1978, Vargo 1980). In addition, genetic variation in susceptibility is clear (Evans 1974) and in the human at least 10%
of the total colo-rectal burden is genetic dependent (Lynch
1977 A & B).

The precise morphologic precursor in the human has been
much debated. In the common experimental model - rat, 1,2
dimethylhydrazine - most carcinomas produced appear to arise
independently of adenoma (Maskens 1981), but the type of tumor, i.e., carcinoma or adenoma, and whether or not carcinomas appear to arise within such adenomas is variable depending on the carcinogen, the microflora, and the genetic background of the animals concerned (Evans 1974, Pour 1978).

Translation of these findings to colo-rectal carcinoma
in man must be interpreted with caution. The tumors so produced tend to occur relatively rapidly, are often multiple,
and are accompanied by tumors of small bowel and other organs.
As Chang (1978) points out, in the animal model a relatively
large amount of carcinogen is given over a short time period,
which is not comparable to the human condition, where induction and progression are slow (Chang 1978).

THE HUMAN MODEL

In the past, debates about pathogenesis of colo-rectal carcinoma in humans have revolved around whether or not it arose in normal mucosa or within adenomatous tissue. More recently, Filipe (1974) and others have described mucosal changes adjacent to or distant from carcinoma consisting of increased length and tortuosity and branching of colonic crypts. (These changes were associated with a shift from sulfated acid mucin secretion to sialic acid mucins, and have been considered by them to be of basic pre-neoplastic nature.) However, similar changes have now been described of mucosa overlying lipomas, metastatic tumors, diverticuli, and endometriosis, and these therefore must be considered non-specific (Rhatigan 1979, Latinsky 1981).

RELATION OF CARCINOMA TO POLYPS

Of the various types of benign polyps, only the hyperplastic and adenomatous are sufficiently common to be significant contenders as carcinoma precursors. The hyperplastic polyp is common and rarely may show an admix of adenoma or carcinoma (Cooper 1979). However, major discrepancies in both its epidemiology and its distribution, which is chiefly rectal, appear to rule it out as a significant factor as a cancer precursor (Correa 1978), a conclusion I share with Spjut (1977), Morson (1977), and others.

RELATION OF ADENOMA OF COLON AND RECTUM TO COLO-RECTAL CARCINOMA

Not all polyps are adenomatous, and not all adenomas polypoid. They may be of microscopic dimensions and unicrystal (Woda 1977). Adenoma may be defined as a benign tumor with crowded elongated nuclei, usually reduction of mucin secretion, and with cell replication present at all levels. Chromosomal abnormalities have been described by myself and others.

Evidence for the origin of colonic cancer in adenoma may be divided into indirect evidence derived from epidemiologic studies and direct evidence, i.e., the observation of minute cancers within adenoma or of adenoma at the periphery of larger carcinomas.

Epidemiologic Studies. There is a rather good parallelism between the incidence of adenomas and carcinomas in low and high incidence areas of the world. Detailed autopsy studies are now available on this point.

Table 1

PREVALENCE OF COLONIC CANCER AND ADENOMAS
BY POPULATIONS
(After Correa, 1978)

| Populations | Colon Cancer Incidence | Prevalence of Adenoma (age 40-59) | |
|---|---|---|---|
| | | Males | Females |
| Hawaiian-Japan. | very high | 63 | 49 |
| N. Orleans-black | high | 35 | 29 |
| Japan (Akita) | intermediate | 35 | 19 |
| Japan (Miyagi) | low | 13 | 11 |
| Colombia (Cali) | low | 10 | 10 |

The distribution of carcinoma and of adenoma within the colon is in reasonable but not total agreement.

Table 2

COMPARISON OF SITE OF ADENOMAS AND CARCINOMA OF COLORECTUM
(Enterline, 1978)

| Source | Cecum + AC% | Transverse % | Desc.% | Sig.+ Rectum% |
|---|---|---|---|---|
| Adenoma-Helwig Autopsy, 1947 | 22 | 15 | 11 | 48 |
| Adenoma-Ecklund, 1974 | 24 | 19 | 11 | 45 |
| Carcinoma-Falterman, 1974 | 18 | 9 | 7 | 65 |

The general conclusion from these and other figures is that there is some excess of adenoma in the right colon and some deficit in the sigmoid and rectum compared with the sites for carcinoma. This has been used as an argument

against the role for adenoma as a carcinoma precursor. However, that would assume that all adenomas are of equal pro-
pensity to develop a malignancy. There is, however, evidence
that the closer an adenoma is to the rectum, the higher the
incidence of areas of dysplasia and of carcinoma within such
adenomas (Ecklund 1974, Shinya 1979).

Table 3

PREMALIGNANT AND MALIGNANT CHANGES IN ADENOMA BY SITE
(After Shinya & Wolff, 1979)

| Site | Total Number | % Ca in Situ | % Invas.Ca |
|------|-------------|--------------|------------|
| Right colon | 752 | 9% | 3% |
| Rectosigmoid | 3,000 | 13% | 6% |

In high incidence countries, adenomas tend to be larger
and hence at greater risk of developing carcinoma than in
low incidence countries such as Colombia and Japan (Correa
1978, Morson 1977, Sato 1976).

Furthermore, in Japan, adenomas from a higher incidence
area for carcinoma (Akita province) were larger and had a
higher incidence of atypia than those from a lower incidence
area (Miyaga province), and a higher per centage of patients
from the higher incidence province had more than one adenoma
(Sato 1976).

Adenomas associated with a separate carcinoma tend to
show more dysplasia, particularly if they are close to the
carcinoma, than do adenomas (Ecklund 1974, Kalus 1972, Silverberg 1970).

If adenomas precede carcinomas, one would expect them
to occur at an earlier age. The peak incidence of adenomas
is estimated to be seven to eight years younger than that of
carcinoma (Wilson 1955, Morson 1978).

Adenocarcinoma is from three to five times as common in
patients with adenoma than in those without. It is even more
common if more than one adenoma is present (Rider 1959). A
careful prospective follow-up study with age and sex matched
controls over a 10-year period has also shown that patients
with adenoma are at higher risk of developing carcinoma

(Brahme 1974).

Table 4

Ten-Year Follow-Up Study of Patients With & Without Adenoma
(After Brahme, 1974)

| Initial Finding | Total # | # With New Adenoma | #With Carcinoma |
|---|---|---|---|
| Adenoma | 115 | 24 | 3 |
| No Adenoma | 115 | 6 | 0 |

The reality of the adenoma-carcinoma sequence does not imply that all adenomas develop carcinoma. Clearly a majority do not within the lifetime of the host. Indeed, some have been observed to remain the same size or even disappear when observed over many years. What are the features that indicate a high risk of carcinoma within an adenoma?

We have already indicated that adenomas associated with a carcinoma, particularly if close to such carcinoma, have a higher incidence of atypical features within them, as do those in the left colon as opposed to the right.

Relation to Size. All studies, including our own, agree that there is a direct correlation of the presence of both in situ carcinoma (dysplasia) and invasive carcinoma to the size of the adenoma. The incidence of invasive carcinoma is 1% or less in those under 1 cm., and rises to 16% or higher in those over 2.5 cm. (Enterline 1978, Shinya 1979, Grinnell 1958).

Relation to Type of Adenoma. Adenomas have been divided by WHO into tubular, villous, and mixed types sometimes called tubulo-villous. The cut-off point between these types, however, has not been uniformly agreed on, and they are not to be thought of as distinct, but rather as points on a spectrum.

The incidence of dysplasia and of invasive carcinoma correlates well with the presence or absence of villi. The large sessile villous adenoma has long been known to have a dismayingly high incidence of carcinoma of up to 50% in some series. Recent figures from Shinya and Wolff's series (1979) of over 3,000 adenomas shows an incidence of carcinoma in villous lesions of all sizes of 9.5%, of mixed adenomas of 8.4%, and of tubular of 2.8%.

Table 5

Incidence of Invasive Carcinoma in Adenoma by Type

| Type | Morson | Enterline | Shinya | Appel |
|------|--------|-----------|--------|-------|
| Tubular | 4% | .6% | 2.8% | 0% |
| Mixed | 23% | 4.0% | 8.4% | 5% |
| Villous | 40% | 48.0% | 9.5% | 8% |

Discrepancies relate largely to cut-off points between the various types. Thus, in Appel's group (1977), one villous element put it in the mixed type, while in Shinya's, an adenoma with villous elements of less than 20% was considered tubular. Morson (1978) and I were considering only the large sessile villous adenomas. In my experience and also that of Shinya, and in Wolff's recent study, the incidence of dysplasia and of invasive carcinoma, however, differs little if the adenomas are matched for size. The fact is that pure tubular adenomas are usually small and very rarely as large as 2 cm., while the purely villous lesions are usually large. Whether or not a given adenoma is pedunculated does not correlate with the incidence of dysplasia or of invasive carcinoma, although it affects the management problem.

It should be borne in mind that, while the incidence of carcinoma in large adenomas is many times that of small adenomas, the number of small adenomas is conversely many times that of large adenomas. While the individual risk of a particular polyp is much smaller, the small adenoma may therefore contribute more than we realize to the ultimate population of adenocarcinomas.

Residual Adenoma in Clinical Carcinoma. A converse of the finding of minute to small carcinomas in adenomas is the finding of adenomatous remnants at the margins of large carcinomas. Morson (1978) found such changes in 60% of Duke A carcinomas, in 20% of Duke B lesions confined to the muscularis, and in 7% of those which had extended into the serosa. Thus, the frequency was inversely proportional to the extent of the carcinoma.

Time Required for Evolution of Carcinoma of the Colon. The rather scanty evidence available suggests that the evolu-

tion of carcinoma from adenoma is a slow process, measured
in years. I have observed a case of carcinoma in an adenoma
in which the carcinoma had extended into the muscularis.
The tumor, in retrospect, was identified on annual films for
a period of at least 8 years. Similar cases have been reported by Morson (1978) and by Marshak (1976), in which carcinoma
was proven from 4 to 13 years later. Kozuka (1975) found a
seven year difference between the average age of typical
adenomas and of those containing carcinoma in situ. Morson
has estimated, from studies of polyposis families, about a
12-year interval from detection of polyps to that of carcinoma. Thus, the average time required for carcinoma to develop is probably at least five years, and more likely much
longer.

Result of Systematic Removal of Polyps During Periodic
Sigmoidoscopic Examinations. If adenomas contribute significantly to later carcinomas, one would expect that systematic
removal of such lesions would result in a reduction of the
incidence of carcinoma. Two large studies suggest that this
is indeed the case. Systematic removal of adenomas in a population of 4,400 patients over a 15-year period by Prager and
co-workers (1974), and of a somewhat smaller group by Gilbert-
son (1974) over a 25-year period, both showed a sharp reduction of carcinoma over the expected figure in the area of the
bowel accessible to polypectomy.

Evidence for "DeNovo" Carcinoma of the Colon and Rectum.
As mentioned, the experimental model has certainly shown that
carcinoma may develop in animals without an intermediary adenoma stage. In South African blacks, though carcinoma is rare,
adenoma is even more so (Segal 1981, Bremmer 1970).

Another possibly unique group is colo-rectal carcinoma
in children. Again, this is a rare occurrence. Chabalko
and Fraumeni (1975) reported that 9 of 13 children under the
age of 10 had non-mucinous carcinomas developing within adenoma. On the other hand, of those older than 10, 21 of 24
were of the colloid type, and only one of these appeared to
arise within an adenoma. One might argue that time in this
older age group permitted overgrowth of preceding adenoma,
but the peculiar dominant colloid type, which is not the most
common of types in adults, suggests that quite likely some
other mechanism of pathogenesis is operative.

Extensive studies in ulcerative colitis of so-called

"pre-cancerous states" have shown that while better differentiated carcinomas arise within adenomatous changes, less differentiated carcinomas may arise in dysplastic areas. It is tempting to hypothesize in this latter group, under conditions of a presumed strong carcinogenic influence, that the adenoma stage, as in many of the experimental models, may be omitted. Spjut (1979) and co-workers have reported five minute carcinomas measuring from 3 to 15 mm., which they have interpreted as de Novo cancers. However, all were stated to show "occasional glands with adenomatous changes at the border." To me, this markedly weakens the argument that they were indeed "de Novo." To be convincing as such, a carcinoma should be extremely small, non-ulcerating, and totally lacking evidence of a bordering adenomatous change. Even then it may be argued that a unicryptal or minute adenoma such as those described by Woda (1977) and others might have been overgrown by carcinoma or dysplasia arising within it.

Lev and Grover (1981) recently reported a study of a series of partial colectomy specimens from patients with carcinoma which were studied by a Swiss role technique permitting assay of large volumes of mucosa. In this series, numerous minute adenomas not otherwise appreciated were found. A few contained foci of dysplasia; however, in one of their cases an area of dysplasia was found quite independent of adenoma which certainly could have been a source of a subsequent cancer. This particular patient had two carcinomas and over 30 adenomatous polyps, again suggesting a strong carcinogenic influence. Shamsuddin (1980) and co-workers have recently described foci of abnormal mucosa in human cancer bearing colons which they believe are similar to the "pre-malignant" epithelium in the rat model. Kino (1980) discovered one micro-carcinoma measuring 800 microns which lacked accompanying adenomatous epithelium. I have also seen one example of a minute area of in situ carcinoma without accompanying adenomatous tissue in a patient with a large nearby cecal carcinoma, through the courtesy of Dr. H. Cooper.

It therefore seems probable that carcinoma "de Novo" may indeed occur through a mechanism of direct dysplasia in exceptional circumstances.

Nonetheless, the evidence to me is overwhelming that the adenoma-carcinoma sequence accounts for the vast majority of colo-rectal carcinoma. The finding, therefore, of an adenoma, or especially of multiple adenomas, identifies patients at higher risk of carcinoma, and intense surveillance and removal of lesions appears justified. Hopefully, this should result in a reduced mortality from colo-rectal carcinoma.

## REFERENCES

Appel MF, Spjut HJ, Estrade RG (1977). The significance of villous component in colonic polyps. Am J Surg 134:770.

Brahme F, Ecklund GL, Norden JG, et. al. (1974). Metachronous colorectal polyps: comparison of development of colorectal polyps and carcinoma in persons with and without histories of polyps. Dis Colon Rectum 17:166.

Bremmer CG, Ackerman LV (1970). Polyps and carcinoma of the large bowel in the South African Bantu. Cancer 26:991.

Chabalko JJ, Fraumeni JF (1975). Colorectal cancer in children: epidemiologic aspects. Dis Colon Rectum 18:1.

Chang WWL (1978). Histogenesis of symmetrical 1,2, dimethylhydrazine induced neoplasms of the colon in the mouse. J Natl Cancer Inst 60:1405.

Cooper HS, Patchefsky AS, Marks G (1979). Adenomatous and carcinomatous changes within hyperplastic colonic epithelium. Dis Colon Rectum 22:152.

Correa P, Haenzel W (1978). The epidemiology of large bowel cancer. In Klein G, Weinhouse S (eds): "Advances in Medical Research, 26," New York, San Francisco, London: Academic Press, p 1.

Correa P (1978). Epidemiology of polyps and cancer. In Morson B (ed): "Pathogenesis of Colorectal Carcinoma," Philadelphia, Toronto, London: W.B. Saunders and Co., chap 11.

Ecklund GL, Lindstron C (1974). Histopathological analysis of benign polyps in patients with carcinoma of the colon and rectum. Gut 15:654.

Enterline HT, Arvan DA (1967). Chromosome constitution of adenoma and carcinoma of the colon. Cancer 20:1746.

Enterline HT (1978). Significance of adenomatous polyps in colon carcinogenesis. In Grundmann (ed): Stuttgart, New York: Fisher Verlag, p 57.

Evans JT, Haushka TS, Mittelman A (1974). Differential susceptibility of four mouse strains to induction of multiple large-bowel neoplasms by 1,2,dimethylhydrazine. J Natl Cancer Inst 52:999.

Filipe MI, Branfort AC (1974). Abnormal patterns of mucus secretions in apparently normal mucosa of large intestine with carcinoma. Cancer 34:282.

Gilbertsen VA (1974). Proctosigmoidoscopy and polypectomy in reducing the incidence of rectal carcinoma. Cancer 34:936.

Graham S, Dayal H, Swanson M (1978). Diet in the epidemiology of cancer of the colon and rectum. J Natl Cancer Inst 61:709.

Grinnell R, Lane H (1958). Benign and malignant polyps and papillary adenomas of the colon and rectum. Surg Gynecol Obstet 106:519.

Hill MJ (1975). Metabolic epidemiology of dietary factors in large bowel cancer. Cancer Res 35:3398.

Kalus M (1972). Carcinoma and adenomatous polyps of the colon and rectum in biopsy and organ tissue culture. Cancer 30:972.

Kino I, Nakamura S (1980). Pathological characteristics of colonic early cancers. Stomach and Intestine 15:357.

Kozuka S, Nogaki M, Ozeki T, et. al. (1975). Pre-malignancy of the mucosal polyp in the large intestine: estimates of periods required for malignant transformation of mucosal polyps. Dis Colon Rectum 18:494.

Latinsky CM, Riddell RH (1981). Patterns of mucin secretion in neoplastic and non-neoplastic diseases of the colon. Hum Pathol 12:923.

Lev R, Grover R (1981). Precursors of human colon carcinoma. Cancer 47:2007.

Lynch HT, Harris RE, Organ CH, et al (1977A). The surgeon, genetics, and cancer control: the cancer family syndrome. Ann Surg 185:435.

Lynch HT, Harris, RE, Bardwell WA, et al (1977B). Management of hereditary site-specific colon cancer. Arch Surg 112:170.

Mark J, Mittelman F, Dencker H, et. al. (1973). The specificity of chromosomal abnormalities in human colonic polyps. Acta Pathol Scan 81:85.

Marshak R, Lindner AE, Maklansky D (1976). Adenomatous polyps of the colon, a rational approach. JAMA 235:2856.

Maskens AP, Dujardin-Loits RM (1981). Experimental adenomas and carcinomas of the large intestine behave as distinct entities. Cancer 47:81.

Morson BC (1977). Polyps and cancer of the large bowel. In: "The Gastrointestinal Tract. International Academy of Pathology Monograph," Wilkins and Wilkins, p 101.

Morson BC (1978). The adenoma-carcinoma sequence. In: "The Pathogenesis of Colorectal Cancer. Major Problems in Pathology, Vol. 10," Philadelphia, London, Toronto: W.B. Saunders Co., chap 6.

Pour P (1978). A new and advantageous model for colo-rectal carcinoma: its comparison with previous models for a common human disease. Cancer (Letters) 4:293.

Prager ED, Swinton NW, Young JL, et. al. (1974). Follow-up studies of patients with benign mucosal polyps discovered by proctosigmoidoscopy. Dis Colon Rectum 17:322.

Reddy BS, Weisburger JH, Narisawa T, et. al. (1974). Colon carcinogenesis in germ-free rats with 1,2,dimethylhydrazine and N-methyl-14[1] nitro-H nitro-soguandine. Cancer Res 34:2368.

Rhatigan RM, Saffos RO (1979). Mucosal hyperplasia in colonic diverticula. Histopathology 3:153.

Rider JA, Kirsner JB, Moeller HC, et. al. (1959). Polyps of the colon and rectum. JAMA 170:633.

Sato E (1976). Adenomatous polyps of large intestine in autopsy and surgical material. Gann 65:295.

Segal I, Cooke SAR, Hamilton DG, et. al. (1981). Polyps and colorectal cancer in South African Blacks. Gut 22:653.

Shamsuddin AKM, Weiss L, Phelps PC, et. al. (1980). Changes in human colon mucosa remote from carcinomas. Lab Invest 42(1):53.

Shinya H, Wolff W (1979). Morphology, anatomic distribution, and cancer potential of colonic polyps. Ann Surg 190:679.

Silverberg SG, (1970). Focally malignant adenomatous polyps of the colon and rectum. Surg Gynecol Obstet 131:103.

Spjut HJ, Estrada RG (1977). The significance of epithelial polyps of the large bowel. In Sommers SC, Rosen PP (eds): "Pathology Annual 1977, Part 1, Vol. 12," New York: Appelton-Century-Crofts, p 147.

Spjut HJ, Frankel NB, Appel MF (1979). The small carcinoma of the large bowel. Am J Surg Pathol 3:39.

Vargo D, Moskovitz M, Floch MH (1980). Faecal bacterial flora in cancer of the colon. Gut 21:701.

Wilson GS, Dale EH, Brines OA (1955). Evaluation of polyps detected in 20,847 routine sigmoidoscopic examinations. Am J Surg 90:834.

Woda BA, Forde K, Lane N (1977). A unicryptal colonic adenoma, the smallest colonic neoplasm yet observed in a non-polyposis individual. Am J Clin Path 68:631.

CONGRESS SYMPOSIA


NUTRITION AND CANCER CAUSATION Burkitt, D., UK, Chairman; Mettlin, C., USA, Co-Chairman; Flag Pavilion A

In Search of Human Colon Carcinogens: Two Approaches to Their Detection and Identification. *Bruce, W. R., Toronto, Ontario, Canada.

Epidemiologic Observation Bearing on the Role of Selected Micronutrients in Carcinogenesis. *Bjelke, E., Bergen, Norway. (By Title Only)

Food Additives and Coffee as Risk Factors. *Newell, G. R., Houston, TX USA.

Dietary Factors in Colon Carcinogenesis with Special Emphasis on the Role of Dietary Fat and Dietary Fibre. *Jensen, O. M., Copenhagen, Denmark.

Dietary Factors in Breast Carcinogenesis. *Modan, B. and Lubin, F., Tel Hshomer, Israel. (By Title Only)

Please note: Papers that are listed as "By Title Only" were presented at the 13th International Cancer Congress, but are not included in these volumes.

**13th International Cancer Congress, Part D**
**Research and Treatment, pages 131–139**
© **1983 Alan R. Liss, Inc., 150 Fifth Avenue, New York, NY 10011**

IN SEARCH OF HUMAN COLON CARCINOGENS:  TWO APPROACHES TO
THEIR DETECTION AND IDENTIFICATION

W. ROBERT BRUCE

LUDWIG INSTITUTE FOR CANCER RESEARCH, TORONTO
BRANCH, 9 EARL STREET, TORONTO, ONT. M4Y 1M4
and
DEPARTMENT OF MEDICAL BIOPHYSICS, UNIVERSITY OF
TORONTO, TORONTO, ONTARIO, CANADA

The relationship between diet and colon cancer poses
a complicated puzzle (1).  Many have sought a solution
through the effects of food on transit time (2), through
the presence of promoters in the diet (3) or formed in the
gastrointestinal tract (4), through studies of the
proliferation of epithelial cells (5) or in the genetic
or familial inheritance of the disease (6).  Our interest
has been directed instead at the nature of the colon
carcinogen - the initiator of the process.  We have sought
possible candidate compounds as carcinogens in two ways.
First we have used the prokaryotic in vitro assay
developed by Ames (7) and more recently we have developed
and used a eukaryotic, colon-specific assay.  This is a
brief review of our work on this aspect of the puzzle.

PROKARYOTIC IN VITRO ASSAY

It was our original supposition that the feces of
individuals at risk for colon cancer contain, or at one
time contained, carcinogenic substances.  That is, that
the colonic epithelial cells of individuals on Western
diets are exposed to carcinogens and that these carcinogens
arise on the lumenal side of the colon.  On the basis of
this supposition we began to look for carcinogens in feces
by extracting feces in various ways and by testing the
extracts with prokaryotic in vitro assays for colon
carcinogens.  We soon found that ether extracts of freeze-
dried feces of many individuals on Western diets contained
a factor that was mutagenically active on Salmonella testor
strain TA-100 without activation (8).  That is that the

feces contained a putative carcinogen. Subsequent studies showed that the mutagenicity was associated with a compound (or related compounds) which had a UV absorption spectrum with maxima at 320, 340 and 365 nm and was extremely sensitive to light, oxygen, and acid (9). The first steps in the purification of this compound were straightforward but with further purification the compound became more and more unstable making the identification of the compound difficult.

Kingstone et al have recently reported that the mutagen is a simple polyunsaturated glyceryl ether (10). We have come to a similar conclusion as is shown in Figure 1 (11). The mutagen is remarkably active. One µg of the compound yields approximately 3000 revertants with TA-100 under standard plate assay conditions. However the mutagen's presence can be even more readily assayed in feces as a consequence of the high extinction coefficient (~ 100,000) of the pentaene moiety. It is because of this property that we have suggested that these compounds be referred to as "fecapentaenes" (11). We have suggested (11) that the mutagenicity of these compounds is a consequence of protonation of the conjugated system and the formation of a relatively stable carbocation that could act as an electrophile.

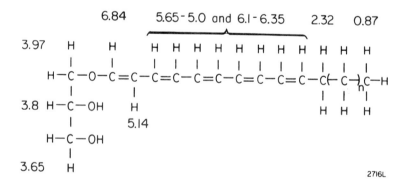

Figure 1 - Proposed Structure of Fecal Mutagen (Fecapentaene) with [1]HNMR spectal assignments.

The origin of the fecapentaenes is not clear at present.
They are not present as such in foods consumed by mutagen
producers (data not shown) or in the ileostomy fluids of
ileostomy patients consuming a wide range of diets (12).
Wilkins et al (13) have shown, however, that the mutagenicity
of mutagenically active feces rises when these specimens
are incubated anaerobically and that this increase is due to
bacterial action. At present it seems plausible that the
mutagen could be produced either de novo by particular fecal
bacteria under certain, as yet to be determined, conditions
or that the mutagen is produced by anaerobic bacteria
acting on compounds present in food that have reached the
colonic cavity.

We have observed that the levels of fecal mutagens are
affected by diet. In pilot studies we observed that
supplemental wheat bran fiber decreased mutagenicity, that
supplementary ascorbic acid and alpha-tocopherol decreased
mutagenicity (14), and that supplementary fat, as milk
fat, produced no consistent change in
mutagenicity (Bright-See and Dion, personal communication).
Further studies with ascorbic acid and alpha-tocopherol
have confirmed that these agents produce an effect on
mutagenicity (15). These investigations were carried out
in two ways. In the first, an active donor was placed on
a constant daily repeating diet that was similar to his
normal intake and fecal mutagenicity was measured daily.
The addition of ascorbic acid (400 mg) and alpha-
tocopherol (400 mg/day) led to an immediate 79% decrease
in fecal mutagenicity which persisted to a limited degree
until more than 30 days following the treatment. In the
second experiment, 24 donors were maintained on a random
self-selected diet. The addition of ascorbic acid and
alpha-tocopherol led to a 74% reduction in the mutagenicity
of the eight active donors, none of the inactive donors
becoming active. While it was observed that the vitamins
had no effect on the sensitivity of the assay system to
the mutagen, it must be noted that the inhibition
observed was only 4-fold and not complete and that the
differences observed were in no way as great as that seen
between active and inactive donors. Perhaps the intake
of these vitamins is one of a number of factors that
differs between individuals that are producers and those
that are not.

While it is usually the case that mutagens of the direct acting variety are carcinogens, it is not clear how important fecapentaenes are with relation to colon cancer in Western society. Ehrich et al (16) have shown that the mutagen is more frequently present in the feces of South African whites than it is amongst the rural or urban South African blacks who have a substantially lower colon cancer incidence. A more direct test of the association of the mutagen with the malignant process, however, has proved less convincing. In a study in New Orleans (17), individuals with and without colonic polyps, recognized precursors to colon cancer, were assessed for the presence of fecal mutagens. Those with polyps were not found to have mutagens present in their feces more frequently than were those without polyps. The absence of association between mutagen and disease could indicate that the mutagen need only be present at the beginning of the carcinogenesis process or that the presence of mutagen in feces indicates only that the carcinogen has not reacted with the colonic epithelial cells. It is also possible that the lack of association means that the fecal mutagen we have studied is not the initiator for colon cancer. A number of other fecal mutagens have been described (18,19,20) though their structures or association with the colon cancer process is not yet known.

EUKARYOTIC, COLON-SPECIFIC ASSAY

There are two possible problems in our use of the prokaryotic, in vitro system to identify human colon carcinogens. The first is that the colon carcinogen is undetectable by the assay system, since these systems do not detect all carcinogens. A battery of tests might be used to get around this problem but would certainly be most cumbersome (21). The second problem is that the approach we have used assumes that the carcinogen reaches the epithelial cells by way of the fecal stream while at least one colon carcinogen in experimental animals is known to reach the colon by the blood stream (22). In order to get around possible limitations of the in vitro, prokaryotic systems applied to fecal extracts, we explored the possibility of colon specific assays in animals instead. We found that it is feasible to assess chemicals for their carcinogenicity to the colon by their ability to induce nuclear aberrations in colonic crypt cells.

The nuclear aberration assay originated in two observations, one from genetics, the other from pathology. Schmid (23) and Heddle (24) had shown some years ago that a small number of erythropoietic cells exposed in vivo to clastogenic agents contained micronuclei and that these resulted from chromosomal fragments unattached to the spindle at metaphase (25). The frequency of micronuclei in reticulocytes has been used as a test system for assessing exposure to genotoxic agents (26). Similar micronuclei have also been reported in the liver (27) and the testes (28) following agents that were clastogenic to these tissues. Maskens (29) has shown, in quantitative analyses of colon pathology after treatment with a carcinogen, that cells of the colonic epithelium frequently contained fragmented and deformed nuclei. These karyorrhectic nuclei could be readily quantitated. These observations from genetic and pathology studies thus led us to carry out a systematic examination of the nuclei of colonic epithelium following dimethylhydrazine, a colon carcinogen, and x-radiation.

We found that in untreated control mice, the frequency of crypts containing aberrations was one in ten, or 0.1. After an exposure to 20 mg/kg DMH (30,31,32) or 100 rads of radiation (33), the frequency rose to 2 or 3 per crypt at 24 hours and decreased to control values at 72 hours. With these agents all aberrations appeared to rise and fall together suggesting that all arose from a general genomic toxicity. While the exact mechanism by which each of these aberrations arise has not been ascertained, it became clear in a comparative study of different pathological lesions following dimethylhydrazine (30) that nuclear aberrations provided the most sensitive and rapid assay for exposure to this carcinogen. What was not known was how specific the effect was. Was it seen with other colon carcinogens?

To answer the question of specificity, we examined the effects of 19 agents of known carcinogenicity on nuclear morphology carrying out our observation at 24 hours following treatment with the agents (31). We found that all the agents known to be colon carcinogens (1,2 dimethylhydrazine, bisoxypropylnitrosamine, 3',2 dimethyl-4-aminobiphenyl, 3 methylcholanthrene orally and methylnitrosourea rectally) produced nuclear aberrations at over 1 aberration per crypt while all the

other agents were without effect excepting benz(a)pyrene
and X rays. Figure 2 illustrates these results for the
colon carcinogen, 1,2-dimethylhydrazine, the non-colon
carcinogen, 1,1-dimethylhydrazine and for hydrazine.
Clearly only 1,2-dimethylhydrazine is active. These
encouraging results prompted us to test the ability of
agents capable of blocking the carcinogenic effect of
dimethylhydrazine in the assay. As anticipated, disulfiram
added to the diet at a concentration of 1/2% led to the
inhibition of the effects of the carcinogen on nuclear
aberrations. These results thus suggested that the
measurement of nuclear aberrations could provide a
sensitive, specific and rapid assay for colon carcinogens.

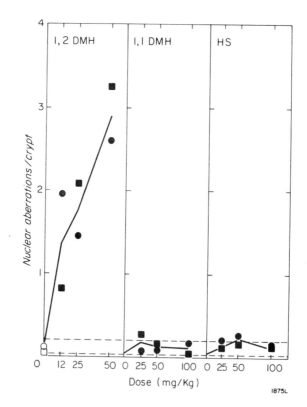

Figure 2 - Frequency of nuclear aberrations in the colonic
crypts of mice injected with graded doses of 1,2-dimethyl-
hydrazine, 1,1-dimethylhydrazine and hydrazine. Symbols
represent experiments with animals of different sexes,
dashed lines limits in control animals.

The nuclear aberration assay can be used in several ways. First, it is possible to introduce into the stomach of the test animals components and fractions of foods from the Western diet and to measure the effects in the colonic epithelium. Second, it is possible to instill into the colon of test animals components or fractions of feces from individuals at risk for colon cancer. Third, and possibly most interesting, it may be possible to carry out studies of nuclear aberrations in the human colon and observe the effect of diet on the colonic epithelium directly. If this can be done simply and without risk, it could provide a direct measure of the factor in Western diet that is the initiator. Such a test could thus greatly aid us in finding the solution to one part of the puzzle, the relationship of diet and colon cancer.

REFERENCES

1. Burkitt DP (1975). Large-bowel cancer: an epidemiologic jigsaw puzzle. J Nat Cancer Inst 54: 3-6.
2. Cummings JH, Jenkins DJA, Wiggins HS (1976). Measurement of mean transit time of dietary residue through the human gut. Gut 17: 210-218.
3. Bull AW, Soullier BK, Wilson PS, Hayden MT, Nigro ND (1979). Promotion of a zoxymethane-induced intestinal cancer by high-fat diet in rats. Cancer Res 39: 4956-4959.
4. Reddy BS, Watanabe K, Weisburger JH, Wynder EL (1977). Promoting effect of bile acids in colon carcinogenesis in germ-free and conventional F344 rats. Cancer Res 37: 3236-3242.
5. Lipkin M, Sherlock P, Bell B (1963). Cell proliferation kinetics in the gastrointestinal tract of man. Gastroenterol 45: 721-729.
6. McConnel RB (1978). Genetic Aspects of Colon Cancer. In Grundmann E (ed): "Colon Cancer", Gustar Fischer Verlag, London, pp. 57-66
7. Ames BN, McCann J, Yamasaki E (1975). Methods for detecting carcinogens and mutagens with the Salmonella/microsome mutagenicity test. Mutat Res 31: 347-363.
8. Bruce WR, Varghese AJ, Furrer R, Land PC. A mutagen in human feces. In: Hiatt H, Watson JD, Winsten JA (eds): "Origins of Human Cancer", Cold Spring Harbor Laboratories, New York, pp. 1641-1644 (1977).

9. Bruce WR, Varghese AJ, Land PC, Krepinsky JF. Properties of a Mutagen Isolated Feces. In Bruce WR et al (eds) "Gastrointestinal Cancer: Endogenous Factors", Banbury Report 7, Cold Spring Harbor Laboratory, New York, pp. 227-238.

10. Kingston GI, Hirai N (1982). Isolation and structure elucidation of a potent mutagen from feces. Abstract. American Chemical Society Annual Meeting #175.

11. Bruce WR, Baptista J, Che T, Furrer R, Gingerich JS, Grey AA, Gupta I, Krepinsky JJ, Yates P (1982). General structures of "fecapentaenes"* - the mutagenic substances in human faeces: a preliminary report. Die Naturwissenschaften (in press).

12. Dion PW (1982). Ph.D. Thesis, University of Toronto.

13. Lederman M, Van Tassel R, West SEH, Ehrich MF, Wilkins TD (1980). In vitro production of human fecal mutagen. Mutat Res 79: 115-124.

14. Bruce WR, Dion PW (1980). Studies relating to a fecal mutagen. Am J Clin Nutr 33: 2511-2512.

15. Dion PW, Bright-See EB, Smith CC, Bruce WR (1982). The effect of dietary ascorbic acid and alpha-tocopherol on fecal mutagenicity. Mutat Res 102: 27-37.

16. Ehrich MF, Aswell JE, Van Tassell RL, Wilkins TD (1979) Mutagens in feces of 3 South African populations at different levels of risk for colon cancer. Mutat Res 64: 231-240.

17. Correa P, Paschal J, Pizzolato P, Pelon W, Lesley DE (1981). Fecal Mutagens and Colorectal polyps: Preliminary Report of an Autopsy Study. In: Bruce WR et al (eds) "Gastrointestinal Cancer: Endogenous Factors", Banbury Report 7, Cold Spring Harbor Laboratory, New York, pp. 119-128.

18. Venitt S (1982). Mutagens in human faeces: are they relevant to cancer of the large bowel. Mutat Res 98: 265-286.

19. Kuhnlein UD, Bergstrom D, Kuhnlein H (1981). Mutagens in feces from vegetarians and non-vegetarians. Mutat Res 85: 1-2.

20. Stemmerman GN, Hayashi T, Ichinotsubo D, Mandel M, Mower H, Rice S, Tomiyasu L (1980). Mutagens in extracts of human gastric mucosa. JNCI 65: 321-326.

21. Heddle JA, Blakey DH, Duncan AMV, Goldberg MT, Wargovich MJ, Bruce WR. Nuclear Anomalies as a Short-Term Assay for Colon Carcinogens. In: Bridges et al (eds) "Indicators of Genotoxic Exposure in Man and Animals". Banbury Report 13, Cold Spring Harbor Laboratory, New York (in press).

22. Rubio CA, Nylander G, Santos M (1980). Experimental colon cancer in the absence of intestinal contents in Sprague-Dawley rats. JNCI 64: 569-572.

23. Schmid W (1975). The micronucleus test. Mutat Res 31: 9-15.

24. Heddle JA (1973). A rapid in vivo test for chromosomal damage. Mutat Res 18: 187-190.

25. Heddle JA, Benz RD, Countryman PI (1978). Measurement of Chromosomal Breakage in Cultured Cells by the Micronucleus Technique. In Evans and Lloyd (eds) "Mutagen-Induced Chromosome Damage in Man", Edinburgh University Press, Edinburgh, pp. 191-200.

26. Heddle JA, Bruce WR (1977). Comparison of Tests for Mutagenicity or Carcinogenicity using Assays for Sperm Abnormalities, Formation of Micronuclei, and Mutations in Salmonella. In Hiatt HH, Watson JD, Winsten JA (eds) "Origins of Human Cancer", Book C Human Risk Assessment, Cold Spring Harbor Laboratory, New York, pp. 1549-1557.

27. Tates AD, Neuteboom I, Hofker M, den Engelse L (1980). A micronucleus technique for detecting clastogenic effects of mutagens/carcinogens (DEN, DMN) in hepato-cytes of rat liver in vivo. Mutat Res 74: 11-20.

28. Lahdetie J, Parvinen M (1981). Meiotic micronuclei induced by x-rays in early spermatids of the rat. Mutat Res 81: 103-115.

29. Maskens AP (1979). Significance of the karyorrhectic index in 1,2-dimethylhydrazine carcinogenesis. Cancer Lett 8: 77-86.

30. Wargovich MJ, Medline A, Bruce WR (1982). Comparative histopathology of precursor lesions to colon cancer in C57BL/6 and CF-1 mice treated with 1,2-dimethylhydrazine. JNCI (submitted for publication).

31. Wargovich MJ, Goldberg MT, Newmark H, Bruce WR (182). Nuclear aberrations as a short-term test for geno-toxocity to the colon: evaluation of 19 agents. JNCI (submitted for publication.

32. Goldberg MT, Blakey DH, Bruce WR (1982). Comparison of the effects of 1,2-dimethylhydrazine and cyclo-phosphamide on micronucleus incidence in bone marrow and colon. Mutat Res (submitted for publication).

33. Blakey DH, Duncan AMV, Wargovich M, Heddle JA (1982). Detection of early lesions in colonic epithelium following treatment by gamma rays or 1,2-dimethyl-hydrazine. Cancer Res (submitted for publication).

13th International Cancer Congress, Part D
Research and Treatment, pages 141–149
© 1983 Alan R. Liss, Inc., 150 Fifth Avenue, New York, NY 10011

# FOOD ADDITIVES AND COFFEE AS RISK FACTORS

Guy R. Newell, M.D.

The University of Texas System Cancer Center
M.D. Anderson Hospital and Tumor Institute
Houston, Texas 77030

## Food Additives

In general, food additives have been subject to careful laboratory screening before they are allowed to be used. Shubik has said, "In spite of the inadequacies of past toxicological surveillance, I believe that intentional food additives have been the best investigated materials" (Shubik 1979). In this group he includes Red dye No.2, cyclamate, saccharin, and nitrites. He further says..."I do not, personally, believe that the public is at any great risk from any intentional food additive, as far as the toxicologist can tell and in so far as carcinogenic risk is concerned" (Shubik 1979).

Chemicals are added to food to preserve it and to give it color, flavor, and consistency. Our complex food distribution system depends entirely on the use of many of these materials. Some definitely carcinogenic chemicals were used but have now been removed, such as butter yellow (DAB), thoiurea, and food presevative AF2 (only in Japan). Of the many additives now in use, Doll and Peto (Doll, Peto 1981) give special consideration to three: saccharin, butylated hydroxytoluene, and nitrites.

Saccharin  Regarding animal and in vitro studies, there is no doubt that saccharin is capable of causing cancer in large doses under special circumstances. However, its mechanism of action is obscure and it is not a powerful animal carcinogen (Congress of the United States, 1977).

Human studies do not show evidence of an association between saccharin use and bladder cancer, either time -trend study, (Armstrong, Doll 1974) studies of diabetics (Armstrong, Doll 1975a, Armstrong, Lea, Adelstein 1976, Kessler 1970) or case-control studies of bladder cancer (Hoover, Strasser 1980, Howe, Burch, Miller, Morrison, Godon, Weldon, Chambers, Fodor, Winsor 1977, Kessler, Clark 1978, Morrison, Buring 1980, Wynder Stellman 1980). Overall results of the five case-control studies are summarized in Table 1.

We have reviewed the status of saccharin carcinogenicity and discussed it in terms of its implications to the public. It is not technically sophisticated to interpret the many subtleties of animal studies or the results of human studies which may have different interpretations by respected scientists (Newell, Boutwell 1981a). The majority of human evidence does not incriminate saccharin as a carcinogen for humans in doses ordinarily consumed; however, there are six points the physician should consider when counseling patients on the safety of saccharin use.

1. Saccharin is a weak carcinogen in second-generation offspring male rats. It is therefore implied by some to be a carcinogen in humans, although it is among the weakest carcinogen ever detected in rats. Thus, prudence would suggest avoiding it, especially if no direct benefit is expected.

2. Most human evidence does not incriminate it as a carcinogen for humans.

3. Subsets of the population may exist that are particularly susceptible to low doses of carcinogens. These individuals cannot be determined by current technology prior to exposure.

4. Individuals are exposed to multiple carcinogens which may act synergistically rather than additively. Again, avoidance where possible to any one of these carcinogens seems prudent.

5. Assessing the benefits of saccharin is difficult at best. A congressional OTA study found no scientific data to prove or disprove that use of a non-nutritive sweetener leads to any health benefits. On the other hand, there is a great perception of benefit by the public at large, centered around diabetics and those attempting to control their weight.

6. Because heavy saccharin use did not occur until the early 1960's, an association with human bladder cancer may not become evident (measurable) for 20 or 30 years.

TABLE 1

Risk of Bladder Cancer with

Use of Artificial Sweeteners

| Authors | Patients No. | Sex | Relative risk with use of: Table-top sweeteners | Diet beverages | Artificial sweeteners any form |
|---|---|---|---|---|---|
| Howe, et al (1977) | 408 | M | 1.6 | 0.8 | - |
| Kessler & Clark (1978) | 365 | M | 0.88 | 0.95 | 0.97 |
| Hoover, et al (1980) | 2,226 | M | 1.04 | 0.95 | 1.08[a] 0.99 |
| Morrison and Buring (1980) | 469 | M | 0.8 | 0.8 | - |
| Wynder and Stellman (1980) | 302 | M | 0.93 | 0.85 | - |
| Howe, et al (1980) | 152 | F | 0.6 | 0.9 | - |
| Kessler & Clark (1978) | 154 | F | 0.91 | 1.00 | 1.00 0.87[a] |
| Hoover, et al (1980) | 744 | F | 1.04 | 0.97 | 1.01 |
| Morrison and Buring (1980) | 197 | F | 1.5 | 1.6 | - |
| Wynder and Stellman (1980) | 65 | F | 0.62 | 0.60 | - |

[a] Specifically saccharin
Adapted from Doll, Peto, 1981

Thus, at issue is the presumed carcinogenicity of saccharin for humans based on animal studies and the perceived benefits by the public of having an artificial sweetener available for use. As a practical recommendation, it seems prudent that pregnant women should not consume saccharin in any dose level, and that children should not be exposed to saccharin from early youth over a lifetime in the doses currently used in soft drinks. Individuals, in general, should not be exposed to a suspect carcinogen unless definite benefit is derived either by the individual or by his/her physician.

Doll and Peto conclude that the proportion of human bladder cancers now attributable to the use of artificial sweeteners in negligible (Doll, Peto 1981).

Butylated hydroxytoluene  This has been used as an antioxidant for many years. This antioxidant property inhibits the formation of active carcinogens in the laboratory (Wattenberg 1978). This might be expected to occur in humans also. No reliable human evidence for or against this is known.

Nitrites  Nitrites have long been used in the meat industry as a food preservative and to prevent botulism. The amount of nitrite reaching the stomach as a food additive is only 10% or less than that reaching it by the natural ingestion of vegetables and fruits (Shubik 1980). Addition of vitamin C can inhibit the reaction of nitrites to nitrosamines and the addition of ascorbic acid to meat cures to prevent nitrosation is now routine (Shubik 1979). We believe that the potential hazard to humans by added nitrites has been exaggerated and that the benefits outweigh the risk (Newell, Boutwell 1981b).

Should patients be concerned that the amount of nitrite they receive in fried bacon or other meat products will cause cancer? In our opinion, probably not, and for the following reasons: Ninety-five percent of nitrites comes from metabolism of naturally occurring ingested nitrates in vegetables. These are impossible to avoid, and there is no known countering agent, although vitamin C may reduce the conversion from nitrate to nitrite. Only 3% to 5% of nitrite comes from all cured meats. Bacon, by law, must be free of preformed nitrosamines in the lowest amount detectable by available technology.

Nitrosamines are not allowed as a food additive in any amount. The benefits of nitrite as a food additive in preventing botulism outweight the potential risks for causing cancer. The animal study incriminating nitrite as causing cancer has been severely criticized by both nongovernment and government scientists. The number of cancers in the United States estimated to be caused by nitrite as an additive is six annually, compared with over 90,000 new cases of cigarette-related cancer or 650,000 total new cancer cases annually.

In summary, because of the uncertainty surrounding nitrites, artificial sweeteners and other food additives, Doll and Peto did not exclude food additives as a source of risk but have attributed to them "a token proportion of less than 1%" (Doll, Peto 1981). Likewise, the National Research Council noted that of the few direct food additives tested and found to be carcinogenic in animals, all except saccharin have been banned from use in the food supply. They concluded that the increasing use of food additives has not contributed significantly to the overall risk of cancer for humans (Diet, Nutition and Cancer 1982).

## Coffee Consumption

Considering the amount of coffee that is consumed in this and other countries, there are surprisingly few human studies of coffee consumption and cancer. In a case-control study conducted in New Orleans in 1958-64 an association between bladder cancer and coffee-drinking was found, but was not statistically significant (Dunham, Rabson, Stewart, Frank, Young 1968). Most studies have included cancer of the lower urinary tract, 90% being bladder cancer. Most of these have been case-control studies (Cole 1971, Howe, Burch, Miller, Cook, Estere, Morrison, Gordon, Chambers, Fodor, Winsor 1980, Mettlin, Graham 1979,Morrison, Buring, Verhoek, Aoki, Leck, Ohno, Obata 1982, Simon, Yen, Cole 1975, Wynder, Goldsmith 1977) and one was a time trend study (Morrison, Buring, Verhoek, Aoki, Leck, Ohno, Obata 1982). They have all shown little or no association between coffee drinking and lower urinary tract cancer. Overall, the observations suggest that any association, if present , is noncausal. These include the nonconsistency of the association, the low strength of the association when present, and the consistent absence of a dose-response relationship.

Morrison et al wrote "If there is a true association of coffee drinking and bladder cancer it is likely to be weak" (Morrison, Buring, Verhoek, Aoki, Leck, Ohno, Obata 1982) and "these results provide little support for an association of coffee drinking with the development of bladder cancer" (Morrison 1978). Similarly, case-comparison studies have found no association between coffee consumption and kidney cancer (Armstrong, Garrod, Doll 1976, Morrison 1978). Correlation studies have shown a correlation between coffee consumption and a variety of cancer types (Armstrong, Doll 1975b, Stocks 1970). No significant credence are placed in these observations by themselves.

Paffenbarger et al reported an increased risk of Hodgkin's disease, myeloid leukemia and lymphatic leukemia among collegians who had been obese, heavy cigarette smokers and coffee drinkers (Paffenbarger, Wing, Hyde 1978a, Paffenbarger, Wing, Hyde 1978b). This has not been confirmed. A prospective study found no evidence to associate coffee drinking with cancer deaths in a population sample from Evans County, Georgia (Heyden, Heyden, Heiss, Hames 1979).

In 1981, MacMahon, et al reported an association between coffee drinking and cancer of the pancreas (MacMahon, Yen, Trichopoulos, Warren, Nardi 1981). The study was criticized on various grounds and the results were both confirmed and disputed by follow-up correspondence. This observation needs to be duplicated by other groups conducting studies specifically designed to test this hypothesis before a causal inference can be made.

In summary, there is little evidence that either food additives or coffee consumption add a significant risk to the burden of cancer in humans.

Armstrong B, Doll R (1976). Bladder cancer mortality in England and Wales in relation to cigarette smoking and saccharin consumption. Br J Prev Soc Med 28:233-240.

Armstrong B, Doll R (1975a). Bladder cancer mortality in diabetics in relation to saccharin consumption and smoking habits. Br J Prev Soc Med 29(2):73-81.

Armstrong B, Lea AJ, Adelstein AM, Donovan JW, White GC, Ruttle S (1976a). Cancer mortality asnd saccharin consumption in diabetics. Br J Prev Soc Med 30(3):151-157.

Armstrong B, Garrod A, Doll R (1976a). A retrospective study of renal cancer with special reference to coffee and animal protein consumption. Br J Cancer 33:127-136.

Armstrong B, Doll R (1975b). Environmental factors and cancer incidence and mortality in different countries with special reference to dietary practices. Int J Cancer 15:617-631.

Cole P (1971). Coffee-drinking and cancer of the lower urinary tract. Lancet 1:1335-1337.

Congress of the United States (1977). Office of Technology Assessment: Cancer Testing Technology and Saccharin. Library of Congress Catalog Card No. 77-600051. Washington, DC. US Government Printing Office, Stock No. 052-003-00471-2.

Diet, Nutrition and Cancer (1982). Committee on Diet, Nutrition and cancer. Assembly of Life Sciences. National Research Council. National Academy Press. Washington, DC.

Doll R, Peto R (1981). The causes of cancer: Quantitative estimates of avoidable risks of cancer in the United States today. J Natl Cancer Inst 66:1191-1308.

Dunham LJ, Rabson AS, Stewart HL, Frank AS, Young JL Jr (1968) Rates, interview, and pathology study of cancer of the urinary bladder in New Orleans, Louisiana. J Natl Cancer Inst. 41:683-709.

Heyden S, Heyden F, Heiss G, Hames CG (1979). Smoking and coffee consumption in three groups: cancer deaths, cardiovascular deaths and living controls. A prospective study in Evans County, Georgia. J Chronic Dis 32:673-677.

Hoover R, Strasser,PH (1980). Progress report to the Food and Drug Administration from the National Cancer Institute concerning the national bladder cancer study. NCI. See also Lancet 1:837-840, 1980.

Howe GR, Burch JD, Miller AB, Morrison B, Gordon P, Weldon L, Chambers LW, Winsor,GM (1977). Artificial sweeteners and human bladder cancer. Lancet 2:578-581.

Howe GR, Burch JD, Miller AB, Cook GM, Esteve J, Morrison B, Gordon P, Chambers LW, Fodor G, Winsor GM (1980). Tobacco use, occupation, coffee, various nutrients, and bladder cancer. J Natl Cancer Inst 64:701-713.

Kessler II (1970). Cancer mortality among diabetics. J Natl Cancer Inst 44:673-686.

Kessler II, Clark JP (1978). Saccharin, cyclamate, and human bladder cancer. No evidence of an association. J Amer Med Assoc 240:349-355.

MacMahon B, Yen S, Trichopoulos D, Warren K, Nardi G (1981). Coffee and cancer of the pancreas. N Engl J Med 304:630-633.

Mettlin C, Graham S (1979). Dietary risk factors in human bladder cancer. Amer J Epidem 110:255-263.

Morrison AS, Buring, JE (1980). Artificial sweeteners and cancer of the lower urinary tract. N Engl J Med 302:537-541.

Morrison AS, Buring JE, Verhoek WG, Aoki K, Leck I, Ohno Y, Obata K (1982). Coffee drinking and cancer of the lower urinary tract. J Natl Cancer Inst 68:91-94.

Morrison AS (1978). Geographic and time trend of coffee imports and bladder cancer. Europ J Cancer 14:51-54.

Newell GR, Boutwell WB (1981a). Counseling patients on saccharin use. Cancer Bull 33:33-34.

Newell GR, Boutwell WB (1981b). Advising patients about nitrites in foods. Cancer Bull 33:180-181.

Paffenbarger RS Jr, Wing AL, Hyde RT (1978a). Characteristics in youth predictive of adult-onset malignant lymphomas, melanomas, and leukemias. J Natl Cancer Inst 60:89-92.

Shubik P (1979). Food additives (natural and synthetic). Cancer 43:1982-1986.

Shubik P (1980). Food additives, contaminants, and cancer. Prev Med 9:197-201.

Simon D, Yen S, Cole P (1975). Coffee drinking and cancer of the lower urinary tract. J Natl Cancer Inst 54:587-591.

Stocks P (1970). Cancer mortality in relation to national consumption of cigarettes, solid fuels, tea and coffee. Brit J Cancer 24:215-225.

Wattenberg LW (1978). Inhibition of chemical carcinogenesis. J Natl Cancer Inst 60:11-18.

Wynder EL, Stellman SD (1980). Artificial sweetener use and bladder cancer. Science 207:1214-1216.

Wynder EL, Goldsmith R (1977). The epidemiology of bladder cancer. Cancer 40:1246-1268.

Wynder EL, Mabuchi K, Whitmore WF Jr (1974). Epidemiology of adenocarcinoma of the kidney. J Natl Cancer Inst 53:1619-1634.

13th International Cancer Congress, Part D
Research and Treatment, pages 151–158
© 1983 Alan R. Liss, Inc., 150 Fifth Avenue, New York, NY 10011

DIETARY FACTORS IN COLON CARCINOGENESIS WITH SPECIAL
EMPHASIS ON THE ROLE OF DIETARY FAT AND DIETARY FIBRE

Ole M. Jensen, M.D.

Director
Danish Cancer Registry
2100 Copenhagen, Denmark

The epidemiological pattern provides ample evidence
that the risk of colon cancer is determined by certain
aspects of diet characteristic of affluent, westernized
populations. The highest incidence rates of the disease
are recorded in North America and Western Europe (Waterhouse
et al., 1976), and such high rates are quickly adopted by
low risk populations that migrate into the areas (Haenszel,
1961). In countries where social class differences may be
an indicator of profound differences in the life-style and
food patterns like in Hong Kong and Columbia the more
affluent parts of society have the highest rates (Crowther
et al., 1976).

Among other dietary items it has been suggested that
both the high fat and meat content of the food of affluent
western societies and the deficiency of roughage - dietary
fibre - are risk determinants of colon cancer. The observation of a low colon cancer mortality and incidence in
population groups like the Seventh Day Adventists (Phillips,
1975; Jensen, 1982) who for religious reasons proscribe to
a lacto-ovo-vegetarian diet, provide additional support for
the association between "westernized" diets and colon cancer. The evidence from descriptive studies has been summarized in Table 1.

DIETARY FAT
Although the first case-control studies (Higginson,
1966; Wynder and Shigematsu, 1967) to test the above hypotheses emerging from descriptive data failed to demonstrate
a role for dietary fat and meat in the aetiology of colon

cancer, Wynder et al. (1969) nevertheless maintained that
fat might be the determining dietary factor. This view obtained numerical support from the highly positive correlation between fat-intake and colon cancer mortality (Armstrong and Doll, 1975).

Table 1:  Selected features of colon cancer epidemiology

| Characteristic | Males | Females |
|---|---|---|
| INTERNATIONAL VARIATION [a] | | |
| Connecticut, USA | 30.1 | 26.1 |
| Ibadan, Nigeria | 1.3 | 1.2 |
| SOCIAL CLASS [b] | | |
| England & Wales, High | 104 | – |
| Low | 110 | – |
| Hong Kong, High | 190 | |
| Low | 110 | |
| MIGRATION [a] | | |
| Miyagi, Japan | 5.6 | 5.4 |
| Hawaii, Japanese | 22.4 | 18.8 |
| RELIGIOUS GROUPS [b] | | |
| Seventh Day Adventists, USA | 61 | 70 |
| Mormons, USA | 62 | 62 |
| Seventh Day Adventists, Denmark | 10 | – |

a)  (Inc./$10^5$) World Standard Population
b)  (SMR) Standardized Mortality Ratio

     The only study of individuals from which fat-intake as
such emerges as a risk factor is the Finnish study by Pernu
(1960) published more than twenty years ago.  A few studies
have shown that meat-intake increases the risk of colon
cancer and such studies have typically been performed in
populations where there is a large variation in dietary
patterns (Haenszel et al., 1973).

     In further support of this fat hypothesis Aries et al.
(1969) suggested that a diet with a high fat content will
increase the bile acid production, and that the bacterial
flora of the large intestine - in particular anaerobes -
are capable of metabolizing the bile acids to secondary

bile acids. The fecal concentration of these metabolites has subsequently been shown to correlate internationally with cancer mortality (Hill et al., 1971), to be higher in colon cancer patients than in controls (Hill et al., 1975) and to promote tumor formation in the colon in animal experiments (Narisawa et al., 1974).

DIETARY FIBRE

In our own studies of populations in Denmark and Finland there was no difference in the average daily intake of fat, and in spite of this the cancer registries report a 3 to 4-fold difference in colon cancer incidence between low risk rural Finland and high risk Copenhagen with rural Denmark and Helsinki taking intermediate incidence rates (IARC, 1977; Jensen et al., 1982). The observations of differences in fibre intake are however in line with the suggestions of Higginson and Oettle (1960) that roughage in the diet may protect against colon cancer. They based their conclusion on the observed rarity of colon cancer in black Africans. This observation was confirmed by Burkitt et al., (1972) who have suggested that the high content of dietary fibre in the African diets compared with European ones would result in a more rapid transit of fecal matter through the bowel and in a larger fecal bulk than in high risk populations. Consequently this should lead to a reduced contact time between carcinogens or co-carcinogens and the mucosal wall of the colon and also result in the carcinogen concentration of the colonic contents being lower due to the dilution in a large fecal volume.

A carefully conducted case-control study in Israel lends support to a protective role of a fibre-rich diet (Modan et al., 1975). In the previously mentioned comparisons of Danish and Finnish men coordinated by the International Agency for Research on Cancer both the original studies in 1977 (IARC, 1977) and the expanded investigations in 1982 (Jensen et al., 1982) show that the intake of dietary fibre follows the colon cancer gradient, Table 2, although slightly different methods were used for measuring dietary fibre intakes in the two surveys. These findings were further supported by a comparison between New York and the same Finnish rural population that was studied by the IARC (Reddy et al., 1978).

Table 2: Trends in colon cancer incidence, dietary and fecal characteristics in Denmark and Finland. Results are given as a proportion of the intake in rural Finland (100%)

| Characteristics studied | Survey | Finland | | Denmark | |
|---|---|---|---|---|---|
| | | Rural | Capital | Rural | Capital |
| Morbidity | | 100 | 254 | 193 | 340 |
| Fat intake. | I a) | 100 | – | – | 87 |
| | II b) | 100 | 77 | 110 | 88 |
| Dietary fibre | I | 100 | – | – | 56 |
| | II | 100 | 79 | 98 | 72 |
| Pentose | I | 100 | – | – | 53 |
| | II | 100 | 74 | 89 | 61 |
| Fat/Pentose | I | 100 | – | – | 189 |
| | II | 100 | 103 | 123 | 145 |
| Fecal weight | I | 100 | – | – | 78 |
| | II | 100 | 90 | 86 | 71 |
| Acid Steroids, total output | I | not available | | | |
| | II | 100 | 106 | 102 | 112 |
| Acid Steroid concentration | I | 100 | – | – | 107 |
| | II | 100 | 124 | 127 | 151 |

a) IARC, 1977
b) Jensen et al., 1982

COMBINED ACTION OF FAT AND FIBRE

It is conceivable that "diet" as a risk factor for cancer may contain components of tumor initiation and promotion, but also that some aspects of diet will tend to counteract such promotional effects and thereby protect against cancer development. It has therefore been proposed that the differences in colon cancer risk between Denmark and Finland, where men for all that we know eat the same amount of fat every day, should be explained by some protective aspect of the Finnish diet. As already indicated its high fibre content is a candidate for having such a protective effect.

The alteration of gut transit time as a mechanism was not however confirmed in our Nordic studies, Table 3, but the combined results of the two surveys were suggestive of a bimodal distribution, and it was previously proposed that there may be a subpopulation (IARC, 1977) whose colon cancer risk is at present unknown. In accordance with this neither do studies of Japanese in Hawaii provide evidence that a rapid transit time is the explanation for the protective action of dietary fibre in colon carcinogenesis (Glober et al., 1977). The bulking effect of dietary fibre was however clear, the fecal volume being inversely related to colon cancer risk in Scandinavia (Table 2).

Table 3:  Mouth-anus transit times in Denmark (Copenhagen) and Finland (rural). Combined results of two surveys [a)]

| Transit (hrs) | Copenhagen | | Rural Finland | |
|---|---|---|---|---|
| | N | % | N | % |
| −29 | 22 | 25.3 | 20 | 23.0 |
| 30–39 | 32 | 36.8 | 42 | 48.3 |
| 40–49 | 7 | 8.0 | 5 | 5.7 |
| 50–59 | 12 | 13.8 | 10 | 11.5 |
| 60− | 14 | 16.1 | 10 | 11.5 |
| Total | 87 | 100.0 | 87 | 100.0 |

a)  IARC, 1977; Jensen et al., 1982

Rather than looking independently at dietary fat and fibre as increasing the risk and protecting against the risk of colon cancer respectively, it may be more relevant to consider an imbalance between these two factors as the determinant of colon cancer risk. In California Dales et al. (1979) found a significantly increased relative risk of colon cancer to be associated only with the combined intake of a high fat, low fibre diet. Similar results emerged from a small case-control study conducted in the Federal Republic of Germany (Esser et al., 1980). In Denmark and Finland the ratio of fat: fibre and in particular fat: pentosans follow closely the colon cancer gradient observed, Table 2.  A joint action of fat and fibre is biologically attractive as the tumor promoting action of the metabolized bile acids is related to their fecal concentration. Other things being equal the concentration of these compounds in the feces will be a result of the bile acid production and output and the fecal volume in which this output is diluted. Indeed, the differences in bile acid concentration between Danish and Finnish men result from the dilution of equal amounts of bile acids in different fecal volumes in these populations. The bile acids are produced in response to the same amounts of dietary fat eaten by the populations and the fecal volume following the differences in dietary fibre intake.

SUMMARY AND CONCLUSIONS

Dietary factors other than fat and fibre have been reported to influence colon cancer risk, in particular a protective effect of cruciferous vegetables (Graham et al., 1978) and an increased risk associated with beer consumption (Breslow and Enstrom, 1974) have been suggested. The role of these dietary aspects is however less well understood than that of fat and fibre; for beer consumption the statistical association has been suggested to be a non-causal nature (Jensen, 1979; Jensen, 1982).

In summary then the epidemiological pattern of colon cancer points to various aspects of diet as a determinant of colon cancer risk. If - as suggested - an imbalance between the intake of fat and fibre is of importance mediated by the fecal concentration of bile acids further studies should attempt to clarify the relative role of these two items in addition to shedding further light on the role of other dietary aspects, for which our present knowledge is even more incomplete. With a view to cancer prevention it may prove more productive to give priority to a search for items that have a protective effect. It may thus be more acceptable to high risk populations to add perhaps only a limited amount of "roughage" to their diets than to reduce the daily fat-intake.

REFERENCES
Aries V, Crowther JS, Drasar BS, Hill MJ, Williams REO (1969). Bacteria and the aetiology of cancer of the large bowel. Gut 10:334.
Armstrong B, Doll R (1975). Environmental factors in cancer incidence and mortality in different countries, with special reference to dietary practices. Int J Cancer 15:617.
Breslow NE, Enstrom JR (1974). Geographic correlations between cancer mortality rates and alcohol tobacco consumption in the United States. JNCI 53:631.

Burkitt DP, Walker ARP, Painter NS (1972). Effect of dietary fibre on stools and transit times, and its role in the causation of the disease. Lancet II:1408.

Crowther JS, Drasar BS, Hill MJ, MacLennan R, Magnin D, Peach S, Teoh-Chan CH (1976). Fecal steroids and bacteria in large bowel cancer in Hong Kong by socio-economic groups. Br J Cancer 34:191.

Esser V, Weithofer G, Bloch R (1980). Zur Bedeutung des Fett und Rohfasergehalts der Nahrung für de Entstehung des Kolonkarzinoms. Z. Gastroenterologie 18:1.

Dales LG, Friedmann GD, Ury HK, Grossman S, Williams SR (1979). A case-control study of relationships of diet and other traits to colo-rectal cancer in American blacks. Am J Epid 109:132.

Glober GA, Nomura A, Kamiana S, Shimada A, Abba BC (1977). Bowel transit time and stool weight in populations with different colon cancer risks. Lancet II:110.

Graham S, Dayal H, Swanson M, Mittelman A, Wilkinson G (1978). Diet in the epidemiology of cancer of the colon and rectum. JNCI 61:709.

Haenszel W (1961). Cancer mortality among the foreign born in the United States. JNCI 26:37.

Haenszel W, Berg W, Segi M, Kurihara M, Loche FB (1973). Large bowel cancer in Hawaiian Japanese. JNCI 51:1765.

Higginson J (1966). Etiological factors in gastrointestinal cancer in Man. JNCI 37:527.

Higginson J, Oettle AG (1960). Cancer incidence in the Bantu and "Cape colored" races of South Africa: Report of a cancer survey in the Transvaal (1953-1955). JNCI 24:589.

Hill MJ, Drasar BS, Aries VC, Crowther JS, Hawksworth G, William REO (1971). Bacteria and the aetiology of cancer of the large bowel. Lancet I:95.

Hill MJ, Drasar BS, Meade TW, Cox AG, Simpson JP, Morson BC (1975). Fecal bile acid and clostridia in patients with cancer of the large bowel. Lancet I:535.

IARC (International Agency for Research on Cancer) Intestinal Microecology Group (1977). Dietary fibre, transit time, faecal bacteria, steroids and colon cancer in two Scandinavian populations. Lancet II:207.

Jensen OM (1982). Cancer risk among Danish Seventh-Day Adventists and other temperance society members. (Submitted for publication).

Jensen OM, MacLennan R, Wahrendorff J, on behalf of the IARC Large Bowel Group (1982). Diet, bowel function, fecal characteristics and large bowel cancer in Denmark and Finland. Nutr Cancer 4:(In press).

Modan B, Barell V, Lubin F, Modan M, Greenberg RA, Graham S (1975). Low-fiber intake as an etiologic factor in cancer of the colon. JNCI 55:15.

Narisawa T, Magadia NE, Weisburger JH, Wynder EL (1974). Promoting effects of bile acid on colon carcinogenesis after intrarectal installation of n-methyl-n-nitro-n-nitrosoguanidine in rats. JNCI 53:1093.

Pernu J (1960). An epidemiological study of cancer of the digestive organs and respiratory systems. A study based on 7078 cases. Ann Med Intern Fenn 49:Supplement 33.

Phillips RL (1975). Role of life-style and dietary habits in risk of cancer among Seventh-Day Adventists. Cancer Research 35:3513.

Reddy BS, Hedges AR, Lakso K, Wynder EL (1978). Metabolic epidemiology of large bowel cancer. Fecal bulk and constituents of high-risk North American and low-risk Finnish population. Cancer 42:2832.

Waterhouse J, Muir C, Correa P, Powell J (1976). Cancer Incidence in Five Continents. Vol. III. IARC Scientific Publications No. 15. Lyon: International Agency for Research on Cancer.

Wynder EL, Kajitani T, Ishikawa S, Dodo H, Takano A (1969). Environmental factors of cancer of the colon and rectum. II. Japanese epidemiological data. Cancer 23:1210.

Wynder EL, Shigematsu T (1967). Environmental factors of cancer of the colon and rectum. Cancer 20:1520.

CONGRESS SYMPOSIA

NUTRITION AND CANCER MANAGEMENT Okada, A., Japan, Chairman; Rhoads, J., USA, Co-Chairman; Olympic Room

Definition of the Nutrition Problems in the Cancer Patient. *Copeland, E. M., III, Houston, TX USA. (By Title Only)

Nutritional Rehabilitation of the Cancer Patient. *Dudrick, S. J., O'Donnell, J. J. and Clague, M. B., Houston, TX USA.

Cyclic Intermittent Parenteral Nutrition (CIPN). The First Adjuvant Therapy for Radio-Chemotherapeutic Combinations in Advanced Ovarian Tumors (AOT). *Joyeux, H., Dubois, J. B., Solassol, C. and Pujol, H., Montpellier, France.

Nutritional Support in Cancer Patient Undergoing Surgery. *Daly, J., New York, NY USA. (By Title Only)

Role of Nutrition Support in the Management of Children with Cancer. *Rickard, K. A., Coates, T. D., Grosfeld, J. L., Weetman, R. M., Provisor, A. J. and Baehner, R. L., Indianapolis, IN USA.

Please note: Papers that are listed as "By Title Only" were presented at the 13th International Cancer Congress, but are not included in these volumes.

**13th International Cancer Congress, Part D**
**Research and Treatment, pages 161–170**
© **1983 Alan R. Liss, Inc., 150 Fifth Avenue, New York, NY 10011**

NUTRITIONAL REHABILITATION OF THE CANCER PATIENT

Stanley J. Dudrick, M.D., Joseph J. O'Donnell, M.D.
and Malcolm B. Clague, M.D.
St. Luke's Episcopal Hospital
M.D. Anderson Hospital and Tumor Institute
Houston, Texas  77030

There is no known pathological process from which a
patient can be expected to recover better when he is malnourished than when he is well nourished, and every patient
requires some form of nutritional support during all phases
of diagnosis, therapy, convalescence and rehabilitation.
Therefore, it is the obligation of all physicians and
surgeons, regardless of their area of special expertise,
to direct their efforts and talents toward the optimal
nutritional support of their patients to the same degree
that they apply their general and specialty management
to the patients' primary pathology.  For the well nourished
patient who has normal function of the gastrointestinal
tract which has not, and will not, be adversely affected
by the primary pathophysiologic disorder and its therapy,
adequate nutritional therapy is usually not a major
problem, and this is the case in a majority of hospitalized
patients.  However, in patients who exhibit signs,
symptoms and/or history of malnutrition prior to hospitalization, or who are likely to develop them during hospitalization as a result of stressful periods of diagnosis and
therapy, a significantly higher morbidity and mortality
can be expected to result if adequate attention has not been
paid to their nutritional maintenance and/or restitution.

In the experience of our nutritional support team
during the past ten years, four indices of evaluation
have proven valuable in making decisions to provide
special forms of nutritional support:  1) History of an
unintentional or unexplained weight loss of 10 pounds or
10% body weight during the previous two months.  2)  Serum

albumin concentration of less than 3.4 gm%. 3) Anergy
to a battery of 4 or 5 standard skin test antigens.
4) An abnormally low total lymphocyte count. If a
patient manifests evidence of any two of these indices,
he is malnourished to a mild or moderate degree; if he
manifests any three of these indices, he is moderately
to severely malnourished; if he manifests all four indices,
he is severely malnourished. Mortality rates during major
therapeutic endeavors can be expected to increase by 15-25%,
25-50% and 50-90% respectively under these conditions of
malnutrition. These are the basic broad criteria by which
our decisions to employ special techniques and substrates
for nutritional support are made.

More specifically, we have developed a nutritional
assessment screening profile consisting of seven indices
of historical, biochemical and anthropometric criteria
which is generally obtained on all surgical patients in
order to establish the nutritional status of the patient in
an objective and reproducible manner. They include
weight, triceps skinfold thickness, mid-arm circumference,
creatinine/height index, serum albumin, total lymphocyte
count and % weight change from usual weight. When a
patient exhibits abnormalities to any of the indices in
the screening profile, a more extensive nutritional
assessment profile which evaluates 14 indices is obtained
in order to define more clearly the nature and magnitude
of the patient's nutritional defects. The additional
indices in the comprehensive assessment are: retinol binding protein, serum transferrin, serum prealbumin, serum
osmolarity, skin tests, % weight change since admission
and nitrogen balance. A team of nurses, dietitians and
physicians are involved in this process. An official
interpretation of the nutritional status of the patient
and recommendations for his nutritional management are
then made by the dietitian and physician and recorded on
the patient's chart.

If the patient is able to eat, he receives dietary
consultation and special attention to his nutritional
requirements via the oral route. If the patient is
unable to eat adequately or not at all, but if his gastrointestinal tract is functional, he is then fed by an
intestinal tube placed preferentially through the nose,
but at times inserted at operation directly into the
stomach or small bowel. If the patient cannot eat,

should not eat, will not eat, cannot eat enough or has a special metabolic problem, it may be necessary to feed him entirely or supplementally via parenteral nutrition techniques. Great progress has been made in the development of many feeding alternatives and substrates during the past decade so that the physician or surgeon and the nutrition support team now have the means at their disposal currently to nourish virtually every patient adequately despite his pathologic status. Indeed, not to nourish a patient adequately reflects a positive decision to starve the patient or a passive decision to accept starvation as an inevitable result.

In general, it appears that the average nutritionally depleted or complicated surgical patient requires between 2000 and 4000 kcal and approximately 12 to 24 gm of nitrogen of high biological value per day. The nitrogen is given in amounts sufficient to achieve nitrogen equilibrium or a positive nitrogen balance of 1 gram or more per day with the simultaneous delivery of at least 150 non-protein calories per gram of nitrogen administered. Thus, as the nitrogen requirements increase, the administered calories are simultaneously increased proportionately. Additional calories combined with individually tailored physical therapy may be given to cachectic patients in order to attempt to restore fat depots and to achieve ideal body weight and composition. As the patient recovers from his initial stress and enters the convalescent stage, the quantity of nutrients is reduced commensurate with his needs. The primary indication for the use of intravenous hyperalimentation (IVH) is to provide adequate nutrition parenterally as long as necessary when use of the gastrointestinal tract is impractical, inadequate, ill-advised, or impossible. When adequate nutrition cannot be obtained by the alimentary tract in seriously ill patients suffering concomitantly from malnutrition, major surgical trauma, sepsis, other major complications or malignancy, the most critical indications for prolonged IVH exist.

General indications for either enteral or parenteral nutritional support include: 1) patients unable to eat; 2) patients unwilling to eat; 3) patients unable and/or unwilling to eat enough; and 4) patients with specific requirements secondary to individual or multiple organ dysfunction. Patients who are unable to eat include those with severe difficulties in swallowing or with upper gastrointestinal tract fistulas or obstruction. Cancer of the mouth, pharynx, larynx or cervical esophagus may result in painful deglutition and progressive difficulty with ingestion of solid food. Moreover, patients with cancer of the head and neck often have a history of heavy smoking, excessive alcohol intake, and dietary indiscretions which render them protein-calorie malnourished. Since most oncologic therapy usually impairs optimal oral nutritional repletion for a considerable period of time, such patients may embark upon a vicious cycle of compounded malnutrition. Surgical treatment of a patient with head and neck cancer often results in diminished oral intake while perioperative or primary radiation therapy often induces severe stomatitis, mucositis and diminished salivary secretions. These adverse signs and symptoms further aggravate the decreased oral intake and increased weight loss.

Oncology patients are able, but <u>unwilling to eat</u> either because of their primary disease or the side effects of therapy. In virtually all patients with malignancies, some degree of anorexia is encountered. This disturbing symptom is usually related both to the type and stage of the disease. For example, patients with carcinoma of the lung often present with severe anorexia and weight loss out of proportion to their tumor volume, whereas patients with metastatic breast carcinoma usually remain in a relatively normal nutritional state until the malignancy becomes unresponsive to usual therapeutic modalities. Anorexia may be secondary to plasma amino acid imbalances, central nervous system neurotransmitter abnormalities, psychological disturbances or to alterations of taste influenced by trace metal imbalances. Regardless of etiology, anorexia is probably the single most important cause of malnutrition in cancer patients. While the primary malignant process may result in decreased oral intake, most antineoplastic therapies result in severe stomatitis and enteritis which militate against the patient's ingesting adequate quantities of nutrients orally. Xerostomia, the delayed effect of radiation treatment to the oropharyngeal area, is another complication which results in decreased taste sensation and unwillingness to eat.

Inadequate gastric reservoir function, pancreatic insufficiency, bile salt depletion, or other abnormal factors such as blind loop syndrome may result in impaired digestion and absorption in oncology patients. In addition, patients with radiation enteropathy, lymphoma or Whipple's disease constitute a group who are unable or unwilling to eat enough.

Finally there are patients who have specific nutritional requirements secondary to individual organ failure. Patients with simultaneous malignancies and cardiac failure, renal failure, and/or hepatic failure present the ultimate challenge to maintenance or improvement of nutritional status while receiving primary oncologic therapy.

Determination of the method of feeding the patient depends upon the patient's nutritional status, the level and degree of residual gastrointesitnal function and the type and magnitude of treatment employed. Ideally, adequate voluntary oral ingestion of food is the optimal goal for all patients. However, most antineoplastic treatment modalities preclude optimal oral intake. Moreover, poor nutritional status results in lassitude and weakness which further decrease oral ingestion of nutrients. If a patient is unable to meet his daily nutritional requirements voluntarily by oral ingestion of normal foodstuffs, oral nutrient supplementation together with aggressive dietary counselling should be initiated. Alert, well-motivated patients can often be encouraged to increase their daily calorie and protein intake through the ingestion of hospital or commercially prepared supplements. The patient should be encouraged and allowed to make his own dietary selections whenever feasible. It is usually best to chill supplemental nutrient preparations as this improves palatability and patient compliance. However, some patients are not well motivated, they may have increased nutritional requirements, or they are anorectic secondary to the disease and cannot ingest adequate nutrients orally. In this situation, in a patient with intact gastrointestinal tract function, tube feedings should be initiated. Although a functional gastrointestinal tract provides the best means of insuring normal digestion and assimilation of foodstuffs, use of the enteral route is contraindicated in the presence of severe gastrointestinal dysfunction such as intestinal obstruction, upper GI bleeding and/or intractable vomiting or diarrhea. If the gastrointestinal tract is not available for use or if rapid nutritional repletion is deemed vital, parenteral nutrition should be instituted. Table 1 illustrates a typical adult IVH formulation.

Table 1

Adult Intravenous Hyperalimentation Solution

Base Solution
  40-50% dextrose in water                    500 ml
  8.5-10% crystalline amino acids             500 ml

Additives to Each Unit
  Sodium chloride                           40-50 mEq
  Potassium chloride                        20-30 mEq
  Potassium acid phosphate                  15-30 mEq
    (10-20 mM phosphorus)
  Magnesium sulfate                         15-18 mEq

Additives to any One Unit Daily
  Calcium gluconate 10%                       4.5 mEq
  Multivitamin infusion (MVI-12)               10 ml
  Zinc sulfate                               5-10 mg
  Copper sulfate                             1-2 mg
  Iron-dextran (Imferon)                      0.1 ml
  Chromium chloride                         10-20 mcg
  Manganese chloride                          0.5 mg
  Selenium (Sodium selenate)                   60 mcg

Additive to any One Unit Twice Weekly
  Vitamin K                                    10 mg

Intravenous Fat Emulsion 10% or 20%
  500 ml 2-7 times weekly over 4-6 hr       50-100 gm

---

Carbohydrate calories          850 kcal/liter
Protein calories               150 kcal/liter
Fat calories              500-1000 kcal/unit
Nitrogen                   6.5-8.0 gm/liter
Amino Acids                  40-50 gm/liter

The decision to initiate and to maintain adequate total parenteral nutrition should be based upon the achievement of a specific, definable and realistic goal in each patient. It must be borne in mind always that the ultimate aim of the technique is to prolong meaningful life, and not merely to prolong the process of an inevitable death. The primary general goal of intravenous feeding in an individual patient is to provide nutrients adequate in quality and quantity to meet the normal or increased metabolic requirements for: 1) growth and development, 2) regrowth to ideal weight, 3) restoration of function, 4) achievement of homeostasis, 5) positive nitrogen balance, 6) improved response to therapy, 7) repair of tissue, 8) recovery from stress, 9) restoration of immunocompetence, 10) accelerated convalescence and rehabilitation. Another general goal of IVH is to reduce mechanical or secretory activity of the alimentary tract to basal levels in order to achieve a state of bowel rest. By providing nutrients entirely parenterally, the bowel mucosa is not exposed to roughage, peristalsis is not induced by intraluminal bulk, and potent digestive secretions of the gastrointestinal tract are not stimulated mechanically to the usual degree. The bowel is physiologically splinted and is able to repair itself or recover from various pathological processes such as untoward side-effects of chemotherapy or radiotherapy without being further traumatized or stressed by the rigors of digestion, absorption, and excretion. Thus, patients have been able to tolerate larger and/or more frequent doses of chemotherapy.

In patients with fistulas from one portion of the alimentary tract to another, to the skin, or to the urogenital tract, significant reductions in the secretion and volume of fistulous drainage diminish the mechanical and chemical impediments to fistula closure and reduce the number of microorganisms which pass through the fistula and thereby impair healing. In malnourished patients requiring prolonged periods of bowel preparation prior to diagnostic studies and major surgical procedures, IVH has allowed adequate nutrition while keeping the bowel free of particulate matter.

A third general goal of IVH is to provide specially-tailored diets by vein to improve nutritional status without aggravating the metabolic derangements precipitated by pathological conditions affecting the kidneys or liver. Thus, intravenous diets of high biological value can be administered to the nutritional benefit of the patient in renal or hepatic decompensation without significantly elevating the BUN or blood ammonia. A fourth general goal is to reduce the urgency for surgical intervention in patients who might eventually require operation, but in whom prolonged, progressive malnutrition has greatly increased the risk of operation. One can "buy" time for patients in high risk morbidity and mortality categories who are malnourished, who obviously need operations, but who, without aid of IVH, would be in worse condition secondary to delaying operation.

A fifth general goal of IVH is to avoid, reduce or correct protein deficiencies and the complications of hypoproteinemia. The surgeon is not trying to promote muscle synthesis when infusing intravenous amino acids and calorie substrates. The general goal is to provide the protein moieties that are required both for repair of injured tissues and for restoration of serum proteins and tissue proteins. The specific goals are to: 1) increase resistance to blood loss, 2) decrease susceptibility to shock, 3) restore serum and tissue proteins, 4) increase plasma and blood volume, 5) increase resistance to infection, 6) reduce edema both locally at the wound and generally, 7) accelerate wound healing, 8) restore digestive enzymes to normal, 9) reverse the protein deficiency of malabsorption, 10) restore immunocompetence, 11) improve metabolic rate, 12) improve cardiovascular function, 13) decrease weakness and lassitude, 14) reverse mental depression, 15) reduce morbidity and mortality and 16) reduce time and expense of convalescence. The sixth general goal is to achieve a steady, definable metabolic or nutritional state in order to study more precisely the physiological, biochemical, and pharmacologic effects of various parenteral nutrients on metabolism, body composition, body function, and their interrelationships in disease.

Nutritional support of patients receiving oncologic therapy has proven effective in allowing adequate treatment programs to be carried out in patients who otherwise might not have been reasonable candidates for any form of anti-neoplastic therapy. Tumor growth has not been measurably enhanced and septic complications have been minimal when established principles and techniques have been observed. There seems to be a positive correlation between nutritional status and the potential for positive tumor responses to chemotherapy. Moreover, when the patient is well nourished,

there appears to be increased tolerance for certain chemotherapeutic drugs, particularly 5-fluorouracil; the tumor
response to these drugs may be improved primarily because
larger doses can be delivered per unit time. With current
emphasis on immunotherapy, interrelationships between the
immune mechanisms of the body and nutritional status
must continue to be explored. A combination of tumor burden
and malnutrition, coupled with chemotherapy, radiation
therapy, and/or surgery, may render the patient immunologically incompetent. The most potent of these factors in
eradicating established delayed hypersensitivity is
probably malnutrition which, on the other hand, can most
easily be corrected promptly by the proper use of IVH.
Finally, malnutrition is potentially harmful to cancer
patients because a cachectic patient has a narrower safe
therapeutic margin for most chemotherapy and radiation
therapy. The cancericidal doses of these agents may be much
closer to the lethal dose for normal tissues in the malnourished patient than in the well-nourished patient.

Recently considerable experience has been gained in
developing a specially designed patient vest which is comfortable, attractive, and practical for continuous central
venous or enteral feeding on an ambulatory basis. Clinical
results have been most gratifying, and it is anticipated
that further advances in this vital field will contribute
to increased cost-effectiveness, cost-containment, and favorable clinical results in the nutritional management of
cancer patients. A rational approach to therapy of the
malnourished cancer patient is to replenish him nutritionally
with IVH before, during, and/or after all forms of therapy,
whenever this highly desirable goal cannot be accomplished
by means of the alimentary tract. Only then can the
achievement of optimal nutritional and antineoplastic results
be expected. Hopefully, it will eventually be possible to
combine chemical and physical antineoplastic agents with
specific parenteral nutrient substrates to effect a synergism
that will totally eradicate systemic malignancies. Moreover,
it is important to evaluate the use of IVH as an adjunct
to long-term continuous infusion chemotherapy. Multiple
investigative efforts are currently underway in our laboratories in an attempt to unravel these mysteries, particularly
with nutritional manipulation and cell cycle specific chemotherapeutic agents in the study of RNA, DNA, purine, and
pyrimidine metabolism. The ultimate aim is to develop
specific parenteral nutrient regimens which will be supportive

of normal cellular metabolism, but which will be detrimental
to the function and survival of neoplastic cells.

Optimal results from surgical procedures, pharmacologic
therapy, chemotherapy, radiotherapy, respiratory therapy,
physical therapy and other forms of patient care can only be
obtained when the patient is simultaneously maintained in
optimal nutritional condition. The ultimate nutritional
goal is to provide optimal nutrition to all patients under
all conditions at all times.

Copeland EM, MacFadyen BV, Dudrick SJ (1974). Intravenous
   hyperalimentation in cancer patients. J Surg Res 16:241.
Copeland EM, MacFadyen BV, Dudrick SJ (1976). Effect of
   intravenous hyperalimentation on established delayed hypersensitivity in the cancer patient. Ann Surg 184:60.
Copeland EM, Daly JM, Dudrick SJ (1981). Parenteral hyper-
   alimentation of the cancer patient. In Newell G, Ellison
   N (eds): "Nutrition and Cancer: Etiology and Treatment"
   New York:  Raven Press, p 393.
Daly JM, Dudrick SJ, Copeland EM (1980). Intravenous hyper-
   alimentation: effect on delayed hypersensitivity in cancer
   patients. Ann Surg 192:587.
Daly JM, Copeland EM, Dudrick SJ (1981). Nutritional manage-
   ment of patients with head and neck malignancies.  In
   Suen JY, Myers E (eds): "Cancer of the Head and Neck"
   New York, Churchill Livingstone, p 63.
Daly JM, Dudrick SJ (1981). Results of intravenous nutrition:
   results of intravenous nutrition in cancer patients.  In
   Hill GL (ed): "Nutrition in the Surgical Patient" New
   York, Churchill Livingstone, p 191.
Daly JM, Smith G, Frazier OH, Dudrick SJ, Copeland EM (1982).
   Effects of systemic hyperthermia and intrahepatic infusion
   with 5-Fluorouracil. Cancer 49:1112.
Daly JM, Massar E, Giacco G, Frazier OH, Mountain CF, Dudrick
   SJ (1982). Parenteral nutrition in esophageal cancer
   patients.  Ann Surg 196:203.
Dudrick SJ, Copeland EM (1981). Nutritional support of the
   cancer patient.  In Miller TA, Dudrick SJ (eds.): "The
   Management of Difficult Surgical Problems" University
   of Texas, p 201.
Dudrick SJ (1981). A clinical review of nutritional support
   of the patient. J Clin Nutr 34:1191.
Dudrick SJ (1983). Parenteral nutrition.  In Dudrick SJ, Baue
   AE, Eiseman B, MacLean LD, Rowe MI, Sheldon GF (eds):
   "Manual of Preoperative and Postoperative Care," Saunders.

**13th International Cancer Congress, Part D**
**Research and Treatment, pages 171–178**
© **1983 Alan R. Liss, Inc., 150 Fifth Avenue, New York, NY 10011**

CYCLIC INTERMITTENT PARENTERAL NUTRITION (CIPN). THE FIRST
ADJUVANT THERAPY FOR RADIO-CHEMOTHERAPEUTIC COMBINATIONS IN
ADVANCED OVARIAN TUMORS (AOT)

H. Joyeux, J.B. Dubois, C. Solassol, H. Pujol

Cancer Institute
Centre Paul Lamarque - Cliniques St. Eloi
34033 Montpellier Cedex - France

Cancer patients in our unit have been receiving the
most up-to-date parenteral nutrition since 1972 (Joyeux
1981). In order to ameliorate patient tolerance we developed "the artificial gut system" (Solassol 1979) which permits ambulatory or home care nutrition (Joyeux 1980). We
previously showed in two randomized trials the benefits of
intestinal rest through exclusive parenteral nutrition following total abdominal irradiation for peritoneal carcinoma
(Solassol 1979) resulting from advanced (Stages III and IV)
ovarian cancer. Our goal was to facilitate the treatment of
patients with advanced ovarian cancer and to employ randomized trials to evaluate the adjuvant value of nutritional
support at the Centre Paul Lamarque from June 1977 to December 1980.

I. MATERIALS AND METHODS

1°/ Ovarian cancer patients
All 43 patients chosen for this study had already been
diagnosed as adenocarcinoma of the ovary. There were 14
Stage III and 29 Stage IV cancers as evaluated by the FIGO
post-operative criteria. Thirty-one patients (72 %) presented retroperitoneal positives nodes.

2°/ Treatment of advanced ovarian tumors (AOT)
Our therapy was based on the findings in the literature
(Marchant 1981). All patients underwent surgery prior to
radio-chemotherapy.

- Surgical treatment : Our surgical technique centers
around an abdomino-pelvian (regional) approach with maximal
tumor resections. The minimum ablation consisted of total
omentectomy with extraperitoneal radical hysterectomy. Complementary surgery was carried out as a function of parietal
and/or visceral involvement leading to parietal and/or visceral resection.

| | |
|---|---|
| Partial anterior parietal resection | 4 |
| Right colectomy | 7 |
| Sigmoidectomy | 10 |
| Total colectomy | 4 |
| Partial ileoectomy | 12 |
| Total ileoectomy | 4 |
| Anterior rectal resection | 5 |
| Lateral and anterior peritonectomy | 16 |
| Diaphragmatic peritonectomy | 12 |
| Left hepatic lobectomy | 1 |

Table 1. 75 parietal and/or visceral resections were performed on the 43 AOT patients.

In all cases, intra-abdominal lesions were so extensive
that an estimated volume equal or greater than 2 cm remained after regional surgery. Different marker clips were
placed at the points where the most invasive lesions were
found or where we believed that residual tumor was probably
still present.

- Radiation therapy

| | |
|---|---|
| Diaphragm region | 7 |
| Pelvis | 32 |
| Right hypochondrium | 6 |
| Left hypochondrium | 8 |
| Anterior abdominal wall | 4 |
| | 57 |

Table 2. Placement of clips indicating the irradiation
field (s) for each patient (total : 57).

These markers allowed us to begin selective irradiation immediately following the surgical phase i.e. an average 3 to
5 weeks after surgery.
Irradiation therapy employed high energy photons (25 MeV)
delivered by a Sagittaire Linear Accelerator.
Irradiated volume was determined as a function of resi-

dual tumor tissue located by marker clips. Consequently, several fiels may have been irradiated simultaneously for the same patient.

The irradiation schedule was determined as a function of irradiated volume. A typical treatment lasted 4 1/2 to 5 weeks (5 x 1.8 Gy or 5 x 2 Gy per week) for a total delivered dose of 45 to 55 Gy with occasional very limited overdose (up to 58 Gys) for smaller volumes.

Parenteral nutrition was given on each day or every other day during radiotherapy depending on the patients' own ability to take oral alimentation (Joyeux 1980).

- Chemotherapy : Chemotherapy was initiated following a one month convalescent period at home or in a convalescent center ; 1 to 2 months post-irradiation for patients in the radiotherapy phase. All drugs were introduced by deep catheter for patients receiving intermittent cyclic parenteral nutrition. Non CIPN patients received chemotherapy by superficial venous route. Chemotherapy protocol :

Day 1 : Adriamycin (Adriblastine* ): 35 $mg/m^2$ (IV) and Cis-dichlorodiamine platinum (CDDP) (Cis-Platyl* ) : 50 $mg/ m^2$ (IV).

Day 8 to day 21 : per os : Hexamethyl-melamine (H.M.M. or Hexastat* ) : 150 $mg/m^2$ per day, given in 3 to 4 fractions exclusive of meal time.

Treatment was re-initiated on day 29. Each cycle lasted 28 days and was carried to a total permissible dose of 450 $mg/ m^2$ for Adriamycin and 650 $mg/m^2$ for CDDP.

3°/ Nutritional support

The same nutrition was administered to all patients over the entire surgical and radiotherapy phases. Patients were randomized into two groups before proceding to chemotherapy. One group received cyclic parenteral nutrition while the other received none.

A radio-opaque silicon catheter was placed preoperatively in the superior vena cava by cut-down followed and puncture of the internal jugular vein.

Parenteral nutrition was administered continuously for 12 to 18 hours for 4 to 6 days leading up to surgery. This was carried over for 15 post-operative days for all patients.

Daily nutritional support consisted of parenteral normo-alimentation calculated as a function of patient weight, varying from 1500 to 2000 Calories and 6.25 to 12.5 gr nitrogen. Our nutritive mixture was contained in an E.V.A. bag and consisted of glucose, amino acids, lipids (20 % Intra-

lipids), electrolytes and trace-elements (Joyeux 1981).
Cyclic intermittent parenteral nutrition (CIPN) : In
Group I, parenteral nutrition was given in a cyclic fashion
during each chemotherapy cycle. The pre-placed catheter for
all patients on CIPN was left in place unless complications
arose. CIPN was employed over the entire chemotherapy sequence i.e. six days per month for 6 months. For six days
patients were fed "ad libitum", oral feeding consisting
essentially of water and some sugar solutions.
The catheter was rinsed with heparinated physiological
saline after each chemotherapy sequence then closed with
an airtight cap.

4°/ The randomized study
This study was performed from June 1977 to December
1980. Patients were divided into two groups : Group I consisted of patients receiving CIPN ; Group II did not receive CIPN. The mean age for Group I was 48 (range : 32 to 68
years old) ; that of Group II was 52 (range : 34 to 69
years old). The distribution of tumor stages was approximately equal for both groups because Stages III and IV were
randomized separately.

|  | Group I<br>( with CIPN ) | Group II<br>(without CIPN) |
|---|---|---|
| Stage III | 8 | 6 |
| Stage IV | 15 | 14 |
|  | 23 | 20 |

Table 3. Patient distribution in both ramdomized groups.

II. RESULTS

1°/ The complications of artificial feeding
The only complication we encountered was due to the catheter which had to be removed for either mechanical dysfunction or infection.

- In the surgical phase, 4 catheters were removed and
replaced : 1 for obstruction, 3 due to suspected infection
which was confirmed in only 1 case (colibacillus and entero-
coccus).
- Eighteen patients in group I (CIPN) showed no catheter

complications, five did. Two of these five for obstruction during the second and third chemotherapy cycle. The catheter in the 3 remaining patients was removed due to febrile episodes. Infection was confirmed in only one case (Krebsiella).

2°/ Interrupted therapy (IT)
Therapy was discontinued when warranted by the guidelines defined by the W.H.O.
The number and intensity of intolerance to chemo and radiotherapy were significantly higher $(\chi^2 < 5$ %) for Group II (2 out of 12 $IT_3$ patients from Group II were NED whereas all $IT_4$ patients were ED).

|        | Group I (23 patients) (with CIPN) | Group II (20 patients) (without CIPN) |
|--------|:---------------------------------:|:-------------------------------------:|
| $IT_1$ | 6                                 | 0                                     |
| $IT_2$ | 3                                 | 4                                     |
| $IT_3$ | 0                                 | 12                                    |
| $IT_4$ | 0                                 | 4                                     |

Table 4. The number of IT for both groups.

3°/ The median relapse-free interval
Relapse was diagnosed based on : 1) either clinical or paraclinical indications : laboratory tests (carcinoembryonic antigen, CEA) or scanner results (infraclinical extension into the peritoneum, lymph nodes, liver pelvic or retropelvic region ; 2) routine second look at 12 to 18 months after initial surgery. The mean relapse free interval for Group I (23 patients) was 15.4 months measured from the time of initial surgery whereas this interval was only 6.6 months for Group II. This represents a significant difference ($\alpha < 0.05$) between the two groups.

4°/ Mean survival time
Survival at 2, 3 and 5 years was very different for the two patient populations. The difference was not significant at 5 years due to the low number of patients treated in 1977 : 8 patients − 4 in Stage III and 4 in Stage IV.

|          | Stage III | Stage IV |
|----------|:---------:|:--------:|
| Group I  | 2         | 0        |
| Group II | 1         | 0        |

Table 5. : Survival at 5 years.

However, the 2 and 3 year survival was significantly different ( $\chi^2 < 5$ %) for Group I versus Group II for Stage III as well as IV.

|  | | Survival at 2 years | | Survival at 3 years | |
|---|---|---|---|---|---|
|  | | Number | % | Number | % |
| Group I | Stage III | 6 ++++ | 75 | 5 +++ | 62.5 |
| | Stage IV | 8 +++++ | 53.3 | 5 +++ | 33.3 |
| Group II | Stage III | 4 +++ | 66.6 | 2 + | 33.3 |
| | Stage IV | 6 +++ | 42.8 | 2 + | 14.2 |

+ patients still alive at June 1982

$\alpha > 5$ % $\chi^2$ test

DISCUSSION

The anticipated survival for advanced ovarian adenocarcinoma at five years generally ranges from 10 to 35 % (Marchant 1981). The protocols developed to treat this form of cancer are poorly tolerated by the patient, particularly from a digestive and nutritive point of view. The necessity of nutritional support during the pre and post-operative periods of the surgical phase is obvious since advanced ovarian cancers indicate digestive tract resection. The benefit of continuing nutritional support into the radiotherapy phase immediately following surgery has already been shown (Dubois 1974, Dubois 1976, Valerio 1978). The innovative aspect of our protocol is the application of a cyclic parenteral nutrition administered parallel to each chemotherapy cycle. Sequential chemotherapy is therefore linked to sequential parenteral nutrition. CIPN significantly reduces the need to discontinue treatment due to therapeutic complications and/or patient intolerance to chemotherapy (Issell 1978). Group II patients (no CIPN) most often did not complete their chemotherapy whereas Group I did. It logically follows that relapse occurred earlier (p<0.05) in Group II (average : 6.6 months) than Group I (average : 15.4 months). This difference was reiterated during analysis of patient survival. The difference at 5 years was inconclusive due to an insufficient number of patients. Survival at 2 and 3 years was significantly greater in Group I for both Stage III and IV cancers.

CONCLUSION

CIPN should be a routine adjuvant to therapeutic protocols for advanced ovarian adenocarcinomas.The randomized studies presented here show that parenteral nutritional support is the first effective adjuvant for this particular type of tumor.

Dubois JB, Joyeux H, Yakoun M, Pourquier H, Solassol C (1974). Irradiation abdominale totale et nutrition parentérale. In proceedings of Congrès International de Nutrition Parentérale, Montpellier, p 695

Dubois JB, Joyeux H, Yakoun M, Pourquier H, Solassol C (1976). Total abdominal irradiation : an experimental study in the dog. Biomedicine 25:123.

Fuller AF, Griffiths CT (1979). Ovarian cancer cachexia - surgical interactions. Gynecol Oncol 8:301.

Griffiths CT, Fuller AF (1978). Intensive surgical and chemotherapeutic management of advanced ovarian cancer. Surg Cli North Am 58:131.

Issell BF, Valdivieso M, Zaren HA, Dudrick SJ, Freireich EJ, Copeland EW, Bodey GP(1978). Protection against chemotherapy toxicity by IV hyperalimentation. Cancer Treat Rep 62:1139.

Joyeux H, Solassol C (1981). Nutrition Parentérale Prolongée Ambulatoire et à domicile chez des malades atteints de cancer. Gastroenterologie Clin Biol 5:515.

Joyeux H, Solassol C (1980). Home Parenteral Feeding. In Truelove SC, Kennedy HJK (eds) : "Topics in Gastroenterology 8", Blacwell Scientific Publications,p 75.

Marchant DJ (1981). Ovarian carcinoma : staging and surgical treatment. Current concepts in Oncology 3:3.

Ponsky JL, Gauderer MW (1980). Expanded applications of Broviac catheter. Arch Surg 115:324.

Solassol C, Joyeux H (1979). Artificial gut in gastro-intestinal cancer. Front Gastro Intest Res 5:44.

Solassol C, Joyeux H, Dubois JB (1979). TPN with complete nutritive mixtures: An artificial gut in cancer patients. Nutrition and Cancer 1:13.

Valerio D, Overett L, Malcolm A, Blackburn GL (1978). Nutritional support for cancer patients receiving abdominal and pelvic radiotherapy : a randomized prospective clini-

cal experiment of intravenous versus oral feeding.  Surg
Forum 29:145.

13th International Cancer Congress, Part D
Research and Treatment, pages 179–192
© 1983 Alan R. Liss, Inc., 150 Fifth Avenue, New York, NY 10011

ROLE OF NUTRITION SUPPORT IN THE MANAGEMENT OF CHILDREN
WITH CANCER

Karyl A. Rickard, R.D., Ph.D.
Thomas D. Coates, M.D.
Jay L. Grosfeld, M.D.
Robert M. Weetman, M.D.
Arthur J. Provisor, M.D.
Robert L. Baehner, M.D.

Departments of Pediatric Nutrition and
Dietetics, Pediatric Hematology/Oncology,
and Pediatric Surgery
James Whitcomb Riley Hospital for Children
Indiana University School of Medicine
Indianapolis, Indiana   46223

Amid the flourish of technology in modern medicine, we have once again rediscovered information known to Hippocrates in 1200 A.D.:

"...physicians are in the practice of doing the very reverse of what is proper, they all wish, at the commencement of diseases, to starve their patients for two, three, or more days, and then to administer the ptisans (medicines) and drinks; and perhaps it appears to them reasonable that, as a great change has taken place in the body, it should be counteracted by another great change. Now, indeed, to produce a change is no small matter but the change must be affected well and cautiously and after the change the administration of food must be conducted still more so.  "

In our zeal to conquer cancer with extensive surgical procedures and ablative chemotherapy, we have failed to recognize the importance and significance of malnutrition in neoplastic disorders. This problem is further amplified in the growing child where maintenance

of weight actually represents deterioration in
nutritional status. Nutritional status at the time of
diagnosis of neoplastic disease has been clearly
associated with outcome in adults (DeWys et.al. 1980) as
well as children (van Eys 1981; Rickard et.al. In
press). It should come as no surprise to physicians,
therefore, that the rate of weight loss in children who
have Wilms' tumors during their initial, intense
treatment phase would be considered "lethal" (Rickard
et.al. 1979a) when judged by the criteria of Keys in his
classic study of starvation (Keys 1950). During the
past six years, we have evaluated the nutritional status
at the time of diagnosis as well as during the course of
treatment of more than 100 children with cancer.
Based on our experience with this group of young
patients, we developed a nutrition staging system for
use at the time of diagnosis and methods to assess
ongoing changes in nutritional status. In addition, we
formulated a program of nutritional management therapy
as well as supportive care during multimodal treatment
of the child with cancer. The purpose of this paper is
to define criteria to identify protein energy
malnutrition (PEM) and emphasize the importance of
assessment, not only at the time of diagnosis, but also
during therapy. The risks and benefits of enteral
nutrition and total parenteral nutrition (TPN) are
reviewed in relationship to age of patient, specific
tumor type, extent of tumor, multimodal treatment
regimen and intensity of the treatment schedule.

STAGING AND ASSESSMENT OF NUTRITIONAL STATUS

Identification Of PEM (Staging At Diagnosis)

    Among the various methods available for
identification of nutritional depletion at diagnosis,
anthropometric measurements provide information
regarding severity, acuteness and chronicity of PEM in
children with relative ease and low cost. Weight for
height proportionality and weight loss evaluations are
particularly useful in identifying the presence of PEM
when the child is first admitted to the hospital. In
addition, a thorough diet and nutrition history obtained
at this time provides essential information regarding
recent changes in the child's eating habits, highest
past weight and rate of weight gain or loss. Additional

data is obtained to identify socioeconomic and educational factors, food resources and number and ages of siblings which allows us to provide nutritional counseling appropriate to the child's and family's needs. We have found that growth information in the family physician's medical records are often available, and, can be extremely useful for documentation of changes in weight, height and weight to height proportionality. Children are considered to be malnourished if they have a weight loss of greater than or equal to 5%, are less than the 5th percentile weight for height (when height is greater than the 5th percentile for age) or have an albumin concentration less than 3.2 g/dl. A weight loss of 5% appears to be a very conservative estimate of true nutritional depletion. This is particularly true in patients with large solid tumors such as in stage III/IV Wilms' tumor or neuroblastoma where the mass of the tumor itself may account for as much as 3 to 5% of the patient's weight (Rickard unpublished data).

Anthropometric measurements, however, have limitations in sensitivity and specificity. Thus, we depend on certain biochemical determinations such as serum albumin to provide information related to protein nutrition. In the Denver Developmental Study (Trevorrow 1970), 99% of the children in the United States considered to be healthy had a serum albumin concentration greater than 3.2 g/dl. Thus, we have arbitrarily established a critical concentration of less than 3.2 g/dl to be an indicator of PEM.

Patients with cancer are staged as malnourished or not based on the specific criteria for weight loss, weight for height percentile, and serum albumin concentration listed in Table 1.

We have observed that serum transferrin concentrations less than 200 mg/dl are associated with average energy intakes more than 2 S.D. below the mean during the preceding several weeks. Thus, transferrin may be a useful biochemical indicator of low energy intakes and PEM at the time of diagnosis, when food records are unavailable or unlikely to be representative of past eating.

Table 1.  Criteria for staging of nutritional status in
children with cancer

| Stage | | Criteria |
|-------|---|----------|
| Nourished | 1. | Weight for height greater than or equal to the 5th percentile. |
| | 2. | Weight loss less than 5%. |
| | 3. | Albumin concentration greater than or equal to 3.2 g/dl. |
| Malnourished | 1. | Weight for height less than 5th percentile. |
| | 2. | Weight loss greater than or equal to 5%. |
| | 3. | Serum albumin concentration less than 3.2 g/dl. |

In a recent study of 18 children with newly
diagnosed stage IV neuroblastoma, we found a significant
correlation between nutrition staging and time to
relapse (Rickard et.al. In press).  It remains to be
determined whether the patients considered to be
malnourished at diagnosis have a more aggressive or
advanced form of neuroblastoma, or, whether the
nutritional status influenced the outcome.

Ongoing Nutritional Assessment.

Only a limited amount of information exists
regarding sequential changes in anthropometric and
biochemical parameters in relation to a defined energy
(and other nutrient) intake during nutritional depletion
and repletion of young children.  We have found that
there are certain factors that place a patient at a
higher risk for the development of PEM (Table 2).  The
factors were determined by monitoring energy intakes,
weight, weight for height proportionality, skinfold
measurements, and the serum proteins albumin and

transferrin. Tumor types usually associated with these risk factors include stages III and IV Wilms' tumors, advanced neuroblastoma, pelvic rhabdomyosarcoma, acute non-lymphocytic leukemias, brain tumors and some non-Hodgkin's lymphomas.

Table 2  Common risk factors for development of PEM in childhood neoplasms.

Advanced disease at diagnosis or treatment

Lack of tumor response

Abdominal and pelvic irradiation

Intense frequent courses at three or less week intervals of cytotoxic chemotherapy which cause nausea and vomiting, gastrointestinal toxicity, or hepatic toxicity, in the absence of corticosteroids or appetite stimulants

Operative procedures of the abdomen or other abdominal complications such as adynamic ileus, etc.

Psychological depression, absence of supportive health care team, and lack of attention to enteral nutrition

Removal from the home and familiar surroundings, separation from parents and siblings during hospitalization

During our studies, it has become clear that the ongoing monitoring of nutritional status is important. The initiation of multimodal therapy is frequently associated with a marked decrease in oral intake due to anorexia induced from the tumor itself, severe nausea and vomiting related to the chemotherapy, esophageal and gastrointestinal dysfunction related to the irradiation, and postoperative inanition after biopsy, partial or complete removal of the tumor. Nutritional assessments are made at least every three weeks and more often in high risk groups (Table 2). As reported previously (Rickard et.al. 1982) patients with very intense treatment as well as certain tumor types (e.g., pelvic rhabdomyosarcoma, neuroblastoma and some non-Hodgkin's

lymphoma) are at high risk for development of PEM.
Patients with nonmetastatic disease or acute lymphocytic
leukemias are at a lower nutritional risk. Even in the
low risk groups of patients, when complications such as
sepsis occur, the potential for development of PEM is
enhanced. While weight loss and anorexia precede the
initial diagnosis of some tumor types, a decrease in
appetite and energy intake in low risk groups or in high
risk groups during maintenance treatment may herald the
emergence of clinically detectable recurrence (Rickard
et.al. 1980b).

We found that changes in weight, weight for height
proportionality, and subscapular skinfold thickness are
particularly useful indicators of real or impending
nutrition depletion and more useful than some of the
biochemical and immunologic parameters. Sustained
periods of low energy intake usually precede
anthropometric changes. Low energy intakes (more than
two S.D. below the mean of healthy children) and
decreases in skinfold measurements were the first
indicators of nutritional depletion and occurred despite
weight maintenance or a slight weight gain in several
children who had no evidence of edema. Fomon et.al.
(1977) reported a similar phenomenon, i.e. decreases of
24 and 27% in triceps and subscapular fatfold
measurements, respectively, in infants who were fed skim
milk (resulting in a low energy intake) and who gained
at a slow rate. Mobilization of fat reserves probably
provided energy (9 kcal/g fat) which was partially used
to compensate for the energy deficit from a low energy
intake and to synthesize a less costly fat free tissue
(estimated energy cost:1.95 kcal/g, Fomon et.al. 1977).
The sequential monitoring of the skinfold measurements,
particularly the triceps, as a measure of nutritional
status may be more useful in normal or malnourished
children than in obese individuals because of the large
variation in repeated measurements of the latter (Bray
et.al. 1978).

Some pitfalls may be associated with the monitoring
of weight changes as a sole index of nutritional
status. Children who are less than the 5th percentile
weight for height have relatively small losses in weight
(in the absence of an elevated body temperature) in
contrast to the well nourished in spite of equally low

energy intakes. Concomitant fluid changes probably mask some of the tissue wasting observed in malnourished children (Smith 1960; Brozek 1974), and, possibly some metabolic adaptation occurs (Waterlow 1975). The full significance of weight losses is realized in young children when weight for height is plotted sequentially on grids (for those with height greater than 5th percentile for age) and the percent weight loss is calculated. A 2 kg weight loss for a 60 kg teenager (3% weight loss) may not seem impressive, however, the same loss in a 20 kg toddler (10% weight loss) may result in a weight definitely low in relation to height (less than 5th percentile). Thus, relative weight loss (e.g., weight for height) may be more useful than absolute weight losses when considered in relation to skinfold changes and energy intake.

We found that skinfold calipers are valuable in detecting more subtle, subclinical changes in nutritional status during early phases of treatment. Changes greater than 0.3 mm correlated with low energy intakes (more than 2 S.D. below normal) in those patients who initially had subscapular skinfold measurements in the normal range. Changes greater than 0.3 mm are twice the coefficient of variation (method error) which was determined from 265 data sets for each subscapular skinfold measurement obtained by two trained examiners.

Transferrin, prealbumin and retinol binding proteins are three biochemical indicators which may indicate subclinical PEM. Transferrin concentrations reflect severely decreased intakes of energy and/or protein and respond more quickly than albumin concentration to adequate energy and protein provided via TPN (Rickard et.al. 1979b). Changes in albumin concentration in relation to nutrient intake appear to be a useful indicator of mild to moderate PEM in some patients, i.e., decreases are seen which correspond to very low protein and/or energy intakes and are observed sometimes before changes in weight. However, adaptation of albumin concentration (Waterlow 1975) at marginal or low ranges of normal (2.9-3.2 g/dl) has been observed in some children with obvious tissue wasting. Liver complications secondary to disease, cancer treatment and/or TPN may interfere with the synthesis of serum proteins albumin and transferrin.

Additional studies of cellular immune mechanisms in malnourished individuals have indicated loss of lymphocyte function in association with PEM (Rickard et.al. 1980). However, monitoring immune competence as an indicator of nutritional status is fraught with error. In our study (Rickard et.al. 1979a) of children with advanced cancer, lymphocyte counts were severely depressed (less than $500/mm^3$) within three to four weeks of therapy and had no apparent relationship to nutritional repletion. It is more likely that lymphopenia was related to the cytotoxic therapy provided to the child with cancer. Furthermore, the evaluation of recall skin test response is difficult to interpret in relation to the known anergic state previously observed in states of PEM for the same reason as stated above. Other factors which may influence the child's cell mediated response include steroids (Rolley et.al. 1977), radiotherapy (Copeland et.al. 1976), terminal clinical state (Meakins et.al. 1977) and release of toxins from the tumor.

Based upon the continuous assessment of nutritional status, we categorized changes or the lack of changes documented at day 21 from diagnosis as favorable or unfavorable. Children with a favorable nutritional course included those who remained nourished, or, were malnourished at diagnosis and were becoming renourished. Children with an unfavorable nutritional course were those who were nourished and becoming malnourished, and, those who were malnourished and did not improve in nutritional status. In a group of 16 patients with stage IV neuroblastoma, we documented that the unfavorable group of patients had significantly more treatment delays which were associated with drug dose alterations during the first 10 weeks of intense chemotherapy (Rickard et.al. In press).

OPTIONS FOR NUTRITION SUPPORT

Enteral Nutrition

Several modes of nutrition support are available for the pediatric patient. For most children with cancer, provision of nutrients by the enteral route is

the preferred method of feeding the child because
treatment may last several years. An individualized
feeding program which uses favorite, nutritious foods of
the child during treatment-free periods has numerous
practical and psychologic advantages over parenteral
nutrition, including a lower risk of infection and other
catheter related complications, more normal play
activities and lifestyle, and a positive way for the
parent and child to be involved in their own care. In
our experience, however, this type of enteral feeding
program has been ineffective in either preventing or
reversing PEM in the high risk groups of patients during
initial intense treatment. In a study of 21 children
with advanced cancer who received intensive nutrition
counseling and oral nutrition supplementation, 16 had a
decreased energy intake (mean 48 + 24% RDA for kcal) and
dramatic weight loss (mean 16 + 12%) (Rickard et.al.
1979a). A more recent study of children with stage IV
neuroblastoma also emphasized the difficulties inherent
in providing adequate nutrition via the enteral route
when chemotherapy is given at three (or less) week
intervals (Detamore 1980). Energy intakes were very low
(less than the 10th percentile of healthy children)
usually during at least 10 of the 21 days between
chemotherapy courses because patients received
chemotherapy for five days and then required a minimum
of five days to recover appetite. Consequently, most of
the nourished children presented evidence of subclinical
PEM by 21 days from the beginning of treatment, i.e.
weight loss and decreases in subscapular skinfold
measurements.

The use of nasogastric tubes to provide enteral
nutrition is contraindicated in the older infant and
toddler and preschool age groups of children because of
psychologic trauma associated with the insertion and
maintenance of the tube and the potentiation of nausea
during abdominal irradiation and chemotherapy.
Gastrointestinal motility and absorption are impaired
which increase the risk for aspiration pneumonia from
vomiting. Gastrostomy feedings seem to be of limited
value because many patients receive chemotherapy, or,
gastrointestinal or abdominal irradiation which may
impede wound healing.

Enteral nutrition is the method of choice for low

nutritional risk groups as well as the high risk groups
of patients after they have completed intense treatment.
In nine children with Wilms' tumor, ages 1-6 years, who
were followed throughout two years of treatment, the
value of a comprehensive enteral nutrition program,
which included nutrition counseling on a regular basis
and oral nutrition supplements, during maintenance
treatment was documented (Rickard et.al. 1980b). Weight
for height was maintained at greater than the 5th
percentile and subscapular skinfold thickness at greater
than the 10th percentile of healthy children unless
there were complicating factors in the patient's
clinical course.

## Parenteral Nutrition

     In a group of 28 patients who had stages III or IV
solid tumors or second relapse leukemia lymphoma, the
effectiveness of TPN in reversing PEM and restoring
immunity was documented (Rickard et.al. 1979a). TPN
provided at a kilocalorie intake of 100% of the RDA and
2.5-3 g/dl amino acids effectively restored muscle and
fat reserves, increased serum albumin and transferrin to
normal concentrations, and, in most patients, reversed
anergy to recall skin test antigens. A shorter period
of TPN (9-14 days) did not restore an appropriate weight
for height, fat reserves nor albumin concentrations;
however, transferrin concentrations were normalized
relatively early (9-14 days) and quality of life was
improved.

     Theoretically, the administration of high
concentrations of glucose through the peripheral veins
poses more technical problems because of the local
trauma to the blood vessel, whereas the central line of
administration allows provision of greater
concentrations of glucose. Recently, we have been
evaluating the effectiveness of parenteral nutrition
provided by either central or peripheral veins. In our
preliminary evaluation of 19 children with advanced
neuroblastoma or Wilms' tumors, we found that both
routes of administration were effective in reversing PEM
when adequate energy and protein was provided over a 21
to 28 day period (Rickard, unpublished data). Although
anthropometric assessments were similar for the two
study groups, serum transferrin concentrations were

lower in the patients who received partial parenteral nutrition (PPN) with enteral nutrition compared to those who received central administration of nutrients (TPN). However, albumin concentrations were indistinguishable. Both groups experienced an equally high incidence of anemia, fever episodes without documented sepsis, and elevated liver enzyme concentrations; however, the PPN group had a significantly higher incidence of line changes associated with peripheral infiltrations and related psychologic trauma. The effectiveness of PPN was dependent upon an adequate enteral intake which provided additional energy (and other nutrients) to meet the Recommended Dietary Allowances. Even with an apparently adequate energy and protein intake when compared to healthy children, transferrin concentration was not normalized in half the PPN patients.

A summary of the indications and potential benefits as well as potential risks are provided in Table 3.

Table 3  Indications, potential benefits and risks associated with enteral and parenteral nutrition provided to children with cancer.

| | Indications | Benefits | Risks |
|---|---|---|---|
| Enteral Nutrition | Stages I/II tumors Acute lymphocytic Stages III/IV tumors in late maintenance phase of therapy and in remission | Ambulatory Psychologically more appealing More normal play and lifestyle Lower infection risks from catheter | PEM with all associated consequences |
| Parenteral Nutrition | Stages III/IV at diagnosis and during induction therapy Nourished patients with cancer who become malnourished on enteral therapy during induction therapy Acute non-lymphocytic Brain tumors during and after intense therapy | Effective in preventing and reversing PEM during intense treatment Restoration of immune competence Ability to tolerate more treatment Potential for improved tumor response | Catheter complications, e.g. sepsis Pulmonary emboli Anemia Fever |

Bray GA, Greenway FL, Molitch ME, Dahms WT, Atkinson RL, Hamilton K (1978). Use of anthropometric measures to assess weight loss. Am J Clin Nutr 31:769.

Brozek J (1974). From a QUAC stick to a compositional assessment of man's nutritional status. Adv Exp Med Biol 49:151.

Copeland EM, MacFadyen BV, Dudrick FJ (1976). Effect of intravenous hyperalimentation on established delayed hypersensitivity in the cancer patient. Ann Surg 184:60.

Detamore CM (1980). "Nutrition Regimens For Children With Advanced Neuroblastoma." M.S. Thesis, Indianapolis: Indiana University School of Medicine, p 86.

DeWys WD, Begg C, Lavin P, Band P, Bennett J, Bertino J, Cohen M, Douglas H, Engstrom P, Ezdinli E, Horton J, Johnson G, Moertel C, Oken M, Perlia C, Rosenbaum C, Silverstein M, Skeel R, Sponzo R,Tormey D. (1980). Prognostic effect of weight loss prior to chemotherapy in cancer patients. Am J Med 69:491.

Fomon SJ, Filer LJ, Ziegler EE, Bergmann KE, Bergmann RL, (1977). Skim milk in infant feeding. Acta Pediatr Scan 66:17.

Keys A, Brozek J, Henschel A, Mickelsen O, Taylor HL (1950): "The Biology of Human Starvation. Vol II," Minneapolis: The University of Minnesota Press.

Meakins JL, Pietsch JB, Bubenick O, Kelly R, Rode H, Gordon L, MacLean D (1977). Delayed hypersensitivity: Indicator of acquired failure of host defenses in sepsis and trauma. Ann Surg 186:241.

Rickard KA, Grosfeld JL, Kirksey A, Ballantine TVN, Baehner RL (1979a). Reversal of protein-energy malnutrition in children during treatment of advanced neoplastic disease. 190:771.

Rickard KA, Matchett M, Ballantine TVN, Kirksey A, Grosfeld JL, Baehner RL (1979b). Serum transferrin: An early indicator of nutritional status in children with advanced cancer. Surg Forum 30:78.

Rickard KA, Baehner RL, Provisor AJ, Weetman RM, Grosfeld JL (1980a). The effects of hyperalimentation on immune function and tumor growth. In White P (ed): "Nutrition in the 80's," New York: Alan R. Liss, p 339.

Rickard KA, Kirksey A, Bachner RL, Provisor A, Weetman R, Ballantine TVN, Grosfeld JL (1980b). Effectiveness of enteral and parenteral nutrition in the nutritional management of childrens with Wilms' tumors. Am J Clin Nutr 33:2622.

Rickard KA, Baehner RL, Coates TD, Weetman RM, Provisor AJ, Grosfeld JL (1982). Pediatric cancer: Supportive nutritional intervention. Cancer Res Supp 42:766s.

Rickard KA, Detamore CM, Coates TD, Grosfeld JL, Weetman RM, White NM, Provisor AJ, Boxer JL, Loghmani ES, Oei TO, Yu P, Baehner RL. Effect of nutrition staging on treatment delays and outcome in stage IV neuroblastoma. Cancer (In press)

Rolley RT, Widman D, Sterioff S, Williams GM (1977). Immunological monitoring of human transplant recipients with recall antigen skin tests. Surg Forum 38:314.

Smith R (1960). Total body water in malnourished infants. Clin Sci 19:275.

Trevorrow VE (1970). Serum protein. In McCammon A (ed): "Human Growth and Development," Springfield, Illinois: Charles D. Thomas, p 235.

vanEys J (1982). Pediatric cancer: Effects of nutritional status on response to therapy. Cancer Res Supp 42:747s.

Waterlow JC (1975). Adaptation to low-protein intakes. In Olson RE (ed): "Protein-Calorie Malnutrition," New York: Academic Press, p 23.

CONGRESS SYMPOSIA

HYPERTHERMIA Streffer, C., FRG, Chairman;
Dewey, W., USA, Co-Chairman; Rainier Room

Deep Heating Techniques Designed for Hyperthermia
Treatments. *Hunt, J. W., Toronto, Ontario,
Canada. (By Title Only)

The Biological Bases for Hyperthermia.
*Field, S. B., London, England.

The Biological Bases for the Clinical Application
of Hyperthermia as an Adjuvant to Radiotherapy.
*Overgaard, J., Aarhus, Denmark.

Clinical Exploitation of Biological Phenomena
in Combined Radiotherapy (RT) and Local
Hyperthermia (HT). *Arcangeli, G., Rome, Italy.

Impact of Microcirculation and Physiologic
Considerations on Clinical Hyperthermia.
*Bicher, H. I., Van Nuys, CA USA.

Please note: Papers that are listed as "By Title
Only" were presented at the 13th International
Cancer Congress, but are not included in these
volumes.

13th International Cancer Congress, Part D
Research and Treatment, pages 195–204
© 1983 Alan R. Liss, Inc., 150 Fifth Avenue, New York, NY 10011

THE BIOLOGICAL BASES FOR HYPERTHERMIA

S.B. FIELD

MRC CYCLOTRON UNIT
HAMMERSMITH HOSPITAL
LONDON W12 OHS

The disappearance of tumour after high fever was first reported more than a century ago (Busch 1866). Early studies such as these and many others gave sufficient encouragement for methods of local heating to be sought. However the techniques are difficult and interest in the possibility of hyperthermic treatment faded. In the 1960s a firm rationale for using hyperthermia in cancer therapy was developed and this in turn has stimulated further technical achievements, so that cancer therapy by hyperthermia has now become a field of considerable interest.

The present paper will consider the rationale for the use of hyperthermia, biological responses to heat alone or in combination with x rays and some aspects of thermotolerance. The emphasis will be on effects on animals since these may be expected to relate to man although differences may also be anticipated.

Rationale for Clinical Use of Hyperthermia

(1) Because of their more sluggish blood supply some tumours may become hotter than normal tissues in a localised treatment field. There is evidence in man to support this but the extent to which a temperature differential may occur will vary from tumour to tumour and also during the course of a fractionated hyperthermia treatment.
(2) Some neoplastic cells may be intrinsically more sensitive than the normal cells at risk. However this possibility remains the subject of some discussion.

(3)   Tumours may contain cells which are
(a)   hypoxic, which in contrast to x rays seems not to
markedly affect their response to hyperthermia;
(b)   at low pH and nutrient-deficient, both making cells more
sensitive to heat.
(4)   Cells in the DNA synthetic phase are particular sensitive to heat when they are relatively resistant to x rays,
so that a combined treatment with hyperthermia and radiotherapy might be an advantage in some circumstances.
(5)   Combining heat with chemotherapeutic drugs may enhance
the therapeutic effect either by increasing drug uptake or
enhancing sensitivity to the drugs.
     Evidence for these statements is derived from experi-
mental work on cells in vitro and both normal and malignant
tissues in situ (see Field and Bleehen, 1979 for a review).

     On the basis of the above rationale there are many pro-
blems which urgently need to be solved in order that hyperthermia may be used in a rational way.   Clearly an understanding of how normal tissues and tumours respond to hyperthermia given alone or in combination with other modalities
is urgently needed.   Ultimately this must be based on knowledge of the basic mechanisms involved in heat damage and
also in the interaction of hyperthermia with other modalities.

     The effects of heat alone are different from heat used
as a potentiator of other anti-cancer modalities.   Whereas
x rays cause cells to lose reproductive integrity which in
general becomes manifest at mitosis, hyperthermia may cause
immediate cell death and lysis.   Rapid destruction of the
vasculature may result from heating with tissue necrosis
following.   It is therefore important to distinguish between
damage by x rays and hyperthermia and new endpoints are needed
to study the latter.   This is particularly difficult with
cells in vitro and with tumours in vivo because in these
cases the endpoints are a direct result of cell killing,
with no account of the mode of cell death.   The problem is
far less difficult with normal tissues.   Use may be made of
qualitative and temporal differences in response to the
different modalities.   Skin, for example, shows radiation
damage as radio-dermatitis.   The injury is enhanced by moderate hyperthermia but remains qualitatively similar to the
radiation response.   In contrast severe hyperthermia alone
causes rapid tissue necrosis (Law et al, 1978).   The same
is true for intestine in which hyperthermia causes almost
immediate injury to the villi, which being composed of post

mitotic cells are unaffected by x rays (Hume and Marigold 1981). The distinction has also been demonstrated with cartilage (Morris et al, 1977). Thus with normal tissues it is possible to separate the effects of heat and radiation and to study the two separately.

Effects of heat alone

With cells in vitro hyperthermia may be used to produce survival curves which are analogous to those after radiation (Westra and Dewey, 1971). With tissues, however, once the threshold for injury is reached a small increase in hyperthermal treatment (either an increased temperature or longer time of heating) will cause a dramatic increase in the probability of tissue necrosis (Mortiz and Henriques, 1947). It is found that an increase of only approximately 20% in heating time or less than 0.5°C may increase the probability of necrosis from 0 to 100%, (Morris et al, 1977). Clearly very careful control of heat delivery and accurate thermometry is required in clinical practice.

It is important to know the relationship between temperature and treatment time required to produce a given level of tissue injury. Fig.1 shows an analysis for a range of tissues and tumours in vivo.

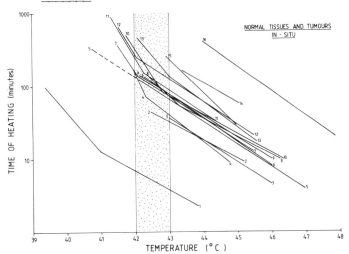

Fig.1. Relationship between heating time and temperature for a given effect on a range of normal tissues and tumours.

It is seen that for temperatures above 43$^O$C a change of 1$^O$C
is equivalent to a change in heating time by a factor of 2,
a value which has consistently been observed in vivo and in
vitro in a wide range of experimental circumstances.    In most
cases the relationship is different for temperatures below
42$^O$C.    In this case    1$^O$C is approximately equivalent to
changing the heating time by a factor of 6.    The change occurs
between 42$^O$C and 43$^O$C but within these limits is variable from
tissue to tissue.    Absolute sensitivity is extremely tissue
dependent covering a factor of 200 in heating times.    The
most sensitive is testis; a whole range of tissues in rodents
lie within a broad band; necrosis of pig and human skin has
been found to be the most resistant.    However with any one
tissue it is possible to relate hyperthermic treatments at
different temperatures using the above relationships.    For
example, if the "break point" is at 42.5$^O$C, 1 hour at 44$^O$C
is equivalent to 14 hours at 42$^O$C or 3½ days at 41$^O$C.

## Interaction between hypthermia and radiation

When radiation is combined with a mild heat treatment
which alone does not cause any visible damage, then the response to radiation may be enhanced.    Table 1 summarises the
ways in which radiation responses are influenced by heating.

TABLE I.

### Influence of hyperthermia on radiation effects

1.   Increases sensitivity to x rays i.e. causes a decrease
     in D$_O$.
2.   Causes a reduction in the capacity for:
       (a)    repair of sublethal damage
       (b)    repair of potentially lethal damage
3.   Selectively enhances effects on the cells in radio-
     resistant phases of the cell cycle e.g. (late S).

The tissue response after combined treatment is normally
qualitatively identical with the radiation response.    It is
therefore possible to compute a thermal enhancement ratio
(TER), namely the ratio of dosages of radiation alone to that
with hyperthermia to produce a given level of damage.    TER
values have been measured for a range of normal tissues in
different laboratories.    It is generally found that for a 1
hour treatment the TER is slightly greater than unity for
41$^O$C, increasing to approximately three by 43$^O$C.    However,
when the results for normal tissues are compared with values

for experimental tumours there does not appear to be a consistently higher thermal enhancement ratio for tumours than for normal tissues (Field et al, 1980). It is important, therefore, to examine whether the rationale for using hyperthermia alone also applies to hyperthermia used to enhance the effect of x rays. It was initially thought that hyperthermia caused a reduction in the oxygen enhancement ratio for x rays but now there is considerable evidence that the ratio is not modified (see Field and Bleehen, 1979). Also whereas pH has a marked effect on direct cell killing, a reduction to pH 6.7 caused no change in the TER (Lunec and Parker, 1980). Other factors have not yet been studied. Table 2 summarises these rationable both for enhancement of radiation damage and for direct thermal injury.

TABLE 2.

Possible reasons for using combinations of hyperthermia and radiation

|  | Enhancement of radiation damage | Direct thermal injury |
|---|---|---|
| Selective heating of Tumours | YES | YES |
| Tumour cells intrinsically more sensitive | ? | DATA CONFLICTING |
| Tumours contain cells at low pH | NO | YES |
| Some tumour cells may be deficient of nutrients | ? | YES |
| Some tumour cells may be hypoxic | NO | YES |

It is seen that if there is selective tumour heating either modality will be clinically useful but the physiological basis for using hyperthermia alone is not generally applicable for heat when used to enhance the effects of x rays.

An important question is whether a combination of hyperthermia and radiation may be found which will give a therapeutic advantage. It is well known that the maximum thermal enhancement ratio is obtained when heat and radiation are given simultaneously. When the two modalities are separated

in time the interaction fades. For hyperthermia given after
irradiation the interaction appears to be reduced to zero
by approximately four hours, when the two modalities appear
to act independently. However, for a number of experimental
tumours it is found that the combination of radiation followed
by hyperthermia four hours later yields a positive thermal
enhancement ratio so that such a combined treatment is more
effective on the tumour than on normal tissues (Field et al,
1980; Overgaard, 1982). The reason for the difference in
response between tumour and normal tissue is believed to be
due to a greater degree of direct damage in the tumour by
virtue of its different environment compared with normal
tissues (Overgaard, 1977).

Thermotolerance

It has been known for a very long time that hyperthermia
renders cells or tissues resistant to a subsequent treatment
with hyperthermia. There are several forms of thermal tolerance which apply either to heat alone, to heat interaction
with radiation or with chemotherapy (Henle and Dethlefsen,
1978; Field and Anderson, 1982). (Table 3). Thermotolerance may be assessed in several different ways.

TABLE 3.

Forms of Thermotolerance

1. Resistance developing during a prolonged heat treatment, usually at temperatures less than approximately
   43°C.
2. Resistance following an acute heat treatment.
3. A reduction in the effect of hyperthermia as a
   radiation sensitizer (i.e. a reduction in the TER).
4. A reduction in the ability of heat to interact with
   themotherapeutic agents.

For example, an acute heat treatment followed later by a test
dose has been used to derive a change in "slope ratio" in
tumours and in normal tissues (Urano et al, 1982; Kamura et
al, 1982; Wheldon et al, 1982) whereas Law et al, 1979 have
simply measured the duration of a test treatment after various
priming doses. It is not quite clear how these may be related,
especially since the slope ratio methods assume that accepted
radiobiological considerations apply to hyperthermia, which
may not be true, especially for normal tissue endpoints.
Further discussion is beyond the scope of this paper. However,

despite the difficulties there are general features.  In
general the peak of tolerance in vivo is reached some time
between one half and two days after hyperthermia.  This is
in marked contrast with the majority of cells in vitro where
the peak of thermal tolerance appears very much earlier.
The maximum extent of thermal tolerance in tissues is such
that a second treatment must be increased by a factor of
between 2 and 5 to overcome the effect.  This is equivalent
to having to increase the temperature of a second treatment
by between 1$^{O}$C and 2$^{O}$C.  The decay of thermotolerance is
relatively slow and is not always complete even by one week.

It is clearly important to study thermal tolerance when
more than a single treatment is given.  In a study using
necrosis of the ear of the mouse it was shown that a test heat
treatment remains the same, independent of the number of prior
treatments up to ten (Law et al, 1983).  Clearly this result
has important implications for fractionated hyperthermia
treatments.

It has been suggested that owing to low pH, thermotolerance may be less in tumours than in normal tissues.  Results
for thermal tolerance in experimental tumours are limited
(Maher et al, 1981; Kamura et al, 1982; Wheldon et al, 1982).
It is clear, however, that thermal tolerance does occur in
tumours and that at the present stage it is difficult to indicate ways in which the phenomenon may be used to clinical
advantage.  Two studies have been made of the therapeutic
ratio (experimental tumour to skin injury) for up to 10 daily
treatments (Overgaard et al, 1980; Urano et al, 1982).  In
general it was found that the "sparing" due to fractionation
of hyperthermia was far greater than for x rays, the effect
being attributed to thermal tolerance.  Although not statistically significant there was a relative therapeutica advantage in multifraction, possibly due to less thermal tolerance
in the tumours.

There is also thermal tolerance for the interaction of
hyperthermia and radiation and this is manifest by a reduction in the thermal enhancement ratio.  It has been shown in
skin that for heat given approximately before x rays a thermal
enhancement ratio of approximately 3 is reduced to about 2 for
ten fractions (Law, 1979).  Effects such as this make it
difficult to compute the thermal enhancement ratio for many
small doses of combined heat and radiation.

## Hyperthermia given at long times after radiotherapy

At the present time hyperthermia will mainly be given
to patients with recurrent tumours after conventional treatment.  It is therefore important to test the heat sensitivity
of tissues at long times after radiotherapy.  This has been
done in the mouse using skin and intestine.  With the intestine a phase of enhanced sensitivity was observed a few days
after radiation therapy, the tissues ultimately returning to
normal sensitivity (Hume and Marigold, 1982).  With skin,
however, the sensitivity increased some days after irradiation
reaching a maximum by 3 months with no indication of a return
to normal (Law and Ahier, 1982).  Clearly it is important to
be aware of the possibility that after radiotherapy some
tissues may be more sensitive to subsequent hyperthermia and
there is at least one clinical report to that effect (Douglas
et al, 1981).

## Conclusions

There are excellent reasons for using hyperthermia in the
treatment of cancer and we are beginning to obtain adequate
knowledge to use it safely and sensibly.  Many centres all
over the world are now using hyperthermia in different ways
and so far there is general optimism about the results.
Clearly an important question is how to design an optimal
treatment.  Our knowledge in this field is progressing but
is still seriously limited and much more information is
required before hyperthermia treatment may be planned on a
rational basis.

Busch W (1866). Uber den Einfluss welchen Heftigere
   Erysipeln Zuweilen auf Organisierte Neubildungen Ausuben.
   Verhandl Naturh Preuss Rhein Westphal 23:28.
Douglas MA, Parks LC, Bebin J (1981). Sudden myelopathy
   secondary to therapeutic total-body hyperthermia after
   spinal-cord irradiation. New England J of Medicine 10:583.
Field SB, Bleehen NM (1979). Hyperthermia in the treatment of
   cancer.  Cancer Treatment Reviews 6:63.
Field SB, Hume SP, Law MP (1980).  The response of tissues to
   heat alone or in combination with radiation.  Proc.of 6th
   Congress of Radiat.Res. Tokyo 1979. Eds.Okada, Imamura,
   Terasima and Yamaguchi. Japanese Ass. of Radiation Research
   pp 847.
Field SB, Anderson RL (1982). Thermotolerance: a review of
   observations and possible mechanisms. J Nat Cancer Inst.

Henle KJ, Dethlefsen LA (1978). Heat fractionation and thermotolerance: a review. Cancer Research 38:1843.

Hume SP, Marigold JCL (1981). The response of mouse intestine to combined hyperthermia and radiation: the contribution of direct thermal damage in assessment of the thermal enhancement ratio. International J Radiat Biol 39:347.

Hume SP, Marigold JCL (1982). Increased hyperthermal response of previously irradiated mouse intestine. Brit J Radiol 55:438.

Kamura T, Nielsen OS, Overgaard J, Andersen AH (1982). Development of thermotolerance during fractionated hyperthermia in a solid tumor in vivo. Cancer Res 42:1744.

Law MP, Ahier RG, Field SB (1978). The response of the mouse ear to heat applied alone or combined with x rays. Brit J Radiol 51:132.

Law MP (1979). Some effects of fractionation on the response of the mouse ear to combined heat and X rays. Radiat Res 80:360.

Law MP, Coultas PC, Field SB (1979). Induced thermal tolerance in the mouse ear. Brit J Radiol 52:308.

Law MP, Ahier RG (1982). Long-term thermal sensitivity of previously irradiated skin. Brit J Radiol (in press).

Law MP, Ahier RG, Somaia S, Field SB (1983). The induction of thermal resistance by fractionated hyperthermia in the ear of the mouse. Submitted to Int J Rad Onc Biol Phys.

Lunec J, Parker R (1980). The influence of pH on the enhancement of radiation damage by hyperthermia. Int J Radiat Biol 38:567.

Maher J, Urano M, Rice L, Suit HD (1981). Thermal resistance in a spontaneous murine tumour. Brit J Radiol 54:1086.

Moritz AR, Henriques FC (1947). Studies of thermal injury. II. The relative importance of time and surface temperature in the causation of cutaneous burns. Amer J Path 23:695.

Morris CC, Myers R, Field SB (1977). The response of the rat tail to hyperthermia. Brit J Radiol 50:576.

Overgaard J (1977). The effect of sequence and time intervals of combined hyperthermia and radiation treatment of a solid mouse mammary adenocarcinoma in vivo. Brit J Radiol 50:763.

Overgaard J (1982). Hyperthermic modification of the radiation response in solid tumours. Proc. 2nd Rome International Symposium "Biological Bases and Clinical Implications of Tumor Radioresistance". Raven Press (in press).

Overgaard J, Suit HD, Walker AM (1980). Multifractionated hyperthermia treatment of malignant and normal tissue in vivo. Cancer Res 40:2045.

Urano M, Rice LC, Montoya V (1982). Studies on fractionated hyperthermia in experimental animal systems. II. Response of mouse tumours to two or more doses. Int J Radiat Res 8:227.

Westra A, Dewey WC (1971). Variation in sensitivity to heat shock during the cell-cycle of Chinese hamster cells in vitro. Int J Radiat Biol 19:467.

Wheldon TE, Hingston EC, Ledda JL (1982). Hyperthermia response and thermotolerance capacity of an experimental rat tumour. Europ J Cancer Clin Oncol (in press).

13th International Cancer Congress, Part D
Research and Treatment, pages 205–216
© 1983 Alan R. Liss, Inc., 150 Fifth Avenue, New York, NY 10011

THE BIOLOGICAL BASES FOR THE CLINICAL APPLICATION OF HYPER-
THERMIA AS AN ADJUVANT TO RADIOTHERAPY

Jens Overgaard, M.D.

The Institute of Cancer Research, Radiumstationen
Nörrebrogade 44, DK-8000   Aarhus C
Denmark

Abundant experimental and early clinical experience
indicate that local hyperthermia has a potential of being
a useful adjuvant to radiotherapy in the treatment of solid
tumours (Dewey et al. 1980, Field & Bleehen 1979, Overgaard
1978, 1982b, Suit & Gerweck 1979). The biological rationale
for this combined therapy has been extensively studied in
experimental models (Field & Bleehen 1979, Overgaard 1980,
1982a), and has created a basis for clinical application
of the two modalities. In the following a series of experiments performed in C3H mammary carcinoma and its surrounding normal skin will be discussed in order to ease the understanding of the biological rationale. However, it should
be noted that there is a general consistency in different
experimental data, and a wider insight into the litterature
can be achieved from several recent reviews (Dethlefsen &
Dewey 1982, Dewey et al. 1980, Field & Bleehen 1979, Overgaard 1982b, Suit & Gerweck 1979).

TYPES OF INTERACTION BETWEEN HEAT AND RADIATION

The biological interaction between heat and radiation
consists at least of two principal different types of interaction (Dewey et al. 1980, Field & Bleehen 1979, Overgaard
1977, 1978, 1980, 1982a, 1982b, Suit & Gerweck 1979).

Firstly, heat has a direct cytotoxic effect. Although
the heat sensitivity varies among the different cells and
tissues, the intrinsic heat sensitivity does not seem to be
higher in malignant cells than in their normal counterparts.
Nevertheless, heat has been able to control experimental
tumours with an acceptable degree of normal tissue damage.

This is because the hyperthermic cytotoxicity is strongly
enhanced by certain environmental conditions, and cells in
areas characterized by nutritional deprivation, chronic
hypoxia and increased acidity, which are typical of the
poorly vascularized parts of solid tumours, are considerably
more heat sensitive than cells in a normal environment. Thus,
a moderate heat treatment, which can be tolerated by well-
vascularized normal tissues, is found to destroy a large
proportion of the cells in many solid tumours. Furthermore, heat itself may enhance such environmental conditions
in tumours by reducing the blood flow. That such heat sensitive chronically hypoxic cells are also the most radioresistant may indirectly influence the response to a combined heat and radiation treatment, since a smaller radiation dose may be adequate to control the remaining oxygenated
cells. Indeed, there is evidence from recent studies that the
number of clonogenic hypoxic cells in a solid tumour can be
markedly reduced after moderate heat treatment which itself
does not induce any severe damage to normal tissue (Overgaard
1981a, Song et al. 1982).

Secondly, hyperthermia has a radiosensitizing effect.
Thus, heating concomitant with radiation result in a direct
radiosensitization, a decreased repair of sublethal and
potential lethal radiation damage, and an enhanced killing
of cells in relatively radioresistant phases of the cell
cycle. However, the oxygen enhancement ratio seems to be
decreased by the combined treatment. The hyperthermic radiosensitization seems neither to be qualitatively nor quanti-
tatively different in malignant and benign  tissues.

THE INFLUENCE OF SEQUENCE AND INTERVAL

Experimental studies on the influence of sequence and
interval  between hyperthermia and radiation indicate that
maximal thermal enhancement occurs with a simultaneous application of heat and radiation (Field & Bleehen 1979, Overgaard
1980, 1982a). This is probably a consequence of the hyperthermic radiosensitization, which is found to be most prominent
with  simultaneous application, and any separation between
the two modalities decreases the radiosensitizing effect
which  completely disappears with intervals longer than 3 to
4 hours (fig. 1).  Unfortunately, simultaneous treatment
gives approximately the same enhancement in tumour and normal
tissue, and will therefore not increase the therapeutic
effect unless the tumour is heated to a higher extent than

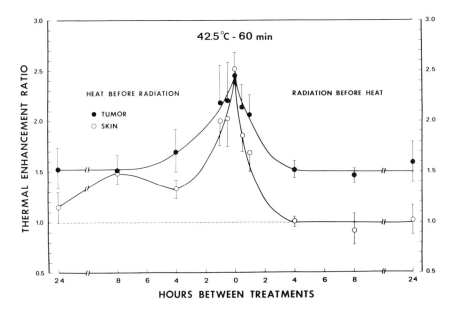

Fig. 1 Thermal enhancement ratio as a function of time interval and sequence between hyperthermia and radiation treatments of a mammary carcinoma and its surrounding skin.

the surrounding tissue. In the normal tissue, sequential treatment with heat given before radiation causes a higher and longer thermal enhancement than with the opposite sequence, where the thermal enhancement in general disappears with intervals greater than 4 hours (Fig. 1) (Field & Bleehen 1979, Overgaard 1982a). However, in most solid tumours, a moderate thermal enhancement persists even with long intervals between the modalities and independent of sequence, a phenomenon which probably is a consequence of the before-mentioned selectively hyperthermic destruction of acidic and chronically hypoxic tumour cells.

Both the hyperthermic radiosensitization and the cytotoxic effect against radioresistant cells increase with increasing heat damage (i.e. combination of temperature and heating time). As seen in figure 2 there is a steep increase in the thermal enhancement ratio (TER) with increasing temperature at a given heating time, but to the same extent in

Fig. 2
Thermal enhancement ratio
after simultaneous or se-
quential treatment at
various temperatures.
Data from Overgaard 1980.

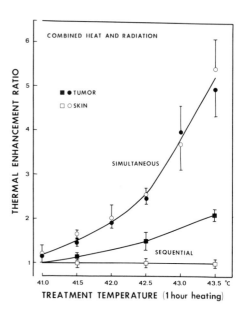

tumour and normal tissue. The enhancement after sequential
treatment, where heat is given four hours after radiation,
is smaller, but occurs only in the tumour, whereas no enhancement is present in the normal tissue.

   Not only do the hyperthermic radiosensitization and
the cytotoxic effect differ with regard to magnitude of the
thermal enhancement in tumours, but also the time-temperature relationship to achieve a given level of thermal enhancement is different (fig. 3). Thus, by simultaneous treatment the radiosensitizing effect shows a time-temperature
relationship in a modified Arrhenius plot corresponding to
839 kJ/mole over the temperature range 41.5 - 43.5° C,
whereas a sequential treatment (the cytotoxic effect) shows
a different time-temperature pattern. At temperatures below
43.0° C there is a steep time-temperature relationship corresponding to 1,210 kJ/mole, whereas at higher temperatures
the relation is less steep with an inactivation energy of
550 kJ/mole. This latter biphasic pattern is similar to the
inactivation energy as observed after heat alone (Field &
Bleehen 1979, Kamura et al. 1982, Overgaard & Suit 1979),
and may give further evidence for the hypothesis that the
effect of sequential radiation and heat is due to an additive effect of the two modalities.

Fig. 3
Time-temperature relationship to produce a TER of 2
with either simultaneous
or sequential treatment
of C3H mammary carcinoma
in vivo.

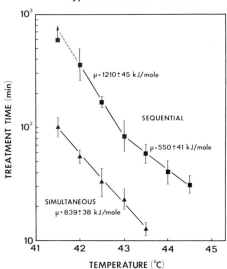

## FRACTIONATED TREATMENT

The clinical application of combined heat and radiation treatment is naturally most likely to be given in fractionated schedules. Unfortunately, there is relativly sparse experimental information about such treatment principles, but it has become evident that fractionated heat treatment alone possesses a potentially very important problem. This is due to the phenomenon known as thermal tolerance (i.e. temporary heat resistance following a prior heat treatment). Recently, this phenomenon has drawn significant attention, since it has become apparent that thermotolerance seems to be a general phenomenon occuring in all normal tissues and tumours studied so far (Field & Anderson 1982). Furthermore, thermotolerance has been found to influence the effect of combined heat and radiation given either simultaneously or sequentially (Nielsen et al. 1982), and that is probably the reason why the few experimental data on fractionated heat and radiation in vivo have given somewhat conflicting data (Overgaard 1982b).

The influence of thermotolerance on the interaction between heat and radiation is most pronounced when radiation and heat is given sequentially (i.e. heat 4 hours after

Fig. 4
Effect of intervals be-
tween fractions on the
tumour growth time (time
to 5 times increase of
tumour volume). The mammary carcinoma was treated
as described by Kamura
et al. 1982.

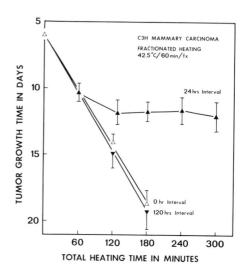

radiation). With such a schedule, where hyperthermia interact with  radiation due to its direct cytotoxic effect against
the radioresistant tumour cells, thermotolerance is expressed
to the same degree after heat alone. Thus, if the intervals
between fractions are such that significant thermotolerance
is present, very long heating times are required to increase
the thermal destruction after heat alone when compared to
the effect of a single fraction (Kamura et al. 1982, Nielsen
& Overgaard 1982). This is illustrated in figure 4, which
shows that in a C3H mammary tumour given 5 fractions of 60
min. at 42.5° C with intervals of 24 hours (i.e. the time
for development of near maximal thermotolerance in this
tumour after such heating) the result  of 5 heat treatments
is not significantly better, than that achieved by a single
fraction. Similarly, daily fractionation with sequentially
combined radiation and heat (42.5° C/ 60 min) does not result
in an improvement of the tumour TER when compared with single
treatment (fig. 5). However, if the intervals between the
fractions are extended to allow the thermotolerance to disappear (in the present example more than 5 days) both the
effect of  heat alone (fig. 4) and the thermal enhancement
with the sequential heat and radiation treatment improves
significantly over that achieved with single-dose (fig. 5).
Thus, with combined sequential heat and radiation treatment
the TER is almost doubled after 5 fractions with 5 days

Fig. 5
Effect of intervals be-
tween fractions on the
thermal enhancement
ratio after treatment
with:
(upper panel):
simultaneous radiation
and heat;
(lower panel):
sequential radiation
and heat.
Principles of experimen-
tal design as described
by Overgaard 1980, 1981b.

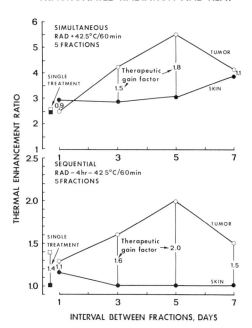

**FRACTIONATED RADIATION AND HEAT**

interval when compared to single dose treatment, or treatment with 5 fractions in 4 days. However, further spacing
between the fractions is likely to reduce the tumour TER
again, but now because the interval has become so long that
the tumour may grow in the interval between the fractions.
Thus, the optimal spacing between fractions seems to be extremely critical for the outcome of the treatment.

A similar effect is seen with simultaneous radiation
and heat treatment (fig. 5). Also here does daily fractionation with 42.5° C for 60 min produce almost the same thermal
enhancement ratio as that found after single dose treatment.
Increasing the fractionation interval to 5 days results in
a TER of 5.5 compared to the 2.5 achieved after single dose
treatment or with 5 fractions in 4 days. Again the spacing
seems to be very important, and an additional increase of
the interval does also after simultaneous treatment tend
to reduce the thermal enhancement due to tumour growth
between fractions. However, in contrast to all previous

studies where simultaneous treatments have shown the same
response in both normal tissue and tumour, the normal tissue
seems to respond differently in the fractionated treatment
schedules depending on the fractionation interval. Thus, in
the present study the skin seems to be less influenced by
the fractionation interval, probably because there is a
different kinetic for the development and decay of thermotolerance between the C3H tumours and the surrounding skin.
In fact, a therapeutic gain with a maximum of 1.8 was achieved
with a 5 days interval, although the same heat treatment was
given to both tumour and the surrounding normal tissue.

It has been questioned whether the kinetic for development and decay of thermotolerance and for the influence of
thermotolerance on the combined heat and radiation treatment follow the same pattern (Law et al. 1979a). This seems
to be the case in the present experiments. Thus, fig. 6
shows that the influence of thermotolerance on the simultaneous treatment with heat and radiation follow the same time
course as the effect of thermotolerance after heat treatment
alone. The same is obviously also the situation when sequential treatment is given.

Fig. 6
Time course of resistan-
ce in a mammary carcino-
ma exposed to heat alone
(43.5° C) and to simulta-
neous heat and radiation
(15 Gy and 43.5° C/ 60
min) induced at various
intervals after prior
heating at 43.5° C/ 30
min. Data as described
by Nielsen & Overgaard
1982.

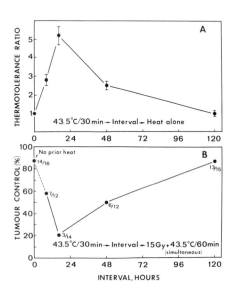

It shall be stressed that the intervals given here only apply to the specific tumour treated at a temperature of 42.5° C for 60 min or with a similar heat treatment resulting in the same hyperthermic damage (Nielsen & Overgaard 1982). Thus,the quantitative magnitude of the shown data may not be general for all the models or clinical situations, but will only tend to illustrate  the enourmous problems related to thermotolerance.

Since thermotolerance reduces both the hyperthermic radiosensitization and the effect of heat when given sequentially with radiation thermotolerance should be avoided in the tumour if maximal interaction is wanted. On the other hand, it would be a preferable situation in normal tissues in order to reduce the amount of damage. Unfortunately, there is a considerable variation in the kinetics and the development of thermotolerance between different tissues (Field & Anderson 1982, Nielsen & Overgaard 1982), and it is currently not possible to predict how thermotolerance will develop in a given tumour or normal tissue. However, both the magnitude and the kinetics of thermotolerance appeared to depend on the heat damage induced by the priming heat treatment (Law et al. 1979b, Nielsen & Overgaard 1982). Thus, in a given tissue thermotolerance will develop later, but reaches a higher maximum if the priming heat treatment is large. This means that if a homogeneous temperature cannot be applied to a given tissue, the different parts will develop thermotolerance, which follows different kinetic patterns. Thus, at the time of the subsequent heat treatment the heterogeneous heated tissue will express different heat sensitivity in different areas. This represents a very important clinical problem, and may also explain why the response to clinical fractionated hyperthermia seems to be almost the same despite different heat treatments and fractionation intervals (Overgaard 1982b).

IMPLICATIONS FOR CLINICAL TREATMENT.

The experimental studies of single dose treatments suggest that two principal different treatment schedules may be useful for clinical treatment, depending on the ability to heat the tumours selectively (Overgaard 1982a, 1982b). Assuming that such selective (or preferential) tumour heating can be obtained, the optimal therapeutic effect will be achieved by simultaneous application of heat and radiation utilizing the hyperthermic radiosensitization. With such a schedule the highest possible heat-treatment should be given, and the limitation will only be the heat damage which may be induced in critical surrounding normal tissue.

If a selective tumour heating cannot be secured, the treatment rationale must be based on a sequential application of radiation hyperthermia utilizing the hyperthermic cytotoxic destruction of chronically hypoxic radioresistant tumour cells. Such treatment should be given with a sequence where hyperthermia is applied at least 3-4 hours after radiation.With such a schedule no enhancement of the radiation response in normal tissues is expected, and an improved therapeutic gain will be the result due to the almost selective destruction of radioresistant tumour cells. The limitation of such treatment is due to the heat tolerance and the surrounding normal tissue. In practice it is likely that such treatment will yield a smaller thermal enhancement in the tumour, but a higher therapeutic effect due to the more selective treatment.

The validity of these treatment principles has been established in early clinical trials (Arcangeli et al. 1982, Overgaard 1981b, 1982b), which have demonstrated that a simultaneous treatment is likely to result in the most pronounced enhancement, but that concomitant heated normal tissue also will show an increased radiation response. The latter can however be avoided if an interval of 3-4 hours is applied between the treatments ; this is likely to result in a smaller thermal enhancement in the tumour, but as mentioned before still with a significant improvement of the therapeutic effect. The evident influence of thermotolerance on the outcome of fractionated treatment makes it impossible to create a biological rationale for a proper use of fractionated combined heat and radiation. This both because all clinical hyperthermia will result in a non-uniform heating and because there is a lack of knowledge about the kinetics and the magnitude of thermotolerance in human tumours and normal tissues. In practice, the best way to overcome the problems of thermotolerance will be a heat treatment with a single or a few but large heat fractions given with an interval which hopefully allows thermotolerance to develop and to decay before the next hyperthermic treatment is given. Since this will happen fastest in the tumour areas given the lowest heat dose a schedule with reasonably long fractionation intervals will probably tend to even the biological heat damage in tumour areas treated at different temperatures.

The tumour area which achieved the smallest heat treatment is the most critical and responsibel for the outcome of the treatment, therefore the presence of thermotolerance in the areas   exposed to    large heat treatment will be of less practical importance.

With the current lack of knowledge the best way to overcome the problems of thermal tolerance in fractionated treatments will be a heat treatment with a single or a few but large heat fractions given with an interval which allows thermal tolerance to develop and decay before the next hyperthermic treatment is given. The use of multiple heat sessions with short intervals may be an unnecessary, costly and not beneficial treatment. Such heat treatment could be combined with conventional radiation if the sequential treatment principle is applied. With simultaneous fractio-nated heating the problem is more complex since an optimal utilisation of the radiosensitizing effect both requires a lack of thermotolerance and a concomitant heat treatment with all radiation fractions (Overgaard 1981b). Therefore in this situation also the radiation must be given with rela-tively large intervals, e.g. once or twice per week.

Evidently, thermotolerance has shown to be the most important biological parameter  of relevance for clinical application of hyperthermia as an adjuvant to radiotherapy. More insight into these problems is therefore strongly required, and further studies in this area should be given the highest priority.

Arcangeli G, Cividalli A, Lovisolo G, Nervi C (1982) Tumor control and normal tissue damage for several sche-dules of combined radiotherapy and local hyperthermia: an updated study. Strahlentherapie 158:378

Dethlefsen LA, Dewey WC (eds) Proceedings of the Third In-ternational Symposium on  Cancer Therapy by Hyperthermia, Drugs  and Radiation. Natl Cancer Inst Monogr 61 (1982)

Dewey WC, Freeman ML et al. (1980) "Cell biology of hyper-thermia and radiation", in Meyn RE, Withers HR, Radiation Biology in Cancer Research, New York, Raven Press, 589

Field SB, Bleehen NM (1979) Hyperthermia in the treatment of cancer. Cancer Treat Rev 6:63

Field SB, Anderson RL (1982) Thermotolerance: a review of observations and possible mechanisms. Natl Cancer Inst Monogr 61:193

Kamura T, Nielsen OS et al.(1982) Development of thermotolerance during fractionated hyperthermia in a solid tumor in vivo. Cancer Res 42:1744

Law MP, Ahier RG et al.(1979b) The effect of prior heat treatment on the thermal enhancement of radiation damage in the mouse ear. Brit J Radiol 52:315

Law MP, Coultas PG et al. (1979b) Induced thermal resistance in the mouse ear. Br J Radiol 52:308

Nielsen OS, Overgaard J. (1982) Importance of preheating temperature and time for the induction of thermotolerance in a solid tumour in vivo. Br J Cancer (in press)

Nielsen OS, Overgaard J et al. (1982) Influence of thermotolerance on the interaction between hyperthermia and radiation in a solid tumour in vivo. Br J. Radiol (in press)

Overgaard J. (1977) Effect of hyperthermia on malignant cells in vivo. A review and hypothesis. Cancer 37:2637

Overgaard J. (1978)"The effect of local hyperthermia alone and in combination with radiation, on solid tumors", in Streffer C et al. Cancer Therapy by Hyperthermia and Radiation, Urban and Schwarzenberg, Baltimore, Munich,49

Overgaard J. (1980) Simultaneous and sequential hyperthermia and radiation treatment of an experimental tumor and its surrounding normal tissue in vivo. Int J Radiat Oncol Biol Phys 6:1507

Overgaard J. (1981a) Effect of hyperthermia on the hypoxic fraction in an experimental mammary carcinoma in vivo. Br J Radiol 54:245

Overgaard J. (1981b) Fractionated radiation and hyperthermia. Experimental and clinical studies. Cancer 48:1116

Overgaard J. (1982a) Influence of sequence and interval on the biological response to combined hyperthermia and radiation. Natl Cancer Inst Monogr 61: 325

Overgaard J. (1982b) "Hyperthermic modification of the radiation response in solid tumors", in Fletcher GH, Nervi C. et al., Biological Bases and Clinical Implications of tumor Radioresistance. Masson Publishing USA, New York.

Overgaard J, Suit HD (1979) Time-Temperature Relationship in Hyperthermic Treatment of Malignant and Normal Tissue in Vivo. Cancer Res. 39:3248

Song WS, Rhee JG et al. (1982) Effect of hyperthermia on hypoxic cell fraction in tumor. Int J Radiat Oncol Biol Phys 8:851

Suit H, Gerweck LE (1979) Potential for hyperthermia and radiation therapy. Cancer Res 39:2290

*** 

Supported by the Danish Cancer Society (grant no. 24/79)

13th International Cancer Congress, Part D
Research and Treatment, pages 217–234
© 1983 Alan R. Liss, Inc., 150 Fifth Avenue, New York, NY 10011

CLINICAL EXPLOITATION OF BIOLOGICAL PHENOMENA IN COMBINED
RADIOTHERAPY (RT) AND LOCAL HYPERTHERMIA (HT)

Giorgio Arcangeli, M.D.,

Head, Radiation Therapy Division
Istituto Medico e di Ricerca Scientifica
00184 Rome, Italy.

The idea of improving the selective response of
malignant tumors to therapeutic treatment by means of
hyperthermia goes back to the beginning of the century
when fever was induced by bacterial toxins. But, apart
from some anecdotic clinical application of heat during
that period, only in the last few years some basic
investigations on its cytotoxic and radiosensitizing mechanism have led to a resurgence of interest in hyperthermia alone or in combination with radiotherapy as a therapeutic modality (Dewey et al., 1977; Dewey et al., 1980;
Field, Bleehen 1979; Overgaard, 1977; Overgaard, 1980a;
Suit, Gerweck, 1979). However, besides physics and technical problems, several other difficulties are encountered in the use of hyperthermia as adjuvant to
radiotherapy.


EXPERIMENTAL STUDIES

In spite of several difficulties and contradic-
tions, some measure of agreement among investigators seem-
s to emerge now on optimum treatment sequence.

Some experimental data by several authors on normal
and tumor tissues (Hill, Denekamp, 1979; Law, 1979; Law
et al., 1977; Law et al., 1979; Myers, Field 1977; Myers,

Field 1979; Overgaard 1980a ; Overgaard 1980b; Stewart, Denekamp 1977; Stewart, Denekamp 1978) are summarized and plotted in figure 1.

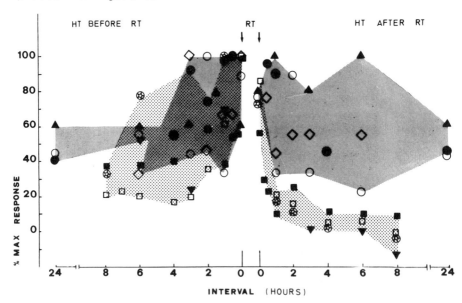

Fig. 1: The time course of the decay of heat radiosensitization in different normal and tumor tissues for hyperthermia given either before or after irradiation. Values have been normalized to the percentage of the maximum response.

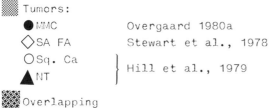

Normal tissues:

☐ Mouse ear skin, 42°C/60 min ⎤ Law, 1979
✪ Mouse ear skin, 43°C/60 min ⎦ Law et al.,1977 and 1979
▼ Mouse foot skin 42.5°C/60 min Stewart et al., 1977
■ Rat cartilage 43°C/60 min    Myers et al., 1977 and 1979.

Tumors:

● MMC        Overgaard 1980a
◇ SA FA      Stewart et al., 1978
○ Sq. Ca     ⎤ Hill et al., 1979
▲ NT         ⎦

Overlapping

With a single treatment at 42-43°C for 60 min, the maximum sensitization in several normal tissues and tumors is obtained when heat and radiation are given simultaneously or in very close sequence. The introduction of an interval between the two modalities decreases the thermal enhancement ratio (TER) to a different extent in tumors and in normal tissues (Denekamp, Stewart 1979; Fowler et al. 1975). When heat is applied after irradiation, there is a sharp separation between tumor and normal tissue TER's with increasing time, suggesting that radiation damage repair is faster in epithelial than in neoplastic cells, so the heating fixes more damage in the tumors than in the normal tissues (Denekamp, Stewart 1979; Fowler et al. 1975). When heat is given before radiation, there is a large area of overlapping between tumor and normal tissue TER's, indicating that the thermal enhancement is not only prolonged but also of the same extent in both normal and neoplastic cells.

Recent studies on mouse tumors (Overgaard 1980a) have supplied further information on optimum fractionation and sequence of hyperthermia and radiation. For instance, they showed that the simultaneous application of radiation and 42.5°C heat, resulted in TER's of similar extent in both tumors and normal tissues, so that no therapeutic gain could be obtained. The best schedule appeared to be the sequential application of the two modalities (i.e., heat delivered 4 h after radiation), each treatment being given at an interval of 72 h. With this schedule the TER's were lower in respect to the simultaneous treatment. However, the enhancement was markedly higher in tumors than in the skin, so that an appreciable therapeutic gain could be obtained.

Other biological problems in thermoradiotherapy concern the correlation of the biological effect with temperature and exposure time. It has been shown that for each degree of temperature increase above 42°C, the exposure time necessary to a complete tumor destruction can be approximately reduced by a half, and that at 50°C the same effect would be obtained by only few minutes heating (Dewey et al. 1977; Dickson 1975; Overgaard and Suit 1979).

However, at temperatures of 45°C or above, the tumor response to combined modalities could be more strictly related to the cytodestructive rather than to the radiosensitizing effect of heat. This is suggested by our

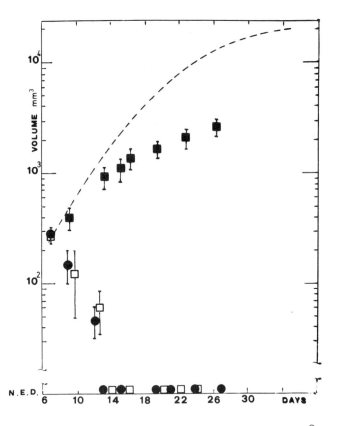

Fig. 2: Mouse fibrosarcoma of less than 600 mm$^3$ treated with hyperthermia (45 ± 0.5°C/45 min) and/or radiotherapy (3 x 10 Gy):

■ Radiotherapy alone
□ Simultaneous combined treatment
● Sequential combined treatment

experiments on a fibrosarcoma of spontaneous origin transplanted in the mouse thigh and treated with implantable
heat applicator(s) at a temperature of 45°C for 45 min (4).
In tumors of less than 600 mm, both simultaneous and
sequential combined treatment induced a tumor reduction
below palpable size during the whole period of observation, while only a small delay in tumor growth was
obtained with radiation alone (fig.2). Figure 3 shows the
response of tumors of more than 600 mm³ to radiation
alone, heat alone and to the combined (simultaneous and
sequential) treatment. Even in these tumors the response
to both simultaneous and sequential treatments appeared to
be similar, though markedly lower than that obtained in
small tumors. Furthermore, the delay slightly longer than
that induced by radiation alone or heat alone suggests

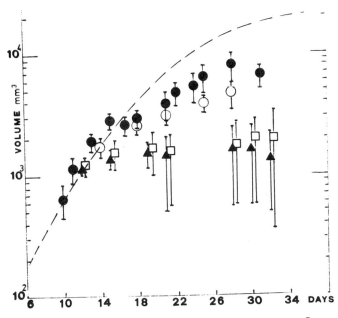

Fig. 3: Mouse fibrosarcoma of more than 600 mm³ treated
with radiotherapy (3 x 10 Gy) and hyperthermia (45 $\pm$
0.5°C/45 min):

○ Radiotherapy alone   ● Hyperthermia alone
□ Simultaneous treatment   ▲ Sequential treatment

that the response to combined treatments could be due, in this case, to an effect essentially additive.

CLINICAL APPLICATION

Most of the recent clinical studies on hyperthermia have focused on the technical problems related to heat delivery and distribution and to temperature monitoring rather than on the clinical demonstration of the potential benefit of such a treatment. Consequently, along with the fact that information on long term response of comparable lesions after single or combined modalities have been rarely reported, probably because most clinical trials have been done on very advanced lesions, the present knowledge about the potential usefulness of hyperthermia as adjuvant to radiotherapy is sparse and it deserves to be more carefully focused.

Patient Selection and Treatment Protocols

This clinical report outlines the results obtained in a series of studies in 57 patients with multiple lesions for a total of 123 lesions, treated with different schedules of fractionated hyperthermia and radiotherapy. Therefore, in each patient, a comparison of the result after single or combined modality was available.

Many of these tumors were failures to conventional treatments, including radiotherapy, and most were, generally, very advanced and/or disseminated.

During the last 5 years 3 studies have been carried out on such patients:

1. Conventional fraction size of radiation combined with moderate hyperthermia: this study was done on 26 patients with a total of 52 multiple neck node metastases from head and neck cancer. Radiation was given to the

whole neck, according to a three fractions per day scheme of 2.0+1.5+1.5 Gy/day, 4 h interval between fractions, 5 days/week (Arcangeli et al. 1980b; Arcangeli et al. 1980-c). A total dose of 60 Gy was delivered in 36 fractions in 16 days, and heat, at a temperature of 42.5°C for 45 minutes was applied, each other day, immediately after the 2nd daily fraction of irradiation, to only 1 lesion per patient, for a total of 7 heating sessions.

2. High fraction size of radiation combined with moderate hyperthermia: 16 patients with a total of 41 lesions have been accrued in this group. The lesions were melanoma recurrences of skin and lymph nodes, cutaneous chest wall recurrences from breast cancer, neck node metastases from head and neck tumors, skin and lymph node metastases from carcinoma of the vulva, skin and scalp nodules from undifferentiated tumors of the lung and of unknown origin (table 1). Radiation was given to involved areas, at a dose of 5 Gy per fraction, twice-a-week, at 72-96 h interval between fractions up to a total of 40 Gy. Heat, at a temperature of 42.5°C for 45 minutes, was applied in connection with each radiation fraction, either immediately after irradiation (simultaneous treatment) or 4 h later (sequential treatment).

TABLE 1

SITES AND HISTOLOGIES OF THE SECOND AND THIRD TRIAL

| HISTOLOGY | SITE | No. OF LESIONS |
|---|---|---|
| Squamous cell carcinoma | Head and neck, lymph nodes | 10 |
|  | Vulva, skin and lymph nodes | 6 |
| Adenocarcinoma | Breast, skin recurrences | 14 |
|  | Lung, skin and lymph nodes recurrences | 8 |
| Melanoma | Recurrences of skin and lymph nodes | 16 |
| Undifferentiated cell carcinoma | Lung, skin and scalp metastases | 12 |
|  | Unknown, skin metastases | 5 |

3. High fraction size of radiation combined with high temperature hyperthermia: 15 patients with a total of 30 lesions have been accrued in this third group. The lesions were miscellaneous but mainly similar to those of the latter group (table 1). Five fractions of 6 Gy were given, twice-a-week, 72-96 h interval, up to a total of 30 Gy, and heat, at a temperature of 45°C for 30 minutes, was applied simultaneously in connection with each radiation fraction.

Treatment Technique

Radiation was given with a 5.7 photon beam by a linear accelerator. All fields were covered with a bolus material of appropriate thickness to secure a full build up on the skin. As already pointed out, total doses ranged from 60 Gy/36 fractions/16 days to 30 Gy/5 fractions/15 days, according to the different treatment protocols.

Heat was delivered by means of various microwave or radiofrequency external applicators and the heating technique and patient set-up have been already described in previous papers (Arcangeli et al. 1980a; Arcangeli et al. 1980 b). Recently, we have used a 2450 MHz generator with newly designed contact or non-contact applicators which will be described in details elsewhere (in preparation). Only in the third trial, in which a temperature of 45°C was attempted, the normal skin surrounding the lesions was actively cooled by means of circulating cold water.

Results

The results of the first trial (conventional fraction size of radiation combined with moderate hyperthermia) are presented in table 2.

A complete response after radiation alone was obtained in 42% lesions (11/26). Addition of heat resulted in an increased degree and speed of tumor control, with 73% lesions (19/26) achieving complete regression. At 12 months, 10/14 (71%) and 5/14 (36%) lesions remained still controlled after combined or single treatment modality, respectively. The unexpected higher tumor control rates at 18 months, 4/7 (57%) and 7/7 (100%) lesions treated with the single or combined modality, respectively, is probably related to the longterm survival of those patients in whom almost all lesions, treated with different modalities, have been controlled. Because of the high death rate during follow-up, the difference between the two modalities is statistically significant ($p \leq 0.05$) only at the end of treatment.

TABLE 2

EFFECT OF MODERATE HYPERTHERMIA ON THE RESPONSE TO RADIATION AT CONVENTIONAL FRACTION SIZE (ACTUARIAL TUMOR CONTROL)

| TREAT. | COMPLETE RESPONSE | | | MOIST DESQUAM. | BLISTERS |
|---|---|---|---|---|---|
| | end RT[3] | 12 months | 18 months | | |
| RT[1] | 11/26(.42) | 5/14(.36) | 4/7(.57) | 10/26(.38) | – |
| RT+HT[2] | 19/26(.73) | 10/14(.71) | 7/7(1.0) | 11/26(.42) | 7/26(.27) |

[1] 42.5°C/45 min, each other day, immediately after the 2nd daily radiation fraction;

[2] 60 Gy/36 F/16 days (3 fractions per day);

[3] Statistical significance: $p \leq 0.05$

Addition of heat did not result in an increased skin radiation reaction: moist desquamation occurred in 38% (10/26) and in 42% (11/26) fields treated with the single and combined modality, respectively. The unexpectedly high incidence of thermal damage (7/26 blisters) occuring in these patients was related to power leakage and over heating of the applicators initially used in this study.

The results of the second trial (high fraction size of radiation combined with moderate hyperthermia) are summarized in table 3.

TABLE 3

EFFECT OF MODERATE HYPERTHERMIA ON THE RESPONSE TO
RADIATION AT HIGH FRACTION SIZE (ACTUARIAL TUMOR CONTROL)

| TREATMENT | COMPLETE RESPONSE | | MOIST | BLISTERS |
|---|---|---|---|---|
| | end RT | 6 months | DESQUAM. | |
| RT[1] | 6/16(.37) | 3/9(.33) | 5/14(.36) | – |
| RT+HT[2] (simul.) | 10/13(.77) | 5/7(.71) | 9/14(.64) | 1/16(.06) |
| RT+HT[3] (sequen.) | 8/12(.67) | 4/7(.57) | 6/13(.46) | 2/15(.13) |

[1] 40 Gy/8 F/25 days (2 fractions per week);

[2] 42.5°C/45 min, immediately after each radiation fraction;

[3] 42.5°C/45 min, 4 h after each radiation fraction;

No statistical significance.

Tumor control was obtained in 37% (6/16) lesions after radiotherapy alone. Combined modalities achieved a better tumor response, especially in the simultaneous treatment group in which a complete clearance was obtained in 77% (10/13) lesions in comparison to 67% (8/12) complete responses obtained after the sequential treatment. The better responses with combined modalities did persist after 6 months follow-up, simultaneous treatment being still the most effective (71% or 5/7 controlled lesions) in comparison with the sequential treatment (57% or 4/7 controlled lesions), which appeared in turn to be better than radiotherapy alone (33% or 3/9 controlled lesions). However, no statistically significant difference could be demonstrated among these groups.

Addition of heat resulted also in an increased skin radiation reaction especially with the simultaneous treatment: moist desquamation occurred in 36% fields treated with radiation alone in comparison with 64% and 46% fields treated with simultaneous and sequential treatments, respectively. A remarkably lower incidence of thermal damage was obtained by employing more carefully designed applicators.

This fact is in contrast with the previous results obtained with conventional fraction sizes of radiation. It may be possible that the killing mechanism plays an important role on heat radiosensitization. In fact, as the size of dose per fraction is reduced, more cell killing results from "single hit" lethal events than from accumulated sublethal injury (Elkind 1976; Withers 1975). Since one of the main mechanism of heat radiosensitization is the impairment of sublethal damage repair (Ben Hur et al. 1974; Gerweck et al. 1975; Kim et al. 1976; Li et al., 1976; Dewey et al. 1980; Suit, Gerweck 1979), it can be deduced that the thermal enhancement of radiation response is higher with high fraction size of radiation, and tends to decrease with low doses per fraction, whether simultaneous or sequential schedule are used. The therapeutic gain, at these low doses, may well be due to the fact that cell killing in tumor may still result from accumulated sublethal injury, or to the direct hyperthermic cytotoxic destruction of the nutritionally deprived acidic and chronically hypoxic radioresistant tumor cells (Gerweck 1977; Kim et al.1975; Shulman, Hall 1974; Dewey et al.1977; Overgaard 1978; Overgaard 1980a; Overgaard, Nielsen 1980).

However, the enhancement of the acute skin radiation effect may not be considered the limiting factor of the simultaneous treatment as the acute skin reaction subside promptly because of the vigorous regeneration of the epithelial cells. On the other hand, one may attempt to cool the surrounding skin during heating. More data are necessary on the occurrence of late irreversible radiation reactions.

The results of the third trial (high fraction size

of radiation combined to high temperature hyperthermia) are reported in table 4.

TABLE 4

EFFECT OF HIGH TEMPERATURE HYPERTHERMIA ON THE RESPONSE
TO RADIATION AT HIGH FRACTION SIZE
(ACTUARIAL TUMOR CONTROL)

| TREATMENT | COMPLETE RESPONSE | | MOIST | NECROSIS |
|---|---|---|---|---|
| | end RT[3] | 6 months | DESQUAM. | |
| RT alone[1] | 5/15(.33) | 2/9(.22) | 4/15(.27) | — |
| RT + HT[2] | 13/15(.87) | 8/9(.89) | 5/15(.33) | 7/11(.64) |

[1] 45°C/30 min, immediately after each radiation fraction. The surrounding normal skin was actively cooled by means of circulating cold water.

[2] 30 Gy/6 F/18 days (2 fractions per week)

[3] Statistical significance: $p = 0.01$.

A complete tumor response was obtained in 33% (5/15) lesions after radiotherapy alone, and in 87% (13/15) lesions after combined modalities. This remarkably higher response in the latter group persisted also after 6 month follow-up when 2/9 (22%) and 8/9 (89%) lesions were still controlled after single or combined modality, respectively. Again, this difference is statistically significant ($p = 0.01$) only at the end of treatment. No increased incidence of skin moist desquamation was observed in the combined versus single modality group (5/15 vs. 4/15), probably because of the active skin cooling and/or lower total doses of radiation employed in this trial.

As expected, the incidence of thermal damage on uncooled skin areas is increased (7/11 necrosis). However, this is a consequence of the necrotic process induced by

the high temperature heating in tumor cells that grossly
involved the overlaying skin. The representative examples
of figure 4 (a-b) shows that the heat induced necrosis is
sharply confined to the tumor area.

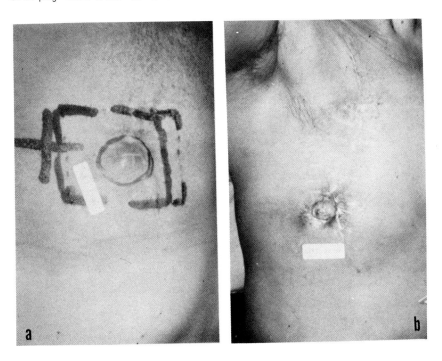

Fig. 4: (a) Patient with a cutaneous chest wall lesion
recurrent after surgery and radiation.
(b): Same patient after combined treatment (30 Gy/5 F + 5
sessions of HT at 45°C/30 min).

Therapeutic Gain

From our results we attempted to estimate the therapeutic gain factor (TGF), usually defined as the ratio of
thermal enhancement ratio (TER) of tumor to TER of skin,
where TER in this study has been defined as the ratio of
percent response (i.e. tumor clearence and moist desquamation) after combined modality to percent response after

radiotherapy alone.

### TABLE 5
### EFFECT OF HYPERTHERMIA ON THE RADIATION RESPONSE
### OF TUMOR AND SKIN

| TREATMENT | TEMPER. °C/min | FRACTION SIZE(Gy) | TUMOR RESP. %C.R. | TER | SKIN RESP. %M.D. | TER | TGF |
|---|---|---|---|---|---|---|---|
| Sim./Seq. | 42.5/45 | 1.5-2 | 73 | 1.74 | 42 | 1.10 | 1.58 |
| Radiat. alone | — | 1.5-2 | 42 | | 38 | | |
| Sequent. | 42.5/45 | 5 | 67 | 1.79 | 46 | 1.28 | 1.40 |
| Simult. | 42.5/45 | 5 | 77 | 2.05 | 64 | 1.78 | 1.15 |
| Radiat. alone | — | 5 | 37.5 | | 36 | | |
| Simult. | *45/30 | 6 | 87 | 2.63 | 33.3 | 1.25 | 2.10 |
| Radiat. alone | — | 6 | 33 | | 26.6 | — | — |

C.R. = Complete tumor response; M.D. = Moist desquamation; TER = Thermal enhancement ratio; TGF = Therapeutic gain factor;
*The normal skin surrounding the tumor was actively cooled by means of circulating cold water.

Table 5 shows percent tumor response and moist desquamation, and the relative TER's and TGF's obtained with the various treatment schedules employed in our studies. Heating tumor and normal tissue to the same temperature, the best TGF (1.58) was obtained when conventional fraction sizes of radiation were used in association with the 42.5°C hyperthermia, indicating that, at these fraction sizes, tumors are still remarkably "sensitized" by heat, while skin is not. TGF values of 1.40 and 1.15 were observed when high fraction sizes of radiation were employed in association with the sequential and simultaneous 42.5°C hyperthermia, respectively. These results are in agreement with other published experimental and clinical findings (Overgaard 1981). When high fraction sizes of radiation were used in association with the simultaneous 45°C hyperthermia, because of the active skin cooling the highes tumor TER (2.63) and TGF (2.10) were obtained. This suggest that this schedule could be very useful in particular clinical situations.

From this clinical evaluation, the following conclusion can be made about the therapeutic effectiveness of the different schedules: simultaneous application of high radiation fraction size and moderate heat resulted in a great enhancement of radiation response, but was apparently of the same extent in both tumor and skin. Therefore, only a slight improvement of the therapeutic ratio was obtained. At the same radiation fraction size, sequential treatment tended to enhance the skin reaction too, but the effect was stronger on tumor, thus indicating an improved therapeutic ratio. Heating tumor and surrounding tissue to the same degree, no increased normal tissue damage was seen after conventional fraction size of radiation, while a significant increase in tumor control was obtained in comparison with radiotherapy alone. Thus, such a schedule clearly indicates a significant improvement of the therapeutic ratio. This ratio could be also significantly improved with high fraction sizes of radiation combined with 45°C hyperthermia, provided tumor to be selectively, or at least preferentially, heated over normal tissue, or skin actively cooled.

Arcangeli G, Barni E, Benassi M, Cividalli A, Creton G, Lovisolo G, Mauro F, Nervi C (1980a). Heating patterns after 27 MHz local hyperthermia. Comparative results in piglet normal tissue and in phantom. In Arcangeli G, Mauro F (eds):"Hyperthermia in Radiation Oncology", Milano: Masson Italia Editori, p 69.

Arcangeli G, Barni E, Cividalli A, Mauro F, Morelli D, Nervi C, Spanò M, Tabocchini A (1980b). Effectiveness of microwave hyperthermia combined with ionizing radiation: Clinical results on neck node metastases. Int J Radiat Oncol Biol Phys 6: 143.

Arcangeli G, Barocas A, Mauro F, Nervi C, Spanò M, Tabocchini A(1980c). Multiple daily fractionation (MDF) radiotherapy in association with hyperthermia and/or misonidazole: Experimental and clinical results. Cancer 45: 2707.

Arcangeli G, Cividalli A, De Vita R, Lovisolo G, Mauro F, Pardini MC (1981). Hyperthermie et irradiation: rôle de la température et du mode d'association. Etude expérimentale chez la souris. Bull Cancer 68: 232.

Ben Hur E, Elkind MM, Bronk BV (1974). Thermally enhanced radioresponse of cultured Chinese hamster cells: Inhibition of repair of sublethal damage and enhancement of lethal damage. Radiat Res 58: 38.

Denekamp J, Stewart F (1979). Evidence for repair capacity in mouse tumors relative to skin. Int J Radiat Oncol Biol Phys 5: 2003.

Dewey WC, Freeman ML, Raaphorst GP, Clark EP, Wong RSL, Highfield DP, Spiro IJ, Tomasovic SP, Denman DL, Coss RA (1980). Cell biology of hyperthermia and radiation. In Meyn RE, Withers HR (eds): "Radiation Biology in Cancer Research", New York: Raven Press, p 589.

Dewey WC, Hopwood LE, Sapareto SA, Gerweck LE (1977). Cellular responses to combinations of hyperthermia and radiation. Radiology 123: 463.

Dickson JA (1975). Hyperthermia and laboratory animal system: Chairman's address. In "Proc. Intl. Symp. on Cancer Therapy by Hyperthermia and Radiation". Washington DC: Am Coll Radiol, p 105.

Elkind MM (1976). Fractionated dose radiotherapy and its relationship to survival curve shape. Cancer Treat Rev 3: 1.

Field SB, Bleehen NM (1979). Hyperthermia in the treatment of cancer. Cancer Treat Rev 6: 63.

Fowler JF, Denekamp J, Sheldon W, Smith AM, Begg AC, Harris SR, Page AL (1975). Sparing effect of X-ray fractionation in mammary tumors and skin reaction in mice. In Alper T (ed): "Survival after Low Doses of Radiation", London: Inst of Physics and Wiley, p 288.

Gerweck LE (1977). Modification of cell lethality at elevated temperatures. The pH effect. Radiat Res 70: 224.

Gerweck LE, Gillette EL, Dewey WC (1975). Effect of heat and radiation on synchronous Chinese hamster cells: Killing and repair. Radiat Res 64: 611.

Hill SA, Denekamp J (1979). The response of six mouse tumours to combined heat and X-rays: Implications for therapy. Brit J Radiol, 52: 209.

Kim SH, Kim JH, Hahn EW (1975). Enhanced killing of hypoxic tumor cells by hyperthermia. Brit J Radiol, 48: 872.

Kim SH, Kim JH, Hahn EW (1976). The enhanced killing of irradiated Hela cells in synchronous culture by hyperthermia. Radiat Res 66: 337.

Law MP (1979). Some effects of fractionation on the response of the mouse ear to combined heat and X-rays. Radiat Res 80: 360.

Law MP, Ahier RG, Field SB (1977). The response of mouse skin to combined hyperthermia and X-rays. Int J Radiat Biol 32: 153.

Law MP, Ahier RG, Field SB (1979). The effect of prior heat treatment on the thermal enhancement of radiation damage in the mouse ear. Brit J Radiol 52: 315.

Li GC, Evans RS, Hahn GM (1976). Modification and inhibition of repair of potentially lethal X – ray damage by hyperthermia. Radiat Res 67: 491.

Myers R, Field SB (1977). The response of the rat tail to combined heat and X rays. Brit J Radiol 50: 581.

Myers R, Field SB (1979). Hyperthermia and oxygen enhancement ratio for damage to baby rat cartilage. Brit J Radiol 52: 415.

Overgaard J (1978). The effect of local hyperthermia alone and in combination with radiation, on solid tumors. In Streffer C et al (eds): "Cancer Therapy by Hyperthermia and Radiation", Baltimore and Munich: Urban & Schwarzemberg p 49.

Overgaard J (1980a). Simultaneous and sequential hyperthermia and radiation treatment of an experimental tumor and its surrounding normal tissue in vivo. Int J Radiat Oncol Biol Phys 6: 1507.

Overgaard J (1980b). Effect of fractionated hyperthermia and radiation on an experimental tumor and its surrounding skin. In Arcangeli G and Mauro F (eds):"Hyperthermia in Radiation Oncology", Milano: Masson Italia Editori, p 241.

Overgaard J (1981). Fractionated radiation and hyperthermia: Experimental and clinical studies. Cancer, 48: 1116.

Overgaard J, Nielsen OS (1980). The role of tissue enviromental factors on the kinetics and morphology of tumor cells exposed to hyperthermia. Ann N Y Acad Sci 335: 254.

Overgaard J, Suit HD (1979). Time-temperature relationship in hyperthermia treatment of malignant and normal tissue in vivo. Cancer Res 39: 3248.

Shulman N, Hall EJ (1974). Hyperthermia: Its effect on proliferative and plateau phase cell cultured. Radiology 113: 209.

Stewart FA, Denekamp J (1977). Sensitization of mouse skin to X irradiation by moderate heating. Radiology 123: 195.

Stewart FA, Denekamp J (1978). The therapeutic advantage of combined heat and X - rays on a mouse fibrosarcoma. Brit J Radiol 51: 307.

Suit HD, Gerweck LE (1979). Potential for hyperthermia and radiation therapy. Cancer Res 39: 2290.

Withers HR (1975). Responses of some normal tissues to low doses of radiation. In Alper T (ed): "Cell Survival after Low Doses of Radiation", London: Inst of Physics and Wiley, p 369.

13th International Cancer Congress, Part D
Research and Treatment, pages 235–245
© 1983 Alan R. Liss, Inc., 150 Fifth Avenue, New York, NY 10011

IMPACT OF MICROCIRCULATION AND PHYSIOLOGIC CONSIDERATIONS ON
CLINICAL HYPERTHERMIA

HAIM I. BICHER, M.D.

Head, Hyperthermia Clinic
Valley Cancer Institute
Western Tumor Medical Group
5522 Sepulveda Blvd; Van Nuys, CA   91405

The initial work of Thomlinson and Gray (1955) demonstrating necrotic regions in tumors at distances greater
than 150 to 200 ц from a capillary and numerous reports of
large hypoxic fractions in tumors (Bicher et.al. 1980; Kallman 1972) confirm that the microvascular network in tumors
is poorly developed and organized when compared to that of
normal tissues.  It is this physiologic difference between
tumor and normal tissue that may provide a therapeutic advantage for a modality such as hyperthermia.

Several general physiologic responses to hyperthermia
have been commonly observed.  These include increased cellular metabolic activity in the heated region and flushing
of the skin overlying the heated area (indicative of increased perfusion of the skin).  The specific responses in
the microenvironment of different organs and tissues (malignant and nonmalignant) to modifications in temperature have
been studied recently in more detail (Bicher, Mitagvaria,
and Hetzel 1980; Reinhold, Blachiewic, and Berg-Blok 1979;
Song 1978).  Examination of several recent publications demonstrates that active investigations of the physiologic phenomena induced by hyperthermia are in progress (Bicher, Mitagvaria, and Hetzel 1980; Berg-Blok 1979; Storm et.al. 1979;
Streffer er al. 1978; Von Ardenne and Reitnauer 1978).  The
studies by Eddy (1980) and by Reinhold, Blachiewicz and Berg
Blok (1978) employing "chamber systems" of different types,
have shown changes in the microvascular network as a function of temperature and exposure time.  The apparent sensitivity of the neovasculature is a critical observation by
these investigators.  Similar results in different test

systems also have been observed by Emami and colleagues(1980) and by Dewhirst and Ozimek(1980).

Knowledge of the effect of hyperthermia on tumor and normal tissue blood flow and the subsequent effects on oxygen tension (p0$_2$) and pH is important not only for the effect of hyperthermia on hypoxic cells at the time of radiation, but also for differential tumor heating.

There is considerable evidence from plethysmography that elevation of normal tissue temperature to 41$^\circ$C is accompanied by considerable increase in blood flow (Lehman 1971). Cater and Silver(1960) reported on changes in tumor oxygen tension with hyperthermia but did not record changes in tumor temperature. They concluded that diathermy had not increased the oxygen tension in the tumor but on the contrary, caused a decrease.

Bicher and co-workers (1980) studying a mouse leg tumor system, reported that tumor blood flow increased at temperatures up to 41$^\circ$C and then progressively decreased. The oxygen tension in the tumor, as measured with a platinum electrode, generally followed the changes in tumor flow, but the exact tumor temperature at which the oxygen tension decreased was not determined. Changes in tissue pH and brain tissue oxygenation were reported earlier by the same author (1978). The studies of Eddy(1980) and Reinhold(1980) employing "chamber systems" have both shown changes in microvascular network as a function of temperature and exposure time. Blood flow and pH changes during hyperthermia have also been reported by Song et al.(1980).

Although blood flow and shifts induced in it by hyperthermia in both tumor and normal tissue are important, several other parameters also have significant roles. Several studies indicate that the pH of interstitial fluid in human and rodent solid tumors is .3 to .5 units lower than the normal tissue pH of about 7.4.

Reduced pH has also been shown to affect the transplantability of tumor cells heated in vitro. In a recent paper,

**This work was partially reported at the 11th European Conference fro Microcirculation,Garmish, 1981(Bibl.Anat.N-20)and the ISOTT meeting in Detroit(1981). Thanks are given to Mr.S. Frinak for technical assistance in part of this work.

Gerweck(1976) has shown that there is a variable influence of pH according to temperature and that there is a critical point in the increased lethality of heat below pH 6.7.

In addition to hyperthermia, Hematopophyrin derivative (HpD) phototherapy is also showing some promise in clinical cancer therapy (Diamond et al. 1972, Dougherty et al. 1978). This type of therapy employs an injectable dye (HpD) which is specifically accumulated in some tumors and/or is specifically cleared from normal tissues. When light of specific wave lengths illuminate the dye of a photochemical reaction takes place yielding the cytoxic agent singlet oxygen (Weishaupt et al. 1976). Although the exact mechanism(s) of tumor inactiviation have yet to be determined, the rapid and dramatic coloration changes observed in tumors following treatment suggest that modification of blood flow with possible concomitant effects of $pO_2$ and pH may play a prominent role (Diamond et.al. 1972).

MATERIALS AND METHODS

Animal system. All in situ studies were carred out in 4th, generation transplants of $C_3H$ mammary adenocarcinoma implanted in the hind leg of $C_3H$ SED-BH mice. This is a syngentic implantable tumor inoculated subcutaneously into recepient mice. Tumors used for experimentation were approximately 8-10 mm in diameter. The mice were anesthetized during microelectrode induction with a combination of Ketamine 40mg/kg I.M. and Thorzine, 50mg/kg I.M.

Oxygen ultramicroelectrodes. The $O_2$ ultramicroelectrodes used were as described by Cater and colleagues(1960) They were made by pulling a glass tube(KG-33, ID 1.5mm OD 2.0mm, Garner Glass Co., Claremont, California), encasing a 20-μ gold wire (Sigmund Cohn Corp., Mt. Bernon, New York) in a David Kopf Model 700 C vertical pipette puller. The exposed gold temp is about 10 μ in diameter, and is coated with a Rhoples(Rhom Haas, Philadelpia, Pa.) membrane as previously described (Bicher 1977). This probe is used as an "external reference" $O_2$ microelectrode.

Electrodes are calibrated as previously described(Bicher et al. 1978) in buttered saline solutions of known $pO_2$ values. The electrodes are 'conditioned' by placing them in buffered saline and applying 0.8V potential for 2 hrs. After this treatment they are usually very stable. The current reading

at zero oxygen tension is very low (residual current) and
the response of the microelectrode to changes of oxygen tension is very rapid.

In these experiments a polarizing voltage of 0.6V has
been used. The relation between current output and oxygen
tension is linear, the current mm Hg being of the order of
magnitude of $0.6 \times 10^{-11}$A.

pH ultramicroelectrodes. Designs for glass pH microelectrodes employed in this study have been developed, most
notably by Hinke(11). The Hinke-type electrode consist of a
pH sensitive glass micrpipette inside of pyrex glass pipette
with the tip of the pH sensitive micropipette extruded from
the pyrex glass pipette. A silver/silver chloride electrode
is inserted into the electrode with an exposed tip has an almost instantaneous response time. This is an advantage over
the other types of microelectrodes in which a recessed tip
may cause a response time of up to several minutes.

Temperature determinations. Tumor and mouse core temperatures were recorded using Copper 0 Constant and micro-
therocouples (tip diameter 30-100 micros-METRA Inc., Encino,
CA) inserted into the tumoral tissue in close proximity to
the microelectrode or in the animal's rectum for core measurements. An Omega Engineering Model 250 Digital Voltmeter
amplifier was used as a link between the micro-thermocouple
and the polygraph. Microwaves of a frequency 2450MHz were
produced by a Raytheon Magnetron and delivered through a
specially designed 2cm square applicator loaded with low
loss dielectric material haveing a dielectric constant of 6.

HpD phototherapy. Tumor-bearing mice were injected
with 20mg/kg HpD and 24 hrs later were exposed to the light
source. The mice were shielded from the light during the 55
min. exposure except for the tumor-bearing region. The light
source was modified Bessler latern slide projector which was
filtered to yield $150,W/cm^2$ at the tumor surface over the
range 600-730 mm.

RESULTS

4 different major experiments were performed. In the
first $pO_2$ distribution after 1 hr. hyperthermia was studied
1, 4 and 24 hrs after treatment. The second experiment was
similar but studied the effect of Phototherapy on $TpO_2$, at

similar time intervals. Experiment 3 studied the effect of hyperthermia on tissue pH, at similar time intervals, while experiment 4 determined and compared the effect of Hyperthermia and phototherapy on tissue pH. All results were expressed in Histogram fashion

Experiment 1: Effect of hyperthermia on $TpO_2$-time correlation. Histograms were obtained before and 1, 4 and 24 hrs after microwave induced hyperthermia (42-43$^{\circ}$C) for 1 hr. These results are shown in Figure 1. There is a progressive shift towards low $pO_2$ values, with all the tumor virtually hypoxic after 24 hrs. No reoxygenation is noted.

Experiment 2: Effect of Phototherapy on $TpO_2$-Time correlation. Histograms were obtained before and 1, 4 and 24 hours after HpD phototherapy (20mg/kg HpD, light, exposure 150mW/cm$^2$ for 55 min.). The $pO_2$ histogram shifts toward the hypoxic region (0.5mm Hg) quickly. However, at 4 hrs.there is an attempt to reoxygenate, as shown by the reappearance of an oxic tail in the 20-40mm Hg region. At 24 hrs. all values are between 0-10mm Hg. These results are shown in Figure 2.

Experiment 3: Effect of Hyperthermia on TpH. Time correlation. Histograms obtained before and 1, 4 and 24 hrs after microwave reduced Hyperthermia (42-43$^{\circ}$C) for 1 hr. Results shown in fig. 3. Note a remarkable shift of the tissue pH values towards acidity with mean TpH changing from 6.74 to 6.21 after heat. TpH remains in that region at 4 and 24 hours.

Experiment 4: Effect of Hyperthermia and Phototherapy on Tissue pH-a correlation. Histograms obtained before 1 hr after microwave induced Hyperthermia, Phototherapy or a combination of both. Note that the pH shift towards acidosis (same as shown in fig. 3) induced by hyperthermia is not present after Phototherapy. This correlation is shown in figure 4.

DISCUSSION

Determination of the mode of tumor inactivation by a treatment modality is critical to its development and future use. It has been shown that hyperthermia may have possible effects on cell survival either alone or in combination with radiation (Gerwick 1977, Overgaard 1976, Rheinhold 1978). It has also been shown to dramatically modify blood flow and

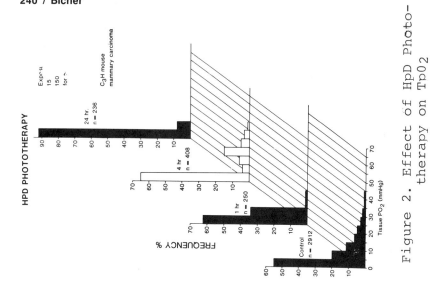

Figure 2. Effect of HpD Phototherapy on TpO2

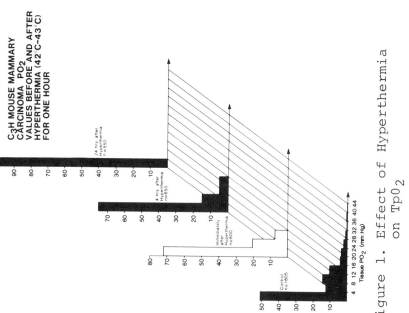

Figure 1. Effect of Hyperthermia
on TpO2

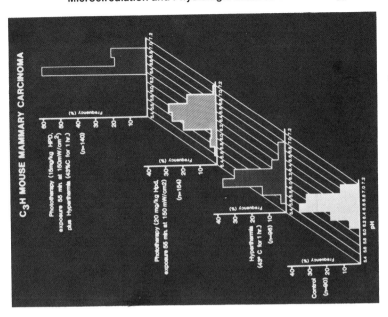

Figure 4. Effect of Phototherapy, Hyperthermia or a combination of both on TpH.

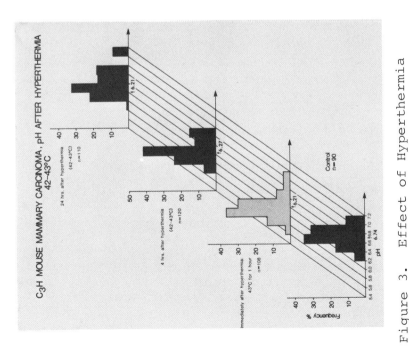

Figure 3. Effect of Hyperthermia on TpH.

oxygenation within tumors (Bicher et al. 1980). The results presented here indicated that a significant reduction in pH is induced by hyperthermia which may result in a significant increase in cell killing with the tumor (Gerwick 1977). It is possible that this observed pH shift is due to a combination of hyperthermia stimulated cellular metabolic activity and the simutaneous reduction in tumor blood flow which is observed at the treatment temperature (Bicher et al. 1980).

The effects seen on pH and $pO_2$ following HpD phototheapy are quite different from those following hyperthermia. It is clear that ther is a sharp reduction in $pO_2$ at all areas within the tumor without any significant shift in pH. Although studies are now in progress, it is possible to speculate on the meaning of the results presented here. Massive coagulation necrosis within tumors is reported to follow HpD phototherapy (Diamond et al 1972). It is likely that the cells most affected by this treatment are the vascular endothelial cells of the tumor microvasculature. Their destruction would result in the observed coagulation necrosis with an abrupt reduction in blood flow. This would result in the low levels of tissue oxygenation reported here. Since there is no cellular metabolic stimulation with this modality and there is direct cytotoxicity (Weishaupt et al. 1976) no dramatic shift in pH would be expected and none was observed.

Further studies are currently in progress to further examine the effects of hyperthermia and HpD phototherapy on tumor microphysiology. Results so far are seen in figure 5.

## MICROPHYSIOLOGY
$C_3H$ Mice Adenocarcinoma Implanted in Leg Muscle
Hyperthermia and Phototherapy

1. $O_2pH$ Inhomogeneities occur in tumor&muscle tissue
2. Important microcirculation changes occur in both Phototherapy & Hyperthermia.
3. One hour $43^\circ C$ Hyperthermia:
   A) Collapses Microcirculation
   B) $O_2$Histogram shifts toward 0-5mm Hg $O_2$ Decrease with time
   C) No Reoxygenation up to 24 hours
   D) pH shifts toward Acidosis
4. Phototherapy: A) Microcirculation Damage
   B) $O_2$ Histogram shifts toward 0-5mm Hg quickly
   C) Reoxygenation at 4 hours
   D) No pH shift

SUMMARY

Changes in tumor tissue oxygenation and acidity were determined using ultramicroelectrodes, and presented in histogram fashion. The effect of Hyperthermia and HpD phototherapy were tested. It was found that both modalities affect tumor microcirculation, causing a marked drop in oxygen availability. Tissue pH is decreased by Hyperthermia, but not by phototherapy. These effects are long lasting at least for 24 hours after treatment.

REFERENCES

1. Bicher, H.I., Increase in brain tissue oxygen availability induced by localized microwave hyperthermia. In Silver Erecinska, and Bicher, Oxygen transport to tissue; Vol. III, pp. 347-353, Plenum Press, NY, 1978.

2. Bicher, H.I. et al. Effects of hyperthermia on normal and tumor microenvironment. Rad. 137:523-530, 1980.

3. Bicher, H.I.; Hetzel,F.W.; and D'Agostino,L. Changes in tumor tissue oxygenation induced by microwave hyperthermia Int. J. Radiat. Oncol. Biol. Phys. 2:157,1977.

4. Bicher, H.I., Mitagvaria, N.; and Hetzel, F.W., Alterations in tumor tissue oxygenation by microwave hyperthermia, Ann, NY Acad. Sci, 335:20-21, 1980.

5. Bicher, H.I. and Ohki, S. Intracellular pH electrode experiments on giant squid axon. Biochem. Biophys. Act. 255:900, 1972.

6. Cater, D. B. and Silver, I.A. Quanitative measurements of oxygen tension in normal tissues and in the tumors of patients before and after radiotherapy, Act. Radio 53:233-256, 1960.

7. Davies, P., and Brink, F. Microelectrodes for measuring local oxygen tension in animal tissue. Rev. Sci. Instrum. 13:524-533, 1942.

8. Dewhirst,M.W. and Ozimek,E.J. Will hyperthermia conquer the elusive hypoxic cell? Radio. 137:811-817, 1980.

9.  Diamond, I., McDonagh,A.F., Wilson C.X., Granelli,S.G. Nielsen,S. and Jaenicke,R. Photodynamic therapy of malignant tumors. Lancet 2:1175-1177, 1972.

10. Dougherty,T.J, Kaufman,J.E., Goldfarb A., Weishaupf,K.R. Boyle,D., and Mittleman, A. Photradiation-therapy for the treatment of malignant tumors. Can. Res.38:2628-2633, 1978.

11. Eddy, H.A. Alterations in tumor microvasculature during hyperthermia Radiology 157:515-521, 1980.

12. Emami,B. etal. Physiological effects of hyperthermia; response of capillary blood flow and capillary under structure to local tumor heating. Rad.137:805-809 1980.

13. England,N.E.:HallbrookT.; Ling,L. Skin and muscle blood flow during regional perfusion with hyperthermia perfusate. ScanJ. Thorc. Cardio. Surg. 8:77-79, 1974.

14. Gerweck,LE. Modification of cell lethality at elevated temperatures: The pH effect. Rad.Res.70224-235, 1977.

15. Gerweck,LE Rottinger, E. Enhancement of mammalian cell sensitivity to hyperthermia by pH alteration, Radiat. Res. 67:508-511, 1976

16. Hinke, J.A. Cation-selective microelectrodes for intracellular use, Glass electrodes for hydrogen and other cations, NY Marcel Dekker, 1973.

17. WeinshauptKR, GomerCJ Dougherty, TJ Identification of singlet oxygen as the cytotoxic agent in photoinactivation of murine tumor. Can. Res. 36, 2326, 1972.

18. Kallman,RF The phenomen of reoxygenation and its implications for fractioned radiotherapy. Rad.105:135-142 1972

19. Lehman,JF Diathermy. In Handbook of physical medicine and rehabilitation eds. Krusen Kouke, Elwood. Philadelphia W.B. Saunders 1971-pp. 273-345.

20. Overgaard, J. Influence of extracellular pH on the viability and morphology of tumor cells exposed to hyperthermia, J.Natl. Can. Inst. 56:1243-1250, 1976.

21. Reinhold, H.S. and Berg-Blok, A.V.D. Features and limitations of the "in vivo" evaluation of tumor response by optical means. Paper read at the 9th L.H. Gray Memorial Conference, Cambridge, Eng. Br. J. Cancer 1980.

22. Reinhold, H.S. Blachiewicz, B. and Berg-Blok, A. V. D. Reoxygenation of tumors in sandwich chambers. Eur. J. Cancer 15:481-489, 1979.

23. Silver, I.A. A Simple microelectrode for measuring $pO_2$ in gas or fluid, Med. Electron, Biol. Eng. 1:547-551, 1963.

24. Song,C.W. Effect of hyperthermia on vascular functions of normal tissues and experimental tumors. J. Nat'l Cancer Inst. 60:711-713, 1978.

25. Song,C.W.,Kang,M.S. and Rhee,J.G. Effect of hyperthermia on vascular function pH and cell survival Radiology 137:795-803, 1980.

26. Storm, F.K. et al. Normal tissue and solid tumor effects of hyperthermia in animal models and clinical trials. Cancer Res. 39:2245-2251, 1979.

27. Streffer, C. et al. Proceedings of the Second International Symposium on Cancer Therapy by Hyperthermia and Radiation, Baltimore and Munich: Urban & Schwarzenberg, 1978, p. 344.

28. Thomlinson, R. H. and Gray, L H. The histological structure of some human lung cancers and the possible implications for radiotherapy. Br. J. Cancer 9:539-549, 1955.

29. Van Ardenne,M., Reitnauer, P.G. Amplification of the selective tumor, acidificaion by local hyperthermia. Natruwissenschaften 65:159-160, 1978.

CONGRESS SYMPOSIA

HIGH LET PARTICLES Catterall, M., UK, Chairman;
Bagshaw, M., USA, Co-Chairman; Opera House

Potential Advantages of High LET Radiation.
*Fowler, J. F., Middlesex, England.

Clinical Experience of Fast Neutron Therapy
in Edinburgh. *Duncan, W., Edinburgh, Scotland.

A Detailed Analysis of the MDAH-TAMVEC Neutron
Therapy Trials for Head and Neck Cancer.
*Hussey, D. H., Maor, M. H. and Fletcher, G. H.,
Houston, TX USA.

Results of PI-Meson Radiotherapy at LAMF.
*Bush, S. E., Albuquerque, NM USA. (By Title
Only)

Heavy Particle Experience in the Treatment of
Human Cancer. *Castro, J. R., Tobias, C. A.,
Saunders, W. M., Chen, G. T. Y., Collier, J. M.,
Lyman, J. T., Woodruff, K. H., Phillips, T. L.,
Grewal-Bahl, R., Char, D. and Carter, S. K.,
Berkeley, CA and Palo Alto, CA USA.

Please note: Papers that are listed as "By Title
Only" were presented at the 13th International
Cancer Congress, but are not included in these
volumes.

13th International Cancer Congress, Part D
Research and Treatment, pages 249–259
© 1983 Alan R. Liss, Inc., 150 Fifth Avenue, New York, NY 10011

POTENTIAL ADVANTAGES OF HIGH LET RADIATION

John F. Fowler, Ph.D., D.Sc., M.D.(Hon),
F.Inst.P., F.A.C.R.(Hon).

Gray Laboratory of the Cancer Research Campaign
Mount Vernon Hospital, Northwood,
Middlesex HA6 2RN, England

INTRODUCTION

There are three potential biological advantages in the use of high LET particles for cancer therapy.

(1) Less radioresistance of hypoxic cells to high LET than to conventional radiotherapy.

(2) Less variation of radiosensitivity around the cell cycle.

(3) Less repair capacity in cells after high LET irradiation.

Each potential advantage is accompanied by snags and both will be discussed in the sequence listed above.

In addition, heavy <u>charged</u> particles provide physical dose distributions which are much better than those of photons or neutrons. This is an important advantage. Lack of space prevents my discussion of these physical distributions here, but they are described by the other authors in this session and in detail in my book (Fowler 1981) and in Raju's (1980).

LESS RADIORESISTANCE OF HYPOXIC CELLS

Most tumors larger than 1 mm in diameter have been

found, in experimental rats and mice, to contain hypoxic cells. Their histological structures and inter-capillary distances are similar to those in human tumors. Some, but not all, of the clinical trials using radiotherapy in hyperbaric oxygen have shown significant increases in local control and long term survival (Watson et al 1978, Henk et al 1977). The lower oxygen enhancement ratios (OER)* obtained with high LET radiation therefore provides a potential advantage. Fig 1 summarises values of OER for various particle beams (Raju 1980, Curtis 1979, Fowler 1981). The values of OER are as low for fast neutrons as for neon ions (the latter in a 10 cm spread peak). The hypoxic gain factors (HGF)*, obtained by dividing the OER for the particle beam into that for X-rays (here assumed to be 2.8), are shown on the right.

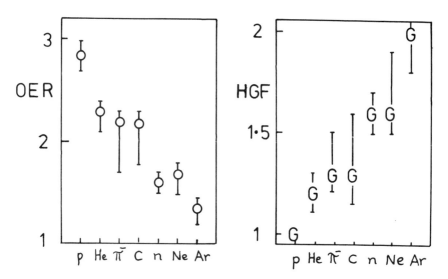

*Fig. 1. Oxygen enhancement ratios and hypoxic gain factors for the particles at the centre of 10 cm spread peaks (Raju 1980, Fowler 1981). p - protons. He - helium ions. $\pi^-$ - negative pi mesons. C - carbon ions. n - fast neutrons. Ne - neon ions. Ar - argon ions.*

---

\*    OER = Radiation dose in absence of oxygen, divided by radiation dose in presence of oxygen, required to produce the same effect.
    HGF = OER of high LET radiation/OER of X-rays.

These HGF factors are, however, theoretical maximum values.  Lower values will be obtained in practice for two reasons.  Firstly, the presence of any euoxic cells in tumors will dilute the disadvantage of hypoxic cells and hence will reduce the HGF, especially at low doses per fraction.  Secondly, any reoxygenation of hypoxic cells during the weeks of treatment will of course also reduce the hypoxic disadvantage.

Fig 2 illustrates the way in which the hypoxic gain factor will be reduced, even to unity (no gain), as the proportion of hypoxic cells in a tumor is decreased from 100 to 0% (Withers and Peters 1979).

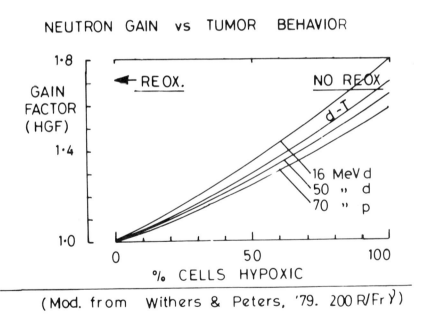

Fig. 2.  The calculated decrease of hypoxic gain factor with decrease in the proportion of hypoxic cells in a tumor (Withers and Peters 1979).

The values of HGF are somewhat higher for lower energy neutrons, as indicated by the four energies of neutron beam shown in Fig 2. The calculations are based on multifraction radiotherapy at 2 grays of photons per fraction, assuming the OER values of Hall and Kellerer (1979). We do not know the rate of reoxygenation in any type of human tumor but it is more likely to be substantial in tumors which shrink rapidly.

This line of reasoning suggests that tumors which do not shrink rapidly are more likely to benefit from measures to overcome the hypoxic cell problem. It would be a major step forward to be able to measure the proportion of hypoxic cells in human tumors. Work with this aim is in progress, some using radioactive nitroimidazoles and some using fluorescent dyes which are fixed in cells by hypoxia only.

## LESS VARIATION OF RADIOSENSITIVITY WITH PHASE OF THE CELL CYCLE

Fig 3 illustrates that the proportion of cells surviving after a dose of neutrons or alpha-particles varies less with phase of the cycle than after X-irradiation (Sinclair 1970, Raju et al 1975). Therefore tumors with a high proportion of radioresistant cells and a low proportion of sensitive cells might be less than adequately treated with X-rays, but with high LET radiation this disadvantage would be less.

If we assume a fixed RBE of 3.0 for relevant normal tissues, so that the dose of neutrons is fixed, then a "kinetic gain factor", KGF, can be defined on the basis of the relative proportion of cells resistant or sensitive to X-rays in the tumor.

$$KGF = \frac{RBE \text{ of tumor}}{RBE \text{ of normal tissue}}$$

insofar as RBE is influenced by the distribution of cells in age through the cycle. The RBE of cells in the S phase is often high, because of the large shoulder on the X-ray survival curve, and the RBE of cells at the $G_1$ S interface is low (e.g. 5.1 and 1.8 respectively, Gragg et al 1978). There may be another peak of RBE during $G_1$ if the $G_1$ phase is long.

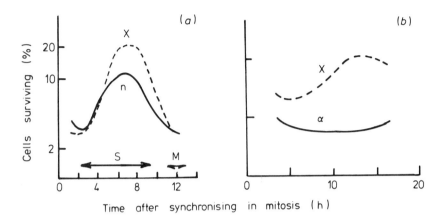

Fig. 3. Measured proportions of mammalian cells surviving in synchronized populations irradiated at different phases of the cell cycle. Dotted curves - low LET X-rays. Full curves - high LET radiation, showing less variation with phase.

The biggest gains will obviously be obtained for tumors which have all their cells in an X-ray-resistant phase. Fig 4 illustrates how the KGF decreases as the proportion of X-ray resistant cells (such as late S) decreases in a hypothetical tumor (Withers and Peters, 1979). Such a change in proportion is called redistribution and will occur more rapidly in a kinetically active tumor, for example a fast-growing tumor. This line of reasoning suggests that slowly growing, rather inert, tumors may benefit most from the kinetic gain factor when neutrons are used. This conclusion is not in contradiction with the requirement for a high hypoxic gain factor, that the tumor should not shrink and reoxygenate too fast. For this reason the HGF is also shown in Fig 4, where a shift to the left represents an "active" type of tumor in which both these advantages of high LET would be diminished.

NEUTRON GAIN vs. TUMOR BEHAVIOR

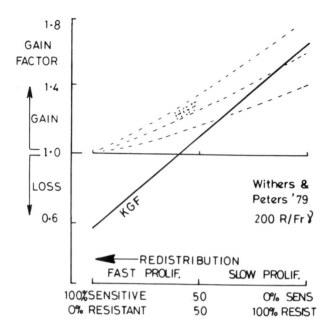

Fig. 4. *Kinetics gain factor (full line) as a function of the proportion of low-LET-resistant cells in a population. As this proportion falls, due to redistribution of cell age through the cycle, before the next dose fraction, KGF obviously decreases. It can fall below 1.0. The dotted lines show the hypoxic gain factors from Fig 2. Both KGF and HGF fall for "kinetically active" tumors.*

It should be noted from Fig 4 that KGF can go below unity. This means that if redistribution, or partial synchrony at the time of the next dose, causes most of the cells to be in a phase that would be <u>sensitive</u> to X-rays, then the use of high LET radiation would of course lead to a therapeutic <u>disadvantage</u>.

There are two possible situations in which the KGF might be high, so that a therapeutic advantage would be expected from the use of high LET radiation:

(1) In very slowly growing tumors with a large proportion of cells in $G_0$ or $G_1$; assuming that cells in these phases are relatively resistant to ordinary low-LET X-rays.

(2) In very fast growing tumors with a large proportion of cells in the S phase, which is resistant to X-rays.

We would not know which of these opposing views to prefer if it were not for a hint from clinical results of neutron treatments of lung metastases at Amsterdam. Higher RBE's were found for the volume reduction of the metastases which grew slowly than for those that grew fast (Van Peperzeel et al 1974). Batterman et al (1981) have obtained further similar results. It therefore seems that very slowly growing tumors should be tested in clinical trials, and that those of intermediate growth rate should be avoided.


LESS REPAIR CAPACITY AFTER HIGH LET IRRADIATION ?

Apart from the possibility of potentiation mentioned below, it is difficult to see how the reduced capacity for intracellular repair of sublethal injury (Elkind-Sutton repair) after high LET radiation can give rise to a therapeutic advantage, unless by chance the reduction is greater in the tumor than in normal tissues. There is no reason for expecting this on any known basis. There is, however, some reason for expecting the opposite, because some authors have reported less repair after X-rays in tumors than in normal tissues (Denekamp and Stewart 1979). Recent clinical evidence suggests that higher RBE's are found for late than for early damage. This goes in the direction of losing, with high LET radiation, an advantage of ordinary photons, that late damage has more repair capability than early damage for small doses per fraction (Withers et al. 1982). This trend has been difficult to detect in animal radiobiology and tends to be seen only for many very small dose fractions (Fowler 1982). It is perhaps significant that the clinical neutron centres that are most pleased with their results are Hammersmith (Catterall 1982) and Fermilab (Cohen 1982). These are centres which use relatively large neutron doses per fraction, 1.3 grays (excluding γ) x 12 and 1.7 grays (including γ) x 12-13 respectively.

Ngo et al have reported <u>potentiation</u> of lethal damage in hamster V79 cells in culture if two doses of ions of LET

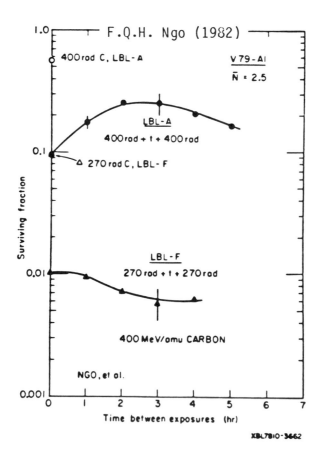

Fig. 5. *The fall in survival when two doses of neon ion irradiation are given demonstrate potentiation. It does not occur if the cells are held at 22°C or 4°C instead (lower curve). The neon ions have an LET of 234 keV/um in the Bragg peak (Ngo 1982).*

greater than 80 keV/um were given (Fig 5). This is the opposite of the repair that is observed between two doses of X-rays or - the point here - charged particles in the plateau region before the Bragg peak is reached. This potentiation was only partially reduced by holding the cells at 4°C so it was assumed to be not entirely due to induced synchrony. It would give a differentially greater cell kill in the peak dose volume than in the overlying plateau region. If the peak volume fitted neatly round the tumor and no vital normal tissues were included, it would augment the known advantages of high local dose and high RBE in the peak volume. A similar potentiation has been observed in vivo for acute intestinal radiation injury (Phillips & Goldstein 1979). However, for a more slowly proliferating normal tissue, mouse lung, significant repair was observed instead of proliferation (Phillips & Goldstein 1979, Curtis 1979, Travis et al, 1982). It can be concluded, on the basis of the present rather few observations, that potentiation can be observed in rapidly proliferating but not in slowly proliferating cell populations. Whether the phenomenon is an advantage in radiotherapy therefore depends upon how exclusively tumors and critical normal tissues fit into those categories.


OPTIONS FOR FUTURE NEUTRON TREATMENTS

In the previous section it was suggested that a large number of small neutron fractions should be avoided, because the sparing of late normal-tissue injury by ordinary X-rays is lost with high LET. This gives the opportunity of using somewhat fewer, rather large, fractions of neutrons (but not larger than Hammersmith or Fermilab have used).

With only about 12 fractions, the opportunity arises to test shorter overall times than usual. These must provide some advantage with respect to killing tumor cells that would proliferate in a longer overall time. There should be no difference in late damage caused by this shortening, although acute damage may be made somewhat more severe. At least the acute damage can be seen and assessed while the optimum dose for the shortened schedule is being worked out in the pilot study. The overall time can be as short as possible consistent with acceptable acute responses in normal tissues (Withers et al 1982).

It is clear that neutron therapy trials should not continue to admit all types of tumor, because this will dilute clinical trials with reoxygenated and/or kinetically active tumors. It was suggested above that very slow growing tumors should be tried. Another basis of selection will emerge when it is possible to measure how many hypoxic cells remain present in tumors during ordinary radiotherapy.

ACKNOWLEDGEMENTS

It is a pleasure to acknowledge stimulating discussions with Drs Alper, Barendsen, Batterman, Breur, Catterall, Cohen, Curtis, Denekamp, Duncan, Field, Hornsey, Ngo, Peters, Phillips, Thames and Withers. I have not agreed with all of them all of the time and they should not be blamed for my present views.

REFERENCES

Batterman JJ, Breur K, Hart, GAM and Van Peperzeel HA (1981). Europ J Cancer 00:000.

Catterall M (1982). Clinical Use of Neutrons - Introduction and the Hammersmith Experience. Proc Workshop on Particle Accelerators in Radiation Therapy - Part III. Int J Rad Oncol Biol Phys (in press).

Cohen L (1982). Clinical Use of Neutrons - the Fermi-Lab Experience, Ibidem.

Curtis SB (1979). The biological properties of high-energy heavy charged particles. In Okada S, Imamura M, Terasima T, Yamaguchi H (eds): "Radiation Research", Tokyo: Japanese Association for Radiation Research, p 780.

Denekamp J and Stewart FA (1979). Evidence for repair capacity in mouse tumours relative to skin. Int J Rad Oncol Biol Phys 5:2003.

Fowler JF (1981). "Nuclear Particles in Cancer Treatment." Bristol: Adam Hilger Press, 178 pp.

Gragg RL, Humphrey RM, Thames HD and Meyn RE (1978). The response of Chinese hamster ovary cells to fast neutron radiotherapy beams. III. Variations in RBE with position in the cell cycle. Radiat Res 76:283.

Hall EJ, Kellerer A (1979). Review of RBE data for cells in culture. In Barendsen GW, Broerse JJ, Breur K (eds): "High LET Radiations in Clinical Radiotherapy," Oxford: Pergamon Press, p 171.

Henk JM, Kunkler PB and Smith CW (1977). Radiotherapy and hyperbaric oxygen in head and neck cancer. The Lancet, July 16th:101.

Ngo FQH, Blakely EA, Tobias CA (1981). Sequential exposures of mammalian cells to low- and high-LET radiations. I. Lethal effects following X-ray and neon-ion irradiation. Radiat Res 87:59.

Ngo FQH (1982). Effects on mammalian cells of fractionated heavy-ion doses, In Skarsgard LD (ed) "International Workshop on Pion and Heavy Ion Radiotherapy". New York: Elsevier North-Holland. (In press).

Phillips TL, Goldstein L (1979). quoted in Curtis (1979).

Raju MR, Tobey RA, Jett JH, Walters RA (1975). Age response for line CHO Chinese hamster cells exposed to X-irradiation and alpha particles from plutonium. Radiat Res 63: 422.

Raju MR (1980). "Heavy Particle Radiotherapy." New York: Academic Press, 500 pp.

Sinclair WK (1970). Dependence of radiosensitivity on cell age. In "Time and Dose Relationships in Radiation Biology as Applied to Radiotherapy," BNL Report 50203 (C 57), p 97.

Travis EL, Curtis SB, Fowler, JF, Phillips TL (1982). Repair observed in mouse lung after fractioned doses of 4cm peak neon ions (in press).

Watson ER, Halnan KE, Dische S, Saunders MI, Cade IS, McEwen JB, Wiernik G, Perrins, DJD, Sutherland I (1978). Hyperbaric oxygen and radiotherapy a Medical Research Council trial in carcinoma of the cervix. Br J Radiol 51:879.

Withers HR, Thames HD and Peters LJ (1982). Biological bases for high RBE values for late effects of neutron irradiation. Proc. Workshop on Particle Accelerators in Radiation Therapy, Part III, Int J Rad Oncol Biol Phys (in press).

Withers HR, Peters LJ (1979). The application of RBE values to clinical trials of high-LET radiations. In Barendsen GW, Broerse JJ, Breur K (eds): "High LET Radiations in Clinical Radiotherapy," Oxford: Pergamon Press, p 257.

Van Peperzeel HA, Breur K, Broerse JJ and Barendsen GW (1974) RBE values of 15 MeV neutrons for responses of pulmonary metastases in patients. Europ J Cancer 10:349.

13th International Cancer Congress, Part D
Research and Treatment, pages 261–265
© 1983 Alan R. Liss, Inc., 150 Fifth Avenue, New York, NY 10011

CLINICAL EXPERIENCE OF FAST NEUTRON THERAPY IN EDINBURGH

William Duncan, F.R.C.S.E.,F.R.C.P.E.,F.R.C.R.

Department of Clinical Oncology
University of Edinburgh
Western General Hospital, Edinburgh, Scotland.

The hospital based neutron beam facility in Edinburgh accommodates a compact cyclotron (CS 30 machine) manufactured by The Cyclotron Corporation. It generates a beam of 15 MeV deuterons which is directed on to a thick beryllium target to provide a spectrum of fast neutrons. The neutrons are then collimated in an isocentric treatment machine capable of 240° rotation or by a similar system of wooden applicators in a fixed horizontal beam. Both treatment arrangements have field defining lights, optical range finders, back pointers and a range of interlocked wedge filters. The radiotherapy techniques that can be employed in this facility are therefore similar to those of most megavoltage X-ray machines. The only real limitation on its application is the relatively poor penetration of the beam which is similar to most 300 kV machines. The dose rate is satisfactory, normally about 40 rads/minute, and the machine has operated reliably during the five years of the clinical programme which began in 1977.

The clinical studies in Edinburgh have been directed to evaluate equally normal tissue reactions and tumour responses, and as much as possible to the comparison of neutrons and photons in randomly controlled trials.

The first trial that was started compared neutron and photon irradiation in the treatment of patients with 'head and neck' cancer. All patients had histologically proved squamous cell carcinoma of the oral cavity, oropharynx, larynx and hypopharynx. The primary objective of the trial was to observe the local tumour control rates after neutrons and photons while keeping similar rates of morbidity. The dose levels employed had therefore been the subject of earlier clinical studies. A slightly higher dose was administered to tumour sites in the oral cavity and oropharynx compared to the larynx and hypopharynx. Also a reduction in dose was made when the field size exceeded 50 cm$^2$. The gamma ray contribution was approximately 7% of the total absorbed dose of neutrons. There was little difficulty in producing a comparable quality of dose distribution in the treatment plans for patients treated by neutrons or photons. A total of 116 patients have been analysed of whom 57 had been randomly selected to receive neutron therapy and 59 photon irradiation. The distribution of T and N categories are similar in the two treatment groups and the groups are also well balanced for age and performance status. There is no significant difference in the complete tumour regression rate observed after neutron therapy (80.2%) and photon therapy (76.4%). At the time of this review a similar number of patients had recurred in both groups and the local tumour control rates are not significantly different, being 52.6% after neutrons and 42.4% after photons. Careful observations were also made of the rate of regression and of recurrence, and both are again similar in both treatment groups. The normal tissue radiation reactions have been evaluated using the RTOG/EORTC scoring system. It is of interest that although it had been considered as a result of preliminary clinical studies that the dose levels employed would produce similar acute mucosal reactions after neutrons or photons, they were on analysis significantly more severe in patients treated by photons ($p < .001$). The acute skin reactions were significantly greater after neutrons ($p < .05$) which was to be expected in view of the skin scarring observed with 4 MV X-rays. However when the numbers of serious late reactions are recorded, they are significantly greater in skin and subcutaneous tissues in patients treated with neutrons ($p < .001$). There was no evidence of a qualitative advantage in tumour regression after neutron irradiation, and there was a real disadvantage in the relative degree of late normal tissue reactions.

The next controlled study undertaken was of patients with cerebral gliomas, after either biopsy or sub-total excision. Eligible patients were stratified by the extent of surgery and by age before randomisation. The treatment involved whole brain irradiation. A target absorbed dose of

13.8 gray (10% gamma) was prescribed for neutrons and 47.5 gray with 4 MV photons; both given in 20 daily fractions. Only 34 patients were randomised, 18 to receive neutron irradiation, 16 to have X-ray therapy. There is no significant difference in survival rates to four years between the neutron and photon-treated groups. Following neutron irradiation two patients developed features of dementia and ataxia that were considered to be the result of demyelinisation induced by irradiation. This was confirmed at autopsy in one of these patients, and in one other there was evidence of white matter degeneration. We believe, therefore, that three of the 18 patients treated by fast neutrons had evidence of radiation myelopathy. None treated by photons exhibited the clinical features or histological appearances of such an effect. The trial was therefore discontinued. The neutron dose level employed was about 5% less than the lower neutron dose given in the Hammersmith trial. It was found, however, that there was still an appreciable incidence of radiation induced brain damage, while in all but one of these patients there was still evidence of residual tumour. These observations are again of a qualitative disadvantage of fast neutrons in respect of normal tissue damage, while no evidence pointed to an enhanced effect on this particular tumour.

In order to examine the responses of another histological type of tumour and other normal tissues, a randomly controlled trial was conducted of patients with transitional cell carcinoma of the bladder. Patients had to have a histologically confirmed bladder cancer suitable for management by radical radiotherapy. Treatment was given in 20 daily fractions for neutrons and photons. The treatment techniques were however quite different because of the comparatively poor penetration of the neutron beam. Six fields were necessary to achieve a satisfactory plan with neutrons, while the technique with photons employed only three fields. The target absorbed doses were 16.5 gray (total dose) with neutrons and 55.0 gray with 4 MV X-rays. 112 patients were recruited to this study, 53 being treated with neutrons and 59 with photons. The distribution of tumour stage and histological grade are similar in the two treatment groups. Patients were assessed by cystoscopy, biopsy and bimanual examination under anaesthesia at approximately six months after the start of radiotherapy. It was observed that the local tumour control was similar after neutrons (50.9%) and photons (48.3%). No qualitative difference was seen following neutron therapy compared to photon therapy in respect of tumour responses. When normal tissue reactions were analysed it was found that there was a significantly greater number of patients with severe acute bladder reactions in the photon group. There was however a larger proportion of patients in the neutron-treated group who had severe late bladder mor- bidity. When bowel reactions were compared there was no significant difference in the distribution of scores for acute effects between the neutron and photon groups. However, again when the degree of the late reactions in the recto-sigmoid were compared, there is a highly significant increase in serious reactions in patients treated with fast neutrons (p $<$ .001). The relative distribution of dose in the pelvis was quite different in the two groups because of the poor penetration of the neutron beam. This imbalance may have contributed to the high level of morbidity experienced in the neutron-treated group. However this fact will not have influenced the very significant disassociation observed between early and late bowel reactions following neutron therapy. The RBE for late effects is clearly much higher than for acute reactions in the large bowel.

The responses of other tumours have also been measured, including adenocarcinoma of the rectum, soft tissue sarcomas, malignant melanoma and salivary gland cancers. Apart from adenoid cystic carcinoma arising in the salivary glands, the tumour control rates observed have been no greater than we would have expected following photon therapy. The treatment of malignant salivary gland tumours, particularly the adenoid cystic carcinoma, requires further careful evaluation by randomly controlled clinical trials to determine if there is a significant qualitative difference in its response to neutrons compared with photons.

With the one possible exception of salivary gland tumours, we have not seen any significant qualitative difference in tumour responses following neutrons compared with photons. There is evidence of a qualitative disadvan- tage in the response of certain normal tissues to fast neutrons. There is a significant increase in the severity of late normal tissue reactions after neutrons compared to those seen following photon irradiation, and in some tissues there is a disassociation of early and late reactions. A particular disadvantage of fast neutrons is the increased absorption in fatty tissue, which probably contributes to increased morbidity in some organs and tissues as well as in subcutaneous tissue.

We have found, therefore, no evidence of an increase in therapeutic ratio which would indicate that neutron therapy is of clinical advantage. The effectiveness of the techniques employed may have been limited by the comparatively poor penetrating quality of the neutron beam in Edinburgh. The next generation of hospital based high energy cyclotrons now being manufactured and installed will better be able to make a definitive assessment of fast neutron therapy compared to results achieved by good megavoltage X-ray therapy.

13th International Cancer Congress, Part D
Research and Treatment, pages 267–277
© 1983 Alan R. Liss, Inc., 150 Fifth Avenue, New York, NY 10011

A DETAILED ANALYSIS OF THE MDAH-TAMVEC NEUTRON THERAPY TRIALS
FOR HEAD AND NECK CANCER

David H. Hussey, M.D., Moshe H. Maor, M.D.,
Gilbert H. Fletcher, M.D.

Department of Radiotherapy
The University of Texas M. D. Anderson Hospital
and Tumor Institute at Houston
Houston, Texas USA 77030

INTRODUCTION

Between October 1972 and March 1980, UT M. D. Anderson
Hospital (MDAH) conducted a series of studies to evaluate the
effectiveness of fast neutron therapy for locally advanced
head and neck cancers. During this period, four clinical
trials were performed: 1) a pilot study using neutrons alone
two or four times weekly, 2) a pilot study using mixed-beam
irradiation, twice weekly with neutrons and three times weekly
with photons, 3) a pilot study of conventional treatment using
surgery or photons or a combination of surgery and photons,
and 4) a randomized trial of mixed-beam or photon irradiation.
The results of these studies have been published previously
(Maor et al. 1981).

In this paper, the head and neck studies are analyzed in
more detail than previously. The objectives were to evaluate
time-dose relationships for neutron therapy and to define a
subset of patients that benefited from this treatment. The
data are analyzed in terms of: 1) site of the primary tumor,
2) stage of the disease, 3) radiation dose delivered, and 4)
site of treatment failure.

MATERIALS AND METHODS

The neutron treatments were delivered with the Texas A&M
University variable energy cyclotron (TAMVEC), using a neutron

beam produced by 50-MeV deuterons incident on a thick beryllium target (50 MeV$_{d \to Be}$).* The photon treatments were delivered with $^{60}$Co gamma rays, occasionally supplemented with
18 MeV x-rays or 6-18 MeV electrons. The dosimetric properties of the 50 MeV$_{d \to Be}$ neutron beam have been described previously (Hussey, Fletcher 1974).

The neutron-beam doses are reported in terms of the
physical dose including both the neutron and the gamma components (rad$_{n\gamma}$). The mixed-beam doses are reported in terms
of the total equivalent dose (rad$_{eq}$), which was determined
by multiplying the neutron physical dose by a relative biological effectiveness (RBE) of 3.1 and adding the result to
the dose delivered with photons. The RBE of 3.1 was determined clinically by comparing the late effects of neutrons
delivered twice weekly with the late effects of photons
delivered in fractions of 200 rad five times weekly (Hussey
et al. 1982).

The standard photon treatment policies at MDAH were
adapted for the neutron therapy program. The same treatment
portals, total equivalent dose, and overall time were employed for neutron and mixed-beam therapy as would have been used
with photon irradiation. The aim was to deliver 6000-6500
rad$_{eq}$ in 6-6½ weeks for moderately advanced tumors and 6500-
7000 rad$_{eq}$ in 6½-7 weeks for massive cancers.

The patients in the neutrons-only pilot study were irradiated with neutrons either twice weekly (160 rad$_{n\gamma}$ per
fraction) or four times weekly (80 rad$_{n\gamma}$ per fraction). A
weekly dose of 320 rad$_{n\gamma}$ is equivalent to 1000 rad delivered
in five fractions per week with $^{60}$Co gamma rays, assuming an
RBE of 3.1 relative to 200-rad $^{60}$Co fractions. The mixed-
beam treatments were delivered with neutrons twice weekly
in 65-rad$_{n\gamma}$ fractions (RBE= 3.1) and with photons three times
weekly in 200-rad fractions.

The field arrangements were determined by the site of
the primary tumor and the distribution of the regional lymph
node metastases. The regional lymphatics of the lower neck
were usually treated with a single anterior $^{60}$Co portal. The

---

* Eleven patients in the neutrons-only pilot study were
treated with a 16 MeV$_{d \to Be}$ neutron beam. For this analysis,
the 16 MeV$_{d \to Be}$ doses have been multiplied by a factor of 1.2,
the ratio of the clinical RBE's (3.7/3.1).

dose to the spinal cord was limited to no more than 4500 $rad_{eq}$ in $4\frac{1}{2}$ weeks using an RBE of 4.1.*

RESULTS

A total of 237 patients with locally advanced head and neck cancers were treated in the MDAH-TAMVEC neutron therapy program. Of these, 142 patients were treated in pilot studies and 95 in the randomized clinical trial. The data were analyzed a uniform 24 months following the initiation of treatment because the duration of follow-up differed for each study.

In the pilot studies, 66 patients were treated with neutrons alone, 31 with mixed-beam irradiation, and 45 with conventional treatment. There was no appreciable difference among the pilot studies with regard to local tumor control or patient survival. However, the complication rate in the mixed-beam pilot study was significantly lower than those observed in the neutrons-only and conventional-treatment pilot studies. None of the patients in the mixed-beam study (0/31) developed major complications, whereas 15% (10/66) of those in the neutrons-only study and 20% (9/45) of those in the conventional-treatment study did. Nine of the ten major complications in the neutrons-only study occurred following treatment with radiotherapy alone. The majority of complications in the conventional-treatment study were at least partly related to surgery, since eight of the nine complications in this group occurred following major surgical procedures.

In the randomized clinical trial, 54 patients were treated with mixed-beam irradiation and 41 with photon irradiation. The preliminary results of this study showed a slight superiority for mixed-beam irradiation, although the difference is not statistically significant. In the mixed-beam group, 46% (25/54) had local tumor control, 7% (4/54) developed major complications, and 35% (15/54) were alive at 2 years; whereas in the photon group, 41% (17/41) had local tumor control, 7% (3/41) developed major complications, and 20% (8/41) were alive at 2 years.

---

* Large-animal radiobiology studies at MDAH-TAMVEC have shown that the RBE for 50 $MeV_{d \to Be}$ neutrons for spinal cord injury is 4.1, a significantly higher value than that obtained for other normal tissues (Hussey et al. 1982).

TABLE 1

COMPARISON OF 2 YEAR LOCAL CONTROL RATES BY PRIMARY SITE
AND TREATMENT MODALITY

| | PILOT STUDIES | | | RANDOM STUDY | |
|---|---|---|---|---|---|
| | Neutrons Only | Mixed Beam | Conventional Treatment | Mixed Beam | Photons |
| Oral cavity | 6/14 (42.9%) | 1/3 | 8/21 (38.1%) | 1/6 | 1/6 |
| Gingiva | 0/1 | 0/1 | | 0/1 | 1/1 |
| Floor of mouth | 3/8 | 0/1 | 4/9 | 1/3 | 0/2 |
| Oral tongue | 3/5 | 1/1 | 2/9 | | 0/3 |
| Hard palate | | | 1/2 | | |
| Buccal mucosa | | | 1/1 | 0/2 | |
| Oropharynx | 13/27 (48.1%) | 9/15 (60%) | 10/16 (62.5%) | 18/36 (50.0%) | 13/29 (44.8%) |
| Tonsillar fossa | 2/7 | | 3/3 | 4/9 | 6/11 |
| Faucial arch | 4/4 | 2/2 | 2/3 | 3/7 | 2/5 |
| Base of tongue | 4/11 | 4/9 | 4/6 | 8/16 | 2/7 |
| Pharyngeal wall | 3/5 | 3/4 | 1/4 | 3/4 | 3/6 |
| Salivary gland | 4/7 | 3/3 | | | |
| Other Primary Sites | 2/7 | 1/2 | 2/6 | 0/3 | 2/3 |
| Nodal metastasis ($T_0$ or $T_X$) | 2/5 | | | 3/4 | 1/1 |
| Recurrent tumor | 1/6 | 0/8 | 0/2 | 3/5 | 0/2 |
| at primary site | 0/2 | 0/4 | 0/1 | 2/2 | 0/1 |
| in nodes | 1/4 | 0/4 | 0/1 | 1/3 | 0/1 |
| TOTAL | 28/66 (42.4%) | 14/31 (45.2%) | 20/45 (44.4%) | 25/54 (46.3%) | 17/41 (41.5%) |

## Analysis by Primary Site

There was a significant difference in the distribution of clinical material by tumor site for the three pilot studies. There were more patients with oral cavity tumors in the conventional-treatment pilot study (47%, 21/45) than in either the neutrons-only (21%, 14/66) or mixed-beam pilot studies (10%, 3/31). On the other hand, a greater percentage of the mixed-beam patients had oropharyngeal tumors. Only 4% (2/45) of the patients in the conventional-treatment study presented with recurrent tumors, compared with 9% (6/66) of those in the neutrons-only study and 26% (8/31) of those in the mixed-beam study. The distribution of clinical material by tumor site was well balanced for the randomized clinical trial, although slightly more patients in the mixed-beam group presented with nodal metastases ($T_0$ or $T_X$) or recurrent tumors.

In general, there were no tumor sites where any one treatment modality showed a clear superiority over the other modalities (Table 1), perhaps because the number of patients in each category was small. In the oral cavity, the local control rate with neutrons alone was the same as that achieved with conventional-treatment, and in the oropharynx, the improvement with mixed-beam irradiation was minimal. The results for faucial arch and pharyngeal wall cancers were slightly better in the neutrons-only and mixed-beam pilot studies than in the conventional-treatment pilot study, and in the randomized trial, the control rate with mixed-beam irradiation for base-of-tongue tumors was slightly better than that achieved with photons. However, the results for tonsillar fossa lesions were slightly better with conventional photon irradiation.

Other sites where there may have been a slight advantage with neutron or mixed-beam irradiation were salivary gland tumors, nodal metastases ($T_0$ or $T_X$), and recurrent tumors. Seven of ten patients with massive salivary gland tumors treated with neutron or mixed-beam irradiation had local control, and six of ten were surviving at 2 years.

TABLE 2

COMPARISON OF THE PILOT STUDY RESULTS AT 2 YEARS

| Pilot Study/Stage[*] | Local Control | | Complications | | Survival | |
|---|---|---|---|---|---|---|
| Neutrons only | 42.4% (28/66) | | 15.2% (10/66) | | 19.7% (13/66) | |
| III | | 60% ( 3/5 ) | | 20% ( 1/5 ) | | 40% ( 2/5 ) |
| IV, or recurrent | | 41% (25/61) | | 14.8% ( 9/61) | | 18% (11/61) |
| Mixed beam | 45.2% (14/31) | | 0% ( 0/31) | | 32.3% (10/31) | |
| III | | 66.7% ( 4/6 ) | | 0% ( 0/6 ) | | 66.7% ( 4/6 ) |
| IV, or recurrent | | 40% (10/25) | | 0% ( 0/25) | | 24% ( 6/25) |
| Conventional treatment | 44.4% (20/45) | | 20% ( 9/45) | | 28.9% (13/45) | |
| III | | 46.7% ( 7/15) | | 20% ( 3/15) | | 33.3% ( 5/15) |
| IV, or recurrent | | 43.3% (13/30) | | 20% ( 6/30) | | 26.7% ( 8/30) |

* AJC staging:
    Stage III = $T_3N_{0-1}M_0$
    Stage IV = $T_3N_{2-3}M_0$, $T_4N_{0-3}M_0$, $T_{X-0}N_3$

TABLE 3

COMPARISON OF THE RANDOMIZED STUDY RESULTS AT 2 YEARS

| Treatment/Stage | Local Control | | Complications | | Survival | |
|---|---|---|---|---|---|---|
| Mixed beam | 46.3% (25/54) | | 7.4% (4/54) | | 35.2% (19/54) | |
| III | | 58.3% (7/12) | | 8.3% (1/12) | | 66.7% (8/12) |
| IV, or recurrent | | 42.9% (18/42) | | 7.1% (3/42) | | 26.2% (11/42) |
| Photons | 41.5% (18/41) | | 7.3% (3/41) | | 19.5% (8/41) | |
| III | | 50% (5/10) | | 10% (1/10) | | 50% (5/10) |
| IV, or recurrent | | 38.7% (12/31) | | 6.5% (2/31) | | 9.7% (3/31) |

## Analysis by Clinical Stage

On the average, the patients in the neutrons-only pilot study had slightly more advanced cancers than those in the mixed-beam pilot study and the patients in the mixed-beam study had more-advanced cancers than those in the conventional-treatment pilot study. Ninety-two percent (61/66) of the patients in the neutrons-only study presented with stage IV or recurrent tumors compared with 81% (25/31) of those in the mixed-beam study and 67% (30/45) of those in the conventional-treatment study. The clinical stage distributions for patients in the two arms of the randomized clinical trial were the same, with three-fourths of the patients in each group presenting with stage IV or recurrent tumors.

The results are listed by clinical stage in Tables 2 and 3. Within each treatment group, the local control and survival rates for stage III tumors were better than those achieved for stage IV or recurrent tumors. However, no treatment modality appeared to be specifically effective for a given stage of the disease. In the randomized clinical trial, mixed-beam irradiation was slightly better than photons for both stage III and stage IV/recurrent tumors. The improvement in local tumor control with mixed-beam irradiation was greater for stage III tumors than for stage IV and recurrent tumors, whereas the improvement in patient survival was greater for stage IV and recurrent tumors (Table 3).

Analysis by Tumor Dose

In general, the doses delivered with neutrons alone varied more than the doses delivered with mixed-beam or photon irradiation. This was because the neutrons-only fractionation schedule was the first to be employed, and the RBE of the 50 MeV$_{d \to Be}$ neutron beam was not then well established. Within each treatment group, the doses varied depending on the site and size of the tumor and its initial response to therapy. Lower doses were employed for patients with smaller tumors and for those whose tumor showed a good initial regression, whereas higher doses were employed for patients with more massive tumors and for those showing poor tumor regression during the course of irradiation.

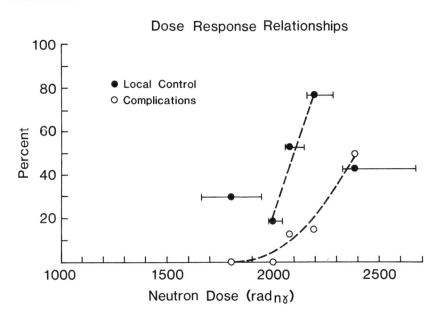

Fig 1. Dose-response relationships for local control and complications for the 66 patients treated with neutrons alone.

A dose-response relationship was noted for local tumor control in the neutrons-only pilot study (Fig 1). Only 19% (3/16) of the patients treated with doses of 1950–2050 rad$_{n\gamma}$ had local tumor control, compared with 53% (8/15) of those treated with 2050–2150 rad$_{n\gamma}$ and 77% (10/13) of those treated

with 2150-2300 rad$_{n\gamma}$.  Similarly, a dose-response relationship
was noted for major complications in this group of patients.
None of the 26 patients (0%) treated with doses less than
2050 rad$_{n\gamma}$ developed major complications, compared with 14%
(4/28) of those treated with doses of 2050-2300 rad$_{n\gamma}$ and 50%
(6/12) of those treated with doses greater than 2300 rad$_{n\gamma}$
(Fig 1).

No dose-response relationship was observed for either
local tumor control or major complications in the mixed-beam
or photon treatment groups.  This is probably because the
clinical material was heterogeneous, and the patients with
more advanced tumors were treated with higher doses.  Although
similar criteria were used to determine the tumor dose for
patients in the neutrons-only study, the doses for that group
also varied because of the uncertainty of the RBE.

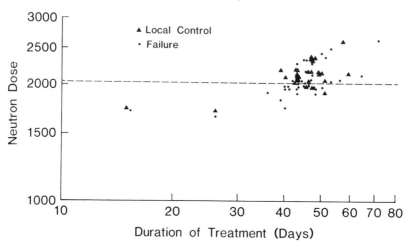

Fig 2.  Time-dose relationship for local control for the
66 patients treated with neutrons alone.

The time-dose relationships for patients treated with
neutrons-only are illustrated in Figures 2 and 3.  The optimum
dose with 50 MeV$_{d \to Be}$ neutrons was ~2100 rad$_{n\gamma}$ in 6½ weeks, but
the range of acceptable neutron doses was narrow.  The local
control rate was poor with doses less than 2050 rad$_{n\gamma}$ (23%,
vs 58% with doses >2050 rad$_{n\gamma}$), and the complication rate was
unacceptable with doses greater than 2150 rad$_{n\gamma}$ (32%, vs 5%
with doses <2150 rad$_{n\gamma}$).

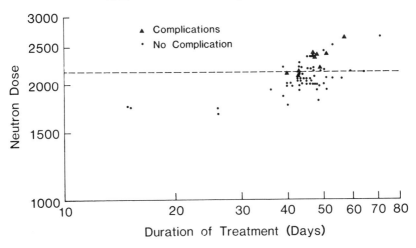

Fig 3. Time-dose relationship for complications for the 66 patients treated with neutrons alone.


Analysis by Site of Failure

The sites of failure are listed by treatment modality in Table 4. There was no significant difference among the treatment groups with regard to the failure rate at the primary site or the incidence of distant metastasis. The failure rates in the regional lymphatics, however, were significantly lower in the groups treated with neutrons alone or with mixed-beam irradiation than in those treated conventionally. In the pilot studies, only 17% (11/66) of patients treated with neutrons alone developed persistent or recurrent disease in the regional lymphatics, compared with 26% (8/31) of those in the mixed-beam study and 38% (17/45) of those in the conventional-treatment pilot study. Likewise, in the random study, only 15% (8/54) of those treated with mixed-beam irradiation had regional failures, compared with 32% (13/41) of those treated with photons. These differences are statistically significant (neutrons only vs conventional-treatment: $\chi^2 = 6.32$, p= .012; mixed-beam vs photons: $\chi^2 = 3.86$, p= .05).

TABLE 4

HEAD AND NECK CANCER: SITES OF FAILURE BY TREATMENT MODALITY

(24 Month Status)

| | PILOT STUDIES | | | RANDOM STUDY | |
|---|---|---|---|---|---|
| | Neutrons Only | Mixed Beam | Conventional Treatment | Mixed Beam | Photons |
| Local Failure | 57.6% (38/66) | 54.8% (17/31) | 55.6% (25/45) | 53.7% (29/54) | 58.5% (24/41) |
| Primary | 48.5% (32/66) | 41.9% (13/31) | 44.4% (20/45) | 42.6% (23/54) | 46.3% (19/41) |
| Regional | 16.7% (11/66) | 25.8% ( 8/31) | 37.8% (17/45) | 14.8% ( 8/54) | 31.7% (13/41) |
| Marginal | 1.5% ( 1/66) | 3.2% ( 1/31) | 0% ( 0/45) | 1.9% ( 1/54) | 4.9% ( 2/41) |
| Distant Metastasis | 18.2% (12/66) | 19.4% ( 6/31) | 28.9% (13/45) | 22.2% (12/54) | 29.3% (12/41) |

* All failures listed. Many patients had failures at more than one site.

TABLE 5

INCIDENCE OF FAILURE IN THE NECK BY INITIAL N STAGE AND TREATMENT MODALITY

| | N STAGE | | | | | | |
|---|---|---|---|---|---|---|---|
| Study/Treatment | $N_{0-X}$ | $N_1$ | $N_2$ | $N_3$ | Neck Recurrence | Primary Recurrence | TOTAL |
| Pilot Studies: | | | | | | | |
| Neutrons only | 2/16 (12.5%) | 0/6 | 1/13 (7.7%) | 5/25 (20.0%) | 3/4 | 0/2 | 11/66 (16.7%) |
| Mixed beam | 1/9 | 0/3 | 1/4 | 2/7 | 3/4 | 1/4 | 8/31 (25.8%) |
| Conventional treatment | 5/16 (31.3%) | 2/6 | 5/15 (33.3%) | 3/6 | 1/1 | 1/1 | 17/45 (37.8%) |
| Random Studies: | | | | | | | |
| Mixed beam | 0/14 | 0/9 | 1/7 | 5/19 (26.3%) | 2/3 | 0/2 | 8/54 (14.8%) |
| Photons | 0/7 | 2/7 | 2/9 | 8/16 (50.0%) | 1/1 | 0/1 | 13/41 (31.7%) |

The incidence of failure in the neck is listed by the initial N stage and treatment modality in Table 5. In the pilot studies, an improvement in the control of neck disease with neutrons-only or mixed-beam irradiation was noted for all stages of neck disease, although the number of patients in each category was small. For the random study, the improvement in the control of neck disease with mixed-beam irradiation was greatest for patients with massive neck disease (stage $N_3$). Only 26% (5/19) of the patients with stage $N_3$ developed recurrence in the neck following mixed-beam irradiation, compared with 50% (8/16) of those treated with photons ($\chi^2$= 2.09, p= .15).

SUMMARY

The local control and survival rates with neutrons-only, mixed-beam, and conventional treatment were similar in the pilot studies, although the complication rate with mixed-beam irradiation was significantly less than that seen with the other treatment modalities. In the randomized trial, the local control and survival rates were better with mixed beam irradiation than with photons although the difference is not statistically significant. In this analysis, there were no tumor sites where any one treatment modality showed a marked superiority over another although neutron and mixed-beam therapy seemed to be most promising for faucial arch, base of tongue, pharyngeal wall, and salivary gland tumors. Analysis of the sites of failure indicated that neutron or mixed-beam therapy may be more effective than conventional radiotherapy in the management of regional lymph-node metastasis. In this study, dose-response relationships for local control and complications were demonstrated for the group treated with 50 MeV$_{d\rightarrow Be}$ neutrons alone. The optimum dose was ~2100 rad$_{n\gamma}$ in 6½ weeks, however, the range of acceptable neutron doses was narrow.

REFERENCES

Maor MH, Hussey DH, Fletcher GH, Jesse RH. (1981). Fast neutron therapy for locally advanced head and neck tumors. Int J Radiat Oncol Biol Phys 7:155.

Hussey DH, Fletcher GH. (1974). Clinical features of 16 and 50 MeV$_d$ Be neutrons. Europ J Cancer 10:357.

Hussey DH, Smathers JB, Meyn RE. (1982). Neutron Therapy. In Bleehen NM, Glatstein E, Haybittle J (eds): Radiation Therapy Planning", New York: Marcel Dekker, Inc., p 393.

13th International Cancer Congress, Part D
Research and Treatment, pages 279–290
© 1983 Alan R. Liss, Inc., 150 Fifth Avenue, New York, NY 10011

# HEAVY PARTICLE EXPERIENCE IN THE TREATMENT OF HUMAN CANCER

Joseph R. Castro, Cornelius A. Tobias, William M.
Saunders, George T.Y. Chen, J. Michael Collier,
John T. Lyman, Kay H. Woodruff, Theodore L. Phillips,
Ranu Grewal-Bahl, Devron Char and Stephen K. Carter

University of California Lawrence Berkeley
Laboratory, Division of Biology and Medicine
University of California School of Medicine,
San Francisco, Department of Radiation Oncology
Northern California Oncology Group, Palo Alto

Supported by NIH/NCI CA19138, CA15184, CA21744, DOE W7405ENG48

One of the attractive areas of radiation oncologic
research is the possibility of improved local and regional
control of resistant tumors through delivery of more effective
radiation therapy to the tumor target volume with lesser dose
to the adjacent normal tissues.

A number of potentially useful modalities are under
study including combinations of debulking surgery and radiotherapy, hyperthermia, and different fractionation schemata
for photon irradiation.

At the University of California Lawrence Berkeley
Laboratory we have been studying another approach, that of
radiotherapy with helium and heavier charged particles which
have several advantageous characteristics for delivery of
cancerocidal therapy to deep seated tumors. These include
greater localization of radiation dose to the target volume
as well as potentially greater effects on tumor cell killing
as compared to normal cell damage. These effects include a
lessening of the radiation protective effect of hypoxia on
tumor cells when exposed to heavier ions such as neon, argon,
or silicon (Blakely 1980; Goldstein 1981; Ngo 1981).

Heavy ions also depress enzymatic repair mechanisms, decrease variations of radiosensitivity during the cell division cycle, cause greater than expected delay in the cell division and decrease the protective effects of neighboring cells in organized systems (Blakely 1979; Raju 1978; Rodriguez 1981).

Potential therapeutic advantage may result from these heavy ions if a significant differential in the above parameters can be found between normal and tumor cells.

Prior to human cancer irradiations, an extensive body of pretherapeutic research into the biology and physics of accelerated stripped nuclei has been carried out in cell, tissue and tumor systems in order to focus on the properties desirable for radiation therapy of human cancers (Roots 1980; Tobias 1973; Tobias 1982).

We have particular interest in silicon ions as a possible therapeutic modality. Like argon, it significantly depresses the oxygen effect to oxygen enhancement ratio (OER) values between 1.4 and 1.6 in the extended parallel opposed Bragg peak. However, the effectiveness at depth of argon ions is limited because of particle fragmentation.

Silicon, therefore, offers an attractive, intermediate combination of enhanced biological effect, low OER and reasonable depth dose characteristics. However, further biological and physical studies as well as preliminary human irradiation studies will be needed in order to verify this opinion.

The goal of the clinical program at Lawrence Berkeley Laboratory (LBL) has been to systematically investigate the potential of improved dose localization through irradiation of selected tumor targets with helium ions, a beam which has little if any biologic enhancement, and to study the combined potential of enhanced biologic effect and dose localization by irradiation with heavier particles such as neon or silicon.

Since the helium ion beam has been used clinically for many years at LBL for pituitary irradiation, we were able to accomplish rapid modification of the beam line and patient positioner in order to begin treatment of human cancers with helium ions in 1975 (Castro 1981; 1980;1980).

Heavier particles have required additional effort and time to be produced in quantities sufficient for patient irradiation and to develop clinical beam delivery techniques.

For both types of particles, steady progress has been made in development of treatment techniques, detailed treatment planning, patient immobilization, dosimetry verification and compensation for tissue inhomogeneities.

Clinical Studies

From 6/75 through 2/82, 419 patients have been irradiated in the heavy charged particle clinical trial, including 27 photon control patients.

Table 1

HEAVY PARTICLE CLINICAL TRIAL PATIENTS
(7/75–03/82)

| Anatomic Region | Helium | Heavy Particle |
|---|---|---|
| Head/Neck | 16 | 14 |
| Intracranial | 28 | 21 |
| Ocular | 62 | -- |
| Thoracic | 41 | 14 |
| Abdomen | 131 | 27 |
| Retroperitoneal | 11 | 3 |
| Pelvis | 18 | 1 |
| Skin & Subcutaneous | 1 | 4 |
| TOTAL: | 308 | 84 |

Low LET Photon Control Patients
(Randomized Pancreas Trial)          27

TOTAL PATIENTS IN TRIAL:          419

Of the heavy charged particle patients, 308 have been treated with helium ions, either solely or in combination with photon irradiation, and 84 have received all or part of their irradiation with one of the heavier particles, either carbon, neon, or argon ions.

Current Treatment Protocols

To accomplish these studies, clinical protocols have been developed with the assistance of interested radiotherapists, biologists, physicists, other physicians and allied scientists in the region and in the Northern California Oncology Group (NCOG) and the Radiation Therapy Group (RTOG).

Through an intergroup agreement between the RTOG and NCOG, the NCOG provides the primary assistance in protocol design, statistical support, quality control, data collection, control patient irradiation and referral of patients. Patients within the geographical area of northern California and northwest Nevada are entered through the NCOG. Patients from other parts of the United States may be entered into the clinical trial through the RTOG.

Patients have been irradiated with heavy ions under the following protocols:

| | |
|---|---|
| LBL-NCOG 3E81/RTOG 79-09 | Localized Squamous Cell Carcinoma of the Esophagus, Nonrandomized (Helium and Heavy Ions) |
| LBL-NCOG 7081/RTOG 79-08 | Localized Ocular Melanoma, Nonrandomized (Helium) |
| LBL-NCOG 0R81/RTOG 79-11 LBL Pilot Studies | Phase I-Phase II Study of Locally Advanced Tumors, Nonrandomized Including Head/Neck Tumors Brain Tumors (Helium and Heavy Ions) |
| LBL-Veterans Administration Surgical Oncology Group (VASOG) | Localized Unresectable Carcinoma of the Pancreas, Nonrandomized (Helium and Heavy Ions) |

Helium Ion Radiotherapy (184-inch Cyclotron)

The aim of the helium ion radiation therapy program has been to test the potential clinical advantage of improved dose localization (Chen 1981).

Dose Localization Studies

Helium ions have been tried in a variety of sites where improved dose localization might constitute a possible advantage including:

1) Selected tumors around the base of the skull and spinal cord as well as in the paranasal sinuses;
2) localized soft tissue sarcomata;
3) carcinoma of the biliary tract (localized);
4) localized metastatic lymph node deposits;
5) ocular melanomata;
6) carcinoma of the pancreas and esophagus.

Tumors at Base of Skull or Juxtaspinal Tumors

For tumors adjacent to critical organs such as the spinal cord or at the base of the brain, we believe that we are able to obtain a higher ratio of tumor dose to normal tissue dose with helium ion radiotherapy than can be delivered with photon radiotherapy.

Doses of 60 to 75 Gray-equivalents have been delivered successfully to the tumor target while keeping spinal cord and brain doses to below tolerance. Tumor control in this group of patients has been excellent to date with a low incidence of normal tissue damage.

Table 2

DOSE LOCALIZATION WITH HELIUM IONS
FOR JUXTASPINAL OR BASE OF SKULL TUMORS

| Site | Status No. | NED | Tumor Dose | Average Survival |
|------|------|-----|-----------|------------------|
| Sacral Chordoma | 4 | 3 | 36-75 GyE | 25 mos |
| Clival Chordoma | 6 | 5 |  |  |
| Base of Skull Meningioma | 2 | 1 | 70 GyE | 7 mos |
| Juxtaspinal Tumors | 6 | 6 | 65 GyE | 23 mos |
| TOTALS: | 18 | 15 (83%) |  |  |

Ocular Melanoma

Uveal melanomas are often small when diagnosed and are potentially curable by a localized treatment modality such as surgery or irradiation. This tumor can be precisely localized for radiotherapy by ultrasound, CT scanning, clinical exam and by a surgical procedure in which the ophthalmologist sutures radio-opaque markers around the base of the tumor.

With precisely delivered charged particle radiotherapy such as with protons or helium ions, a high uniform dose can be delivered to the tumor with little dose to nearby critical structures such as optic disc and fovea centralis unless the tumor is within a few millimeters of them. Doses of 70-80 Gray-equivalents may be delivered in 5 fractions over 7 to 10 days.

As of 3/1/82, we have completed treatment in 62 patients with followup to 49 months. Twenty patients received 70 GyE in 5 fractions with failure to control the tumor in one patient due to unknown causes and in three others from now recognized technical errors or multifocal disease. The average survival in this group is 25 months and 11 of 17 patients retaining their eyes have useful vision.

Forty-two patients received 80 GyE in 5 fractions with failure to control the tumor in one patient. A second patient required enucleation because of glaucoma following irradiation of a very large lesion. The average survival in this group of patients is only 10 months with useful vision preserved in 29 of 40 patients retaining their eyes. Overall, the local control rate is 56/62 or 90%.

Thus, only two patients clearly have local failure without a technical explanation; one occurred at a dose of 70 GyE and the other at 80 GyE.

Normal tissue effects has been mild, most commonly consisting of mild epitheliitis of the eyelid and loss of lashes in those cases where the lid cannot be fully retracted out of the radiation field. Two patients have developed cataracts which are not affecting their vision significantly as yet. About two-thirds of the patients have retained useful vision in the treated eye. One patient, with a very large tumor, had shrinkage of the tumor but severe pain secondary to glaucoma and retinal detachment requiring enucleation.

Further studies to elucidate the best dose and fraction number are under development particularly for lesions close to critical structures such as the optic nerve or fovea centralis.

In addition to the avove mentioned sites, dose localization with helium ion irradiation has proven of value in patients with localized soft tissue sarcoma, metastatic disease in paraaortic lymph nodes and localized carcinoma of the biliary tract.

Although not statistically proven in a prospective randomized trial, our observation is that the improved dose localization with charged particles will be of great value for selected tumor target sites providing sufficient increase in tumor dose relative to normal tissues can be achieved.

For tumors like carcinoma of the esophagus and pancreas, the increase in delivered dose with helium ion radiotherapy does not appear sufficient to result in any significant improvement in local control. It appears that for large tumors, increases in tumor dose over standard radiotherapy must be greater than 10-20% to give any chance of significantly improving local control. This is possible with small, localized tumors such as ocular melanomat or juxtaspinal tumors where high doses can be safely given with excellent results. For other more difficult tumor sites, use of heavier particles such as neon or silicon may offer a chance of increased biological potential as well as some slight improvement from dose localization (Castro 1980).

Carcinoma of the Pancreas

Irradiation of patients with localized, unresectable carcinoma of the pancreas has been carried on at Lawrence Berkeley Laboratory since 1976 beginning with helium ions and now progressing to the use of neon particles. With the increasing incidence of this disease in industrialized nations and the potential for local and regional control using radiotherapy, we were interested in determining if patients with localized disease could be controlled by delivering a relatively high dose to the tumor with reduced irradiation of adjacent normal structures. This goal seems achievable with charged particle radiotherapy.

A pilot study of helium ion irradiation was accomplished in which 35 patients received a minimum of 50 GyE (usually 60) given in 2.0 GyE per fraction, 4 fractions per week. With this dose we have achieved local and regional control in about 15% of patients with several patients surviving for long periods without recurrence of disease. The average survival was about 11 months although many patients in the study had advanced disease.

The results were not sufficient to clearly show improvement over standard irradiation so that a randomized trial between helium therapy plus 5-FU and photon therapy plus 5-FU was begun in 1978.

Although this study did not accumulate enough patients in each arm for statistical significance, no difference in survival between the two arms was found. There was a small trend to a longer time interval before local failure in the helium arm but the difference was not statistically significant. A high incidence of liver metastases was encountered in both arms of the study despite careful pretherapeutic evaluation and the chemotherapy. Because it did not appear likely that any major difference between the two arms would develop even if the study was continued to statistical significance, we elected to discontinue this study in favor of proceeding to trials with a heavier particle, namely neon ions.

We expect to shortly begin Phase I studies of neon ion irradiation of patients with carcinoma of the pancreas in which we expect to also utilize multidrug chemotherapy. An eventual prospective controlled study is envisioned to compare with standard and helium ion results.

It seems clear that increased efforts to achieve both local control of pancreatic tumors as well as liver metastases is needed in order to make a significant impact on this disease. To date, our overall experience with this disease using helium and heavy ions has not as yet achieved sufficient local control and survival to clearly be of value. Of 95 patients completing therapy between 1975 and 1981 with all or part of their therapy with helium or heavy ions, only 15% had local/regional control of their disease with 7% surviving an average of 15 months to date free of disease (Castro 1982).

Carcinoma of the Esophagus

Twenty-four patients have now been accrued in a Phase II nonrandomized prospective study for helium and heavy ion irradiation of localized carcinoma of the esophagus.

The tumor dose was initially 60 GyE given at 2.0 GyE per fraction over a period of 7-8 weeks, but was raised in increments to the present level of 69.75 GyE given at 2.25 GyE per fraction in 7½-9 weeks.

Of the initial 24 patients, only six had local control of their tumor. The average survival was 9 months in the helium treated patients.

Table 3

CA of Esophagus

|  | Phase I | Phase II (Helium) | Phase II (Neon) |
|---|---|---|---|
| # of pts | 10 | 22 | 2 |
| NED, Alive | 0 | 1 | 0 |
| Expired NED, ID | 2 | 1 | 0 |
| Expired, NED Complication | 1 | 1 | 0 |
| Failure in XRT Field | 7/10 (70%) | 17/22 (77%) | 1/2 |
| Average Survival | 14 mos | 9 mos | 13 mos |

As these results did not appear any better than those obtained with megavoltage radiotherapy, we have started a Phase II trial using neon ion irradiation. The superior biological potential of this beam over helium ions may afford an improvement in local control. If a significant improvement over the helium results is seen, a prospective randomized study may be needed.

Phase I-II Studies with Neon and Silicon Ions

The goals of the Phase I-II neon and silicon studies are:

1) Evaluation of the potential of improved dose localization.
2) Evaluation of acute and subacute response of normal tissues such as mucosa, skin, and intestine.
3) Initial evaluation of tumor response.
4) Clinical evaluation of the physical and biological dose distributions.
5) Development of effective treatment techniques.
6) Design and implementation of Phase III clinical trials.

Phase I:

Establish maximum tolerable heavy charged particle dose using dose fractions of 2.0-3.0 GyE through treatment of:

Metastatic skin and subcutaneous nodules
Ca esophagus
Ca pancreas
Ca head/neck
Ca stomach
Glioma, brain

Phase II:

Establish levels of local control in specific tumors using maximum tolerable dose as determined in Phase I.

Phase III:

Establish definite superiority of modality (randomized or single arm).

It is our hope to complete the Phase I studies for neon and silicon ions this year so that Phase II and III studies can begin as soon as possible.

The target sites under consideration for possible Phase III heavy particle studies include glioblastoma, advanced upper aero-digestive tract tumors, carcinoma of the esophagus, pancreas, stomach and lung as well as possibly advanced pelvic lesions such as carcinoma of the bladder, prostate or rectum (inoperable).

The final decision regarding Phase III trials is dependent on several factors including additional radiobiological data on silicon ions especially with reference to entrance region versus spread peak biological effectiveness, Phase I and II studies of these sites, availability of patients and planned improvements in beam delivery and treatment techniques.

We fully expect this process to require an additional five years to complete so that a definitive answer to the possible place of these beams in clinical radiotherapy can be determined.

Blakely EA, Ngo FQH, Chang PY, Lommel L and Tobias CA (1980). Silicon: radiobiological cellular survival and the oxygen effect. Lawrence Berkeley Laboratory Report LBL-11220 p 119.

Blakely EA, Tobias CA, Ngo FQH, Yang TCH, Smith KC and Lyman JT (1979). Inactivation of human kidney cells by high energy monoenergetic heavy ion beams. Radiat Res 80:122.

Castro JR (1981). Particle therapy: the first forty years. Seminars in Oncology 8:1:103.

Castro JR, Hendrickson C, Quivey JM, Saunders WM, Hannigan JF, Silverberg IJ and Torti FM (1981). Heavy charged particle radiotherapy for localized esophageal squamous cell carcinoma. Proceedings of Am Soc Clin Oncol 22:450.

Castro JR, Quivey JM, Lyman JT, Chen GTY, Phillips TL, Tobias CA (1980). Radiotherapy with heavy charged particles at Lawrence Berkeley Laboratory. J Canadian Assoc Radiol 31:30.

Castro JR, Quviey JM, Lyman JT, Chen GTY, Phillips TL, Tobias CA and Alpen EL (1980). Current status of clinical particle radiotherapy at Lawrence Berkeley Laboratory. Cancer 46:633.

Castro JR, Saunders WM, Quivey JM, Chen GTY, Collier JM, Woodruff KH, Lyman JT, Twomey P, Frey C and Phillips TL (1982). Clinical problems in radiotherapy of the pancreas. Presented at the annual meeting of the American Radium Society, San Antonio, Texas.

Chen GTY, Castro JR and Quivey JM (1981). Heavy charged particle radiotherapy. Ann Rev of Biophys and Bioeng 10:419.

Goldstein LS, Phillips TL, Fu KK, Ross GY and Kane LJ (1981). Biological effects of accelerated heavy ions: I. Single doses in normal tissues, tumors and cell in vitro. Radiat Res 86:529.

Ngo FQH, Blakely EA and Tobias CA (1981). Sequential exposures of mammalian cells to low and high-LET radiations: I. Lethal effects following X-ray and neon ion irradiation. Radiat Res 87:59.

Raju MR, Bain E, Carpenter SG, Cox RA and Robertson JB (1978). A heavy particle comparative study. Part II. Cell survival versus depth. British J Radiol 51:704.

Rodriguez A and Alpen EA (1981). Cell survival in spheroids irradiated with heavy ion beams. Radiat Res 85:24.

Roots R, Yang T, Craise L, Blakely EA and Tobias CA (1980). Rate of rejoining of DNA breaks induced by accelerated carbon and neon ions in the spread Bragg peak. Radiat Res 38:203.

Tobias CA (1973). Pretherapeutic investigations with accelerated heavy ions. Radiology 108:145.

Tobias CA, Blakely EA, Alpen EL, Castro JR, Ainsworth EJ, Curtis SB, Ngo FQH, Rodriguez A, Roots RJ, Tenforde TS and Yang TCH (1982). Molecular and cellular radiobiology of heavy ions. Presented at the CROS/RTOG PART III Intl Particle Workshop, Houston, Texas.

CONGRESS SYMPOSIA

RADIATION SENSITIZERS AND PROTECTORS Breccia, A.,
Italy, Chairman; Phillips, T., USA, Co-Chairman;
Playhouse

Improved Hypoxic Cell Radiation and Chemosenitizers.
*Adams, G. E., Stratford, I. J. and Sheldon, P. W.,
Sutton, England. (By Title Only)

Clinical Trials with Hypoxic Cell Sensitizers:
The European Experience. *Dische, S.,
Middlesex, England.

Clinical Trials with Hypoxic Cell Sensitizers:
The U.S.A. Experience. *Phillips, T. L.,
Wasserman, T. H., Brady, L. W. and Stetz, J.,
San Francisco, CA USA, St. Louis, MO USA and
Philadelphia, PA USA. (By Title Only)

The Topical Use of Misonidazole in Bladder
Cancer. *Awwad, H. K., El Moneim, H. A.,
El Baki, H. A., Omar, S., El Merzabani, M., and
Farag, H. I., Cairo, Egypt.

Phase I Studies of WR2721 Administered Before
Radiotherapy and Alkylating Agents. *Kligerman,
M.M., Turrisi, A., Glover, D., Yuhas, J. and
Glick, J., Philadelphia, PA USA. (By Title Only)

Please note: Papers that are listed as "By Title
Only" were presented at the 13th International
Cancer Congress, but are not included in these
volumes.

13th International Cancer Congress, Part D
Research and Treatment, pages 293–303
© 1983 Alan R. Liss, Inc., 150 Fifth Avenue, New York, NY 10011

# CLINICAL TRIALS WITH HYPOXIC CELL SENSITIZERS - THE EUROPEAN EXPERIENCE

Stanley Dische, M.D., F.R.C.R.

Marie Curie Research Wing for Oncology,
Regional Radiotherapy Center,
Mount Vernon Hospital,
Northwood, Middlesex HA6 2RN, England.

After nearly 8 years of clinical experience with misonidazole results so far observed in randomized controlled clinical trials can be reviewed. In 8 out of 12 studies in head and neck cancer a margin of benefit has been shown following treatment, but in some this has subsequently been lost. In carcinoma of bladder, uterine cervix and bronchus and in glioblastoma, the large majority of studies show no benefit. The limit as to the total dose of misonidazole which may be given because of the risk of neurotoxicity is probably a major factor leading to these disappointing results. A more efficient radiosensitizing drug will show the extent to which such agents will improve radiotherapy and so also the true importance of hypoxia as a cause of failure in clinical radiotherapy.

On November 1st, 1974, a patient with multiple metastases from carcinoma of cervix received misonidazole as an hypoxic cell sensitizer (Gray, et al., 1976). Nodules were irradiated with and without the sensitizer and the regression and regrowth compared (Thomlinson, et al., 1976). This patient presented a particularly suitable model, there being many subcutaneous nodules within a relatively narrow range of size and shape. An enhancement of overall radiation effect by 20% was determined and in later calculations it was estimated that the proportion of hypoxic cells in these tumor nodules was of the order of 20% (Denekamp, Fowler and Dische, 1977). An increased response was noted in tumor irradiated with misonidazole in 3 of 4 cases where this type of analysis could be made (Thomlinson, et al., 1976).

Further tumor nodule studies have been performed, including one using radiotherapy given in 10 fractions, and these have also demonstrated evidence for an increased effect with misonidazole (Dawes, et al., 1978; Ash, et al., 1980).

The nodule studies were important for they confirmed that hypoxic cells did exist in human tumors and could be sensitized. However, the main objective for the introduction of hypoxic cell sensitizing agents into clinical radiotherapy was to improve the rate of local tumor cure above that currently obtained by conventional radiotherapy when much higher radiation doses are given during multi-fraction courses.

The neurotoxicity of misonidazole which was observed in 1975 led to further clinical studies to determine a safe dose regime (Dische, et al., 1977). The dose limit of 12g per meter square of surface area when misonidazole is given over at least 17 days was established by 1977 and randomized controlled clinical trials started soon afterwards (Dische, et al., 1978).

Now, in 1982, over 5000 patients have been included in some 120 randomized controlled clinical trials with misonidazole and the drug has been given to over 3000 patients. With our knowledge as to the incidence of neurotoxicity we can calculate that at least some 750 cases of peripheral neuropathy have been induced. What have we to show for all this effort and this toxicity? Most of the trials are still continuing and only in some have we interim, let alone definitive results. Those results of randomized controlled trials performed outside North America which are available will be considered.

The dose limit of 12g per meter square of surface area has led to a variety of different patterns of administration designed to overcome this serious limitation of dose. (Fig. 1). First, misonidazole may be given with every treatment in a multi-fraction course of radiotherapy. Necessarily the dose which may be given each day is a small one. Radiotherapy may be given with sensitizer in a small number of fractions when a much higher dose of misonidazole may be given, and because of the high radiation dose we can also expect a greater effect upon hypoxic cells. A variation upon this is to give such doses combined with misonidazole at the beginning or at the end, or both at the beginning and at the end, of a normally fractionated course of radiotherapy. In another application, a

single large dose of misonidazole is given weekly with a large dose
of radiation; smaller doses of radiation are given alone on most
of the other days of the week.   A further variation of this is to
administer a big dose once a week, but to give radiotherapy twice
on that day and again early on the following morning so as to take
advantage of any remaining concentration of drug.   Finally, the
dose of misonidazole may be given before multiple treatments in
one day so that the highest mean concentration of misonidazole may
be attained throughout a course of radiotherapy, or where this is
combined with a 'split-course' during the first or second phases.
All these variants have been used in randomized controlled clinical
trials.

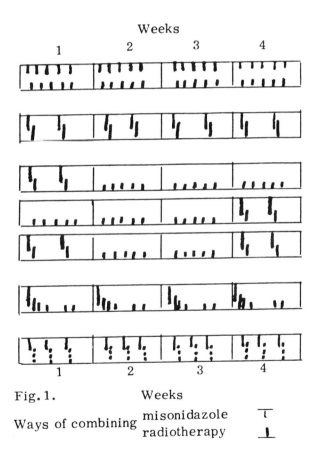

Fig. 1.

Ways of combining misonidazole    radiotherapy

The sensitization which may be achieved depends, of course, on the number of fractions into which misonidazole is distributed. If we go by serum concentrations at the time of treatment, we can see a range of values for sensitization (Table 1).

| Fractionation | Dose g/sq. m | Plateau Plasma Concentration | | Probable levels in hypoxic tumour cells | |
|---|---|---|---|---|---|
| | | μg/ml | Enhancement | μg/g | Enhancement |
| 6 | 2 | 80 | 1.65 | 40 | 1.50 |
| 10 | 1.2 | 50 | 1.55 | 25 | 1.40 |
| 20 | 0.6 | 24 | 1.40 | 12 | 1.20 |
| 24 | 0.5 | 20 | 1.35 | 10 | 1.20 |
| 30 | 0.4 | 16 | 1.25 | 8 | 1.15 |

Table 1. Plateau plasma and levels in hypoxic tumor cells if 50% of the plasma is achieved when misonidazole is given in different fractionation regimes using the dose limit of 12g per meter square of surface area. Also shown are the enhancement ratios for hypoxic cells relating to the concentrations achieved.

These fall far short of the 2.5 - 3.0 for a full sensitization of totally hypoxic cells and the figure decreases further when we consider that the concentration in tumors is lower than that in the serum. For vascularized tumor showing no necrosis, the mean concentration is of the order of 80% but we can expect that the concentration in the hypoxic cells will be lower than the average concentration through the tumor. At worst it may be of the order of 50% and we can see the order of sensitization efficiencies so generated (Table 1). It is no wonder, therefore, that we can be concerned as to the efficiency of misonidazole when given using the current dose limitation.

In those clinical trials in head and neck cancer performed outside North America some results, usually of an interim nature, are available concerning 12 (Table 2).

| Senior Worker/ Title | Location | Case Material | Total No. | Total Dose $g/m^2$ | Assessment of local tumour control |
|---|---|---|---|---|---|
| Sealy | Cape Town South Africa | Advanced oral ca. | 97 | 12 | Early months – benefit to miso. Lost at 1 year |
| Sealy | Cape Town S. Africa | Advanced oral ca. | 64 | 12 | Margin favours miso. |
| Bataini | Paris France | Oral cavity Oropharynx | 84 | 14 | Margin favours miso. (not sig.) |
| DAHANCA | Denmark | Pharynx Larynx | 153 | 11 | Margin favours miso. (not sig.) |
| Arcangeli | Rome Italy | Secondary ca. Neck nodes (mult. lesions) | 25 | 12 | Benefit to miso. |
| MEDICAL RESEARCH COUNCIL | United Kingdom | Oral Pharyngeal Laryngeal | 164 | 12 | No benefit |
| Cattan | Rheims France | Advanced head & neck tumour | 71 | 12 | No benefit |
| Giaux | Lille France | Bucco - pharyngeal | 56 | 12 | Early margin in favour of miso. Lost in further F.U. |
| Bataini | Paris France | Larynx Hypopharynx | 65 | 14 | No benefit |
| MEDICAL RESEARCH COUNCIL | United Kingdom | Oral Pharyngeal Laryngeal | 93 | 12 | No benefit |
| DAHANCA | Denmark | Pharynx Larynx | 143 | 11 | Margin favours miso. (not sig.) |
| Gil-Goyarre | Madrid Spain | Head & neck (incl. some ca. cervix) | 40 | 15 | Early benefit to miso. (P= <0.05) |

Table 2.  Head & Neck (excl. North America)

Of course there are wide differences between the studies. Some are performed in one institution, others at many centers and the misonidazole and radiation protocols differ widely. In 8 of the 12 a margin of improved local control has been seen in the first year and this, in some, reaches statistical significance. However, in several trials this advantage is lost at later times and in most only follow-up will determine the importance of this observation. Looking at the many different regimes employed there is none that stands out as being of particular promise.

In carcinoma of the bladder (Table 3) and in carcinoma of the cervix (Table 4) no benefit has been shown, while in carcinoma of the bronchus (Table 5) there is only a suggestion of improved immediate response without improvement in survival in one of the 4 studies.

| Senior Worker | Location | Case Material | Total No. | Total Dose $g/m^2$ | Assessment of local tumour control |
|---|---|---|---|---|---|
| Basutti | Bologna Italy | $T_3$ $N_x$ $M_o$ | 36 | 12 | Improved response at end of treatment |
| Dische | London England | $T_3$ & $T_4$ $N_x$ $M_o$ | 41 | 12 | No benefit |

Table 3.  Bladder (excl. North America)

| Senior Worker / Title | Location | Case Material | Total No. | Total Dose g/m² | Assessment of local tumour control |
|---|---|---|---|---|---|
| MEDICAL RESEARCH COUNCIL | United Kingdom | Stage III | 153 | 12 | No benefit |
| Scandinavian Trial | Norway Denmark Sweden Finland | Stages IIB, III and IVA | 341 | 12 | No benefit |

Table 4. Cervix (excl. North America)

| Senior Worker | Location | Case Material | Total No. | Total Dose g/m² | Assessment of local tumour control |
|---|---|---|---|---|---|
| Saunders | London England | Locally advanced non oat cell ca. | 62 | 12 | No benefit |
| Basutti | Bologna Italy | Locally advanced non oat cell ca. | 33 | 12 | No benefit |
| Kjaer | Copenhagen Denmark | Inoperable squamous cell ca. | 67 | 12 | No benefit. Trend to poorer survival with misonidazole |
| Mäntylä | Jyväskylä Finland | Inoperable ca. | 46 | 15 | Small improvement in immediate tumour shrinkage |

Table 5. Bronchus (excl. North America)

In the management of glioblastoma we have 4 studies to consider and only in one, the smallest of them, has benefit been shown (Table 6).

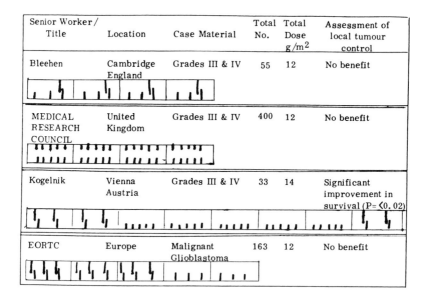

| Senior Worker / Title | Location | Case Material | Total No. | Total Dose g/m² | Assessment of local tumour control |
|---|---|---|---|---|---|
| Bleehen | Cambridge England | Grades III & IV | 55 | 12 | No benefit |
| MEDICAL RESEARCH COUNCIL | United Kingdom | Grades III & IV | 400 | 12 | No benefit |
| Kogelnik | Vienna Austria | Grades III & IV | 33 | 14 | Significant improvement in survival (P= <0.02) |
| EORTC | Europe | Malignant Glioblastoma | 163 | 12 | No benefit |

Table 6. Glioblastoma (excl. North America)

This trial differs in its pattern of radiation dose and administration of misonidazole from the remainder. A doubling of survival has been shown and the control group shows a survival similar to those included in the other studies. This improvement is impressive, although considerable reservations must be made because of the small numbers. Where so many trials take place chance can certainly lead to one of them giving evidence of benefit.

We have, therefore, to record a series of disappointing results. Only in head and neck tumors has any evidence for an increase in radiation effect upon tumor been attained and this has been a relatively modest improvement in immediate local tumor control. Long term follow-up is required in some of the studies to determine whether the degree of benefit would justify the use of a drug which has a real morbidity in the form of neurotoxicity.

We can contrast this dismal pattern of result with the great success of misonidazole in improving tumor control in practically every animal tumor system which is used in the laboratory. Obviously the conditions under which drugs are employed clinically differ greatly from those in the laboratory. A much smaller total dose of misonidazole is used and this must be distributed over the many treatments making up the course.

Does the oxygen effect exist at the 200 cGy dose increment so commonly used in clinical radiotherapy and in a number of the trials? Evidence in the biological laboratory is sparse and contradictory and it remains a point of controversy among our colleagues. There is, however, clear evidence from the effects in normal tissues seen in clinical trials of hyperbaric oxygen that such an effect does occur with a 200 cGy dose increment (Dische et al., 1982).

When misonidazole is given throughout a conventional fractionated course of radiotherapy, only low levels of drug may be reached in hypoxic tumor cells. There have been advocates of administration only at the beginning or at the end of a course of radiotherapy. There are those who feel that unless the drug is combined with a very high radiation dose - high, that is, in relation to the normal 200 cGy dose increment per day - then insufficient sensitization will be achieved. It is possible that we are not employing misonidazole at the time when there is the greatest concentration of hypoxic cells, but unfortunately we have only supposition and theory and no practical technique to guide us as to the best time to employ it.

A further alternative is that after a fractionated course of radiotherapy hypoxia is not a common cause of radiation failure. Obviously every tumor coming to us for treatment contains hypoxic cells, but fractionation may allow even more efficient reoxygenation than occurs in the animal tumor. However, the wide variety of human malignant disease makes it possible that there are subgroups where hypoxia is particularly important as a cause of failure after fractionated radiotherapy and if we could identify these then we would have the type of cases most sensitive to the determination of the efficiency of an hypoxic cell sensitizer.

Analyses of the data in hyperbaric oxygen trials in carcinoma of the cervix have shown support of this suggestion for patients who were so anemic prior to treatment that they required a blood transfusion formed a special group as regards response to treatment (Dische et al. , 1982). Despite all cases being transfused to above a 10g Hb level prior to radiotherapy, those treated in air showed poor local tumor control while those treated in hyperbaric oxygen did extremely well. The most favored explanation is that the type of tumor which most readily bleeds to give rise to anemia is also one where the vascular supply does not facilitate reoxygenation and where hypoxia is indeed a dominant problem, even when anemia is restored and a multi-fraction course of radiotherapy given. There is, unfortunately, no method now available to us for direct observation of the changes in the hypoxic fraction during a course of radiotherapy. We are greatly in need of methods to identify those groups of cases where hypoxia is a real problem, so that we can conduct our trials of sensitizers in groups where benefit may most readily be shown.

In summary, therefore, the initial reports concerning the value of misonidazole in clinical radiotherapy available to us in Europe and the rest of the world are not encouraging. This drug may have a limited place as an adjuvant in clinical radiotherapy, but we need an improved hypoxic cell sensitizer, preferably showing at least a 5-fold advantage over misonidazole. With it we will be able to determine the benefit to be gained in clinical radiotherapy with use of an effective sensitizer. Further, we will learn the importance of hypoxia as a problem at the end of a fractionated course of radiotherapy. Such work will be much facilitated if we can also identify the patients most likely to benefit.

I wish to thank Roche Products Ltd. for their close co-operation in the gathering of trial data.

## REFERENCES

Ash DV (1980). Growth delay studies in patients with multiple metastases. Br J Cancer 41: Suppl IV 17.

Dawes PJDK, Peckham MJ, Steel GG (1978). The response of human tumour metastases to radiation and misonidazole. Br J Cancer 37: Suppl III 290.

Denekamp J, Fowler JF, Dische S (1977). The proportion of hypoxic cells in a human tumour. Int J Radiat Oncol Biol Phys 2: 1227.

Dische S, Saunders MI, Lee ME, Adams GE, Flockhart IR (1977). Clinical testing of the radiosensitizer Ro 07-0582: Experience with multiple doses. Br J Cancer 35: 567.

Dische S, Saunders MI, Flockhart IR (1978). The optimum regime for the administration of misonidazole and the establishment of multi-centre clinical trials. Br J Cancer 37: Suppl III 318.

Dische S, Anderson PJ, Sealy R, Watson ER (1982). Carcinoma of the cervix - anaemia, radiotherapy and hyperbaric oxygen. Br J Radiol. (Awaiting publication).

Gray AJ, Dische S, Adams GE, Flockhart IR, Foster JL (1976). Clinical testing of the radiosensitizer Ro 07-0582. I. Dose tolerance, serum and tumour concentrations. Clin Radiol 27: 151.

Thomlinson RH, Dische S, Gray AJ, Errington LM (1976). Clinical testing of the radiosensitizer Ro 07-0582. III. Response of tumours. Clin Radiol 27: 127.

13th International Cancer Congress, Part D
Research and Treatment, pages 305–316
© 1983 Alan R. Liss, Inc., 150 Fifth Avenue, New York, NY 10011

# THE TOPICAL USE OF MISONIDAZOLE IN BLADDER CANCER

Hassan K. Awwad, H. Abd El Moneim, H. Abd El Baki,
S. Omar, M. El Merzabani, H. I. Farag.
Radiotherapy Department
National Cancer Institute
Kasr El Aini Street, Fom El Khalig
Cairo, Egypt

The essential problem associated with the clinical use of misonidazole(MIS) is that it cannot be given orally under optimum conditions; neurotoxicity being the most important dose-limiting factor. Attempts have to made in order to optimize the oral use of MIS. One approach is to use the drug in association with unconventional fractionation regimes which permit the administration of relatively large individual drug doses. The topical use of MIS is another means of attainment of relatively high local concentrations while circumventing systemic toxicity provided that no significant absorption into the general circulation occurs. The intravesical route of administration is taken as a prototype of the topical use of the drug.

## DETERMINATION OF MIS CONCENTRATION IN BLADDER TISSUE AND TUMOR AFTER INTRAVESICAL AND ORAL ADMINISTRATION

Material and Drug Administration

Patients with T3 bladder cancer eligible for radical cystectomy were included. All tumors were associated with bilharzial cystitis and they were all of the solid protuberent type. Three groups of patients were studied.

The first group included four patients- two with squamous cell cancer (SQC) and two with transitional cell tumors (TCC). Patients of this group were given MIS orally in a dose of 3 g/m². The drug was dissolved in 150 ml distilled water and the patient was instructed to sip the solution slowly, on an empty stomach, over a period of approximately 15 minutes. Surgery was started 2.5 hours after injestion. The time of ligation of both vascular pedicles was carefully recorded. The time interval between drug injestion and vascular ligation varied between 3.5 and 4 hours. A venous blood sample was taken from the antecubital vein at time of ligation of the second vascular pedicle. The tissue and tumor concentrations of MIS were related to the drug concentration of this blood sample.

The second group included nine patients in whom the drug was administered intravesically. Six patients had SQC and three had TCC. The day prior to surgery the patients were prepared by bladder washing using a solution of 1/1000 EDTA and Triton. Repeated administration of 100 ml of this solution was done until the wash became clear. This was followed by introduction of 100 ml of 1/1000 trypsin solution which was kept into the bladder for 10-15 minutes to be repeated three times. On the morning of surgery the patient was instructed to evacuate his bladder. In four patients the MIS solution used consisted of 2.5 g dissolved in 50 ml of distilled water. In the remaining five patients 10 mg of $^{14}$C-labelled MIS was added to the same solution. The added radioactivity amounted to 38 μCi (1410 KBQ) and the final specific activity (SA) was 38 μCi/2.51 g(562 KBQ/g).

The third group comprised two patients in whom a combination of the oral and intravesical routes was used. Drug dosage, patients preparation and time schedule of drug administration and surgery were the same as mentioned above. $^{14}$C-labelled MIS of the above mentioned SA was used for the intravesical route.


Tissue Sampling

The cystectomy specimens were immediately frozen and kept at - 20°C until analyzed.

The concentration of MIS was determined in tissue aliquots cut from cystectomy specimens. Carefully weighed one gram pieces were taken from the following parts: 1-superficial part of the tumor; 2- deep part of the tumor; 3- the perivesical tissue; 4- a repressentative lymph node from the external iliac group; 5- mucosa away from the tumor; 6- occasionally the prostate, seminal vesicles and ovaries.

The removed piece was cut and minced using a scissor and a pair of sharp scalpels. For the determination of MIS tissue concentration one of two methods was used: the spectrophotometric or the radioisotopic method.

## The Spectrophotometric Method for Determination of MIS Concentration in Tissues

This method was used for determination of the concentration of MIS in tissues after either oral or intra-vesical use. The minced tissue fragments were left for 24 h in 9 ml ethanol with gentle shaking on an electric shaker. After centrifugation 5 ml of the supernatent fluid were pipetted in the spectrophotometer cuvette. The extinction was then read at 312 nm using a "Pye Unicam" UV spectrophotometer, (SP-500, series 2).

A standard calibration curve was determined using MIS concentrations of 5, 10, 25, 100 µg/ml ethanol.

## The Radioisotopic Method for Determination of the Concentration of MIS in Tissues

This was used for determination of the tissue concentration of MIS after intravesical administration.

The tissue fragments were immersed in 10 ml ethanol for 24 h with continuous shaking over a mechanical shaker. After centrifugation 2 ml of the supernatent fluid were pipetted and evaporated over

a sand bath. The residue was dissolved in 1 ml methanol + 2 ml hyamine + 14 ml of the scintillation fluid having the composition: (POPOP 50 mg + POP 4 g
dissolved in one liter toluene). Mixing was done
in the counting vial of the liquid scintillation
counter (SC-722 automatic dual scaler/spectrometer,
ICN Pharmaceuticals, Belgium). The count rate (C1)
was then determined. An internal standard solution
was prepared by dissolving 1 mg of the labelled
compound in 100 ml methanol. The vial was recounted
after adding an aliquot of 50 µl of the standard
solution. If the count rate obtained was C2 then
the differences (C2-C1) represented the count rate
due to the internal standard added ($1.9 \times 10^{-3}$ uCi)
when counted with the same counting efficiency as
that used for counting the tissue extract. To determine this efficiency 50 ul of the internal standard solution were mixed in a counting vial with 1 ml
methanol + 2 ml hyamine + 14 ml scintillation fluid.
If the count rate obtained was C3 then the counting
efficiency (E) is given as:

$$E=(C2-C1)/C3 \times 1.9 \times 10^{-3}$$

The activity in 2 ml tissue extract is then calculated as $(C1/E)\mu Ci$ and the drug concentration in
tissue is given as:

$$5 \times (C1/E) SAxx \ 10^6 \ \mu g \ MIS/g \ tissue$$

Determination of MIS Concentration in Plasma

The plasma concentration of MIS was measured
using a spectrophotometric method at 312 nm (Urtasun,
Strurmawind, Razin, Band and Chapman 1974). The
patients samples were read against blanks made up
of the plasma of the same subject obtained from
blood withdrawn before drug administration. A Calibration standard was prepared by adding a known MIS
quantity to the patient's own control sample.

Results

Table 1 gives the tissue concentration of MIS
after intravesical administration. It can be seen
that: 1-MIS concentration within the mucosa was
consistently lower than in the superficial part of

the tumor ;2-2 concentratio gradient existed across
the tumor down to the perivesical tissue (Fig.1);
3-Significant concentrations were found in lymph
nodes with a mean value of $47\pm14$ µg/g which was approximately 50% of the concentration in the perivesical tissue; 4-The prostate and seminal vesicles were
examined in one patient only and the drug concentration amounted to 30 and 28 µg/g respectively;
5-The drug could not be detected in the blood of any
of the nine patients.

| Pat. → | 1 | 2 | 3 | 4 | 5 | 6 | 7 | 8 | 9 | Mean+SD |
|---|---|---|---|---|---|---|---|---|---|---|
| Mucosa | 92 | 450 | 121 | 390 | 478 | 405 | 520 | 321 | 382 | 351±150 |
| Sup.T. | 192 | 1670 | 133 | 530 | 576 | 1142 | 576 | 529 | 780 | 680±475 |
| Deep T | 72 | 127 | 93 | 50 | 85 | 289 | 98 | 182 | 90 | 120± 73 |
| Peri.V | 62 | 107 | 102 | 65 | 71 | 82 | 95 | 64 | 72 | 80± 17 |
| L.N. | 42 | – | 78 | 42 | 55 | 41 | 50 | 42 | 29 | 47± 14 |
| Pros. | 30 | – | – | – | – | – | – | – | – | – |
| Sem.V. | 28 | – | – | – | – | – | – | – | – | – |
| Ovary | – | 29 | 28 | – | – | – | – | – | – | – |

Pat.=Patient; Sup.T.=Superficial tumor; Deep T=Deep
tumor; Peri.V.=Perivesical tissue; L.N.=Lymp nodes;
Sem.V. =Seminal vesicles.

Table 1  Tissue concentration 1.5-2 hours after
intravesical administration (µg/g of tissues).

The tissue distribution after oral use (Table 2;Fig.
1b) was much more uniform.  The average concentration  within the tumor amounted to 58-108% of the
blood level. It is worthnoting that the pelvic nodes
had a somewhat greater concentration than that within the tumor and blood in all patients.

| Pat. → | 1 | 2 | 3 | 4 | Mean+SD |
|---|---|---|---|---|---|
| Blood | 84(100) | 115(100) | 92(100) | 97(100) | 97±13 |
| Tumor | 49( 58) | 105( 91) | 87( 95) | 105(108) | 87±26 |
| Peri.V | 78( 93) | 138(120) | 90( 98) | 117(121) | 106±27 |
| Mucosa | 43( 51) | 101( 88) | 82( 89) | 103(106) | 82±28 |
| L.N. | 98(117) | 149(130) | 109(119) | 149(154) | 126±27 |

N.B. The figures between brackets represent per cent
     of blood level.

Table 2  Tissue concentration 3.5 hours after oral
use of 3 g per meter square. For abreviations see
footnotes of Table 1.

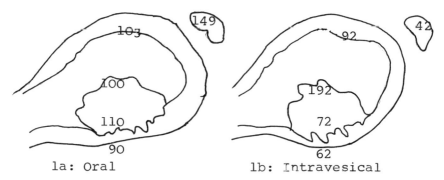

la: Oral                        lb: Intravesical

Fig.la: Tissue distribution of MIS 3.5 hours after
an oral dose of 3 g per meter square. A fairly uniform distribution is noted with a somewhat higher
concentration in nodes. Fig. lb: Tissue distribution of MIS 2 hours after intravesical administration of 2.5 g dissolved in 50 ml of distilled water.
A concentration gradient across the tumor and down
to the perivesical tissue is noted. The mucosal
concentration is lower than that of the superficial
part of the tumor.

| Patient⟶ | 1 | | | 2 | | |
|---|---|---|---|---|---|---|
| | Total | I.Ves. | Oral | Total | I.Ves. | Oral |
| Blood | 77 | 0 | 77 | 92 | 0 | 92 |
| Mucosa | 550 | 480 | 70 | 540 | 459 | 90 |
| Sup.T. | 696 | 606 | 90 | 610 | 530 | 80 |
| Deep T. | 18 | 110 | 72 | 217 | 127 | 90 |
| Peri.V. | 141 | 72 | 69 | 198 | 109 | 89 |

Table 3: Tissue concentration after combined oral
and intravesical use. Cystectomy was performed 3.5
hours after oral administration of 3 g per meter
square and two hours after intravesical instillation of 2.51 g of the drug labelled with [14]C. For
abreviations see footnotes of Table 1.

     The drug distribution after a combination of
oral and intravesical administration is given in
Table 3. The spectrophotometric method described
above gave the tissue concentration of the drug
resulting from both routes. The concentration resulting from the intravesical route alone was derived by dividing the concentration of radioactivity
in tissues (μCi/g) by th SA of the instilled solut-

ion as given above. The difference between the total concentration and that due to intravesical administration represented the contribution of the oral dose. The tissue concentrations given in Table 3 for intravesical and oral administration are similar to those given in Tables 1 and 2 respectively. It appears therefore that the total concentration represented the sum of the concentration resulting from both routes.

DISCUSSION

Passive movement of water and solutes across the mammalian bladder epithelium was demonstrated (Hayes and Leaf 1962). The permeability of the mammalian bladder is estimated to be 100 times greater than that of skin. Permeability was also shown to increase as a result of cystitis and presence of dedifferentiated tumors though well differentiated tumors did not influence permeability (Fellows and Marshall 1972). Increased permeability could be also induced by the administration of chemical agents such as cyclophosphamide (Turnbull 1971). Such agents are believed to act through destruction of the junction between epithelial cells and break of continuity of the surface membrane of cells lining the lumen (Turnbull 1971; Hicks 1966). Similar lack of tight junction between surface tumor cells was shown to occur in case of dedifferentiated tumors but not in association with well differentiated papillary tumors (Cooper 1975), this may explain the increased permeability associated with dedifferentiation.

The present study demonstrated that MIS could diffuse into both the bladder mucosa and into bladder tumors. However the drug concentration within the superficial parts of tumors was considtently greater than that within the mucosa. This can be taken to indicate a break of the mucosal barrier to diffusion in the region occupied by the tumor,

Studies of the capillary vascular bed in carcinoma of urinary bladder could give an indication of the magnitude of hypoxia. The vascular bed of bilharzial and non-bilharzial bladder cancer could be

histochemically demonstrated by an alkaline phosphatase technique staining the capillary endothelium
in a thick frozen section (Omar, Shalaby and Ibrahim
1975; Mocktar, El Bolkaini, Abd El Baki and Awwad
1981). The normal bladder epithelium and bengin hyperplastic lesions found in association with bilharzial cystitis showed an abundant capillary network
with uniform shape and regular distribution. This
contrasted with the scarce distribution with wide
intercapillary distances in case of carcinoma in
bilharzial bladder. However different histological
types of carcinoma in bilharzial bladder showed
degrees of vascular inadequancy. Transitional cell
bilharzial bladder cancer had a more adequate capillary network compared with the squamous cell bilharzial variety. Moreover the intercapillary distances tended to increase with the degree of de-diffe-
rentiation. It is also interesting to note that the
non-bilharzial transitional cell bladder cancer
tended to have a more adequate capillary network.

The use of an efficient hypoxic cell radiosensitizer is expected, in the light of the above findings, to result in a net therapeutic gain. It is
unlikely that a significant   enhancement of the
radiation damage of the bladder mucosa is produced
since an efficient microcirculation could be demonstrated even in presence of bilharzial infection.

The intravesical route of administration represents a prototype of the topical use of MIS.  It
also offers means of optimizing the use of MIS through complete elimination of the risk of neurotoxicity. However practical considerations and comfort
of the patient do not permit the use of the intravesical route in association with conventional daily
fractionation. Hence the main domain of applicability of this route is in schedules involving the
adminstration of few large fractions. Such regimens
do not make full use of the spontaneous reoxygenation properties of human solid tumors. The use of a
hypoxic cell radiosensitzer may make up for this
deficiency.

Short concentrated preoperative radiotherapy
regimens proved to reduce the risk of local recurr-

ence in tumors with deep infiltration into the bladder wall (Whitmore 1980). The objective of preoperative irradiation in such tumors is to sterilize the
deep infiltrating margins of the tumor which represent a high risk of local recurrence. Hence the
penetration of radiosensitizers into these parts
and into the perivesical tissues had to be evaluated.
The intravesical administration resulted into in a
concentration of MIS of the order of 100 ug/ml in
the deep part of the tumor and perivesical tissue.
A similar concentration could be attained in these
regions after an oral use. However the concentration
of the drug in blood was nil after intravesical administration compared with a peak value of 32(ug/ml)
per (g/meter square) in case of the oral use. Hence
no neurotoxicity is expected after topical application.

The spectrophotometric and radioiostopic methods used in the present study do not resolve MIS
from its demethylated metabolite. A number of measurements were made using a high pressure liquid
chromatography  technique. A single peak only could
be resolved. This seems to indicate that no drug
degradation occurred during drug diffusion into the
bladder wall.

The fact that the intravesical route was associated with a much higher concentration in the superficial parts of the tumor does not seem to represent an dvantage over the oral route when properat-
ive irradiation is used. Though the superficial components represent the main bulk of the tumor, yet
they are completely removed during surgery and are
most unlikely to contribute to the risk of local
recurrence. Attempts were made to increase the drug
concentration in the deep infiltrating margins and
perivesical tissues by increasing the drug concentration in instilled solution with the help of solub-
ilizing agents such as Tween 80 (Awwad et al.1980).
However concentrations higher than that used in the
present studies caused bladder irritation and were
not tolerated. Hence a combination of the oral and
the intravesical route was considered as a mean of
augmenting the drug concentration. The present study
confirmed that the drug concentration was additive

and a concentration of about 200 ug/g could well be attained in the deep part of the tumor and peri-vesical tissues. Unfortunately the increase in the SER corresponding to this increase in drug tissue concentration is not great due to the shape of curve relating the SER to drug concentration which tends to flatten up at higher concentrations (Adams 1979). The combined route would increase the ER from 1.7 to 1.85 though the tissue concentration is increased by a factor of 2.0. However the combined route may have two additional merits. First-a higher concent-ration in pelvic lymph nodes may be attained as is clearly shown in tables 1,2 and 3. Second-the higher concentration and the relatively long contact time with tumor cells may have an additional advantage other than sensitization of hypoxic cells. Under such conditions drug cytoxicity has a better chance to operate and this may add to the ultimate thera-peutic gain (Whitmore, Gulyas and Varghese 1978).

A clinical trial is currently underway testing the therapeutic gain obtained by the use of oral, intravesical or combined administration of MIS as a preoperative measure in T3 bladder cancer. In addit-ion to this trial other methods of topical applic-ation of MIS are investigated. One promising area is the topical application in ulcerated skin tumors where penetration can be helped by the use of an appropriate solvent.

SUMMARY

Penetration studies of MIS after intravesical administration showed adequate concentrations with a gradient across the tumor. After instillation of 2.5 g in 50 ml water the concentration in the deep parts of the tumor amounted to about 100 ug per ml. This corresponds to a SER for hypoxic cell of the order of 1.7. A more uniform tissue distribution of the drug was noted 3.5 hours after an oral dose of 3 g/meter square. The concentration in the deep parts of the tumor and perivesical tissue was of the order of 100 ug/g. The concentration in these regions are relevant to preoperative irradiation which aims at sterilizing the deep infiltrating margings. The intravesical use with or without oral augmentation is suitable for use in association with concentrated preoperative radiotherapy regimens. The topical use of MIS in such regimens markedly reduces the risk of neurotoxicity. The tissue concentration resulting from the two routes proved to be additive. The higher concentration in lymph nodes after the oral route the greater concentration and prolonged contact after combined adminstration may have therapeutic merits.

1-Awwad HK, El Merzabani MM, El Badawy SA, Ezzat S, Akoush H, Abdel Moneim H, Said A, Soliman O, Khafagy M, Burgers M (1980) Misoniadazole in the preoperative and radical radiotherapy of bladder cancer. Cancer Clin Trials 3:275.

2-Cooper EH (1975) Biology of human bladder cancer. In: Cooper EH, Williams RE Eds The biology and clinical management of bladder cancer. Blackwell Scientific publications, Oxford London Edinburgh Melbourne p.37.

3-Fellows GJ, Marshall DH (1972) The permeability of the bladder epithelium to water and sodium. Invest Urol 9:339.

4-Hayes RM, Leaf A (1962) Studies on the movement of water through the isolated toad bladder and its modification by vasopressin. J Gen Physiol 45:902.

5-Hicks RM (1966) Permeability of the rat transitional epithelium keratinization and the barrier to water. J Cell Biol 28:21.

6-Mocktar NM, El Bolkainy, El Baky H, Awwad H (1981) Quantitation of tumour vacularity in Bilharzial bladder cancer. Med J Cairo University 49:419.

7-Omar AH, Shalaby MA, Ibrahim AH (1975) The capillary vascular bed in carcinoma of the urinary bladder. E Afr Med J 52:35.

8-Turnbull, GJ (1971) Investigation of the ultrastructure and function of the bladder epithelium Ph D Thesis, University of Leeds.

9-Whitmore WF (1980) Integrated irradiation and cystectomy for bladder cancer. Br J Urol 52:1.

10-Whitmore GF, Gulyas S, Vargnese AJ (1978) Sensitizing and toxicity properties of misonidazole and its derivatives. Br J Cancer 37 (Suppl III): 115.

11-Ultrasun RC, Sturmawind J, Razin H, Band TR, Chapman JD (1974) High dose metronidazole: a preliminary pharmacological study prior to its investigational use in clinical radiotherapy. Br J Radiol 47:297.

CONGRESS SYMPOSIA

ONCOLOGIC EMERGENCIES Besznyak, I., Hungary,
Chairman; Scanlon, E., USA, Co-Chairman;
Playhouse

The Management of Malignant Effusion.
*Yarbro, J. W., Columbia, MO USA.  (By Title Only)

Neurological Emergencies in Cancer Patients.
*Cairncross, J. G., London, Ontario, Canada.

Neoplasia Associated Superior Vena Cava Syndrome.
*Presant, C. A., Perez, C. A., Bertrand, M. and
Klein, L., Los Angeles, CA USA and Duarte, CA USA
and St. Louis, MO USA.

Oncologic Emergencies in Gastro-Intestinal Cancer.
*Gentil, F., Sao Paulo, Brazil.  (By Title Only)

Oncologic Emergencies: Metabolic Derangements
of Clinical Importance.  *Myers, W. P. L. and
Isaacs, M., New York, NY USA.

Malignant Effusions as Oncologic Emergencies.
*Hausheer, F. and Yarbro, J. W., Columbia, MO USA.

Please note: Papers that are listed as "By Title
Only" were presented at the 13th International
Cancer Congress, but are not included in these
volumes.

13th International Cancer Congress, Part D
Research and Treatment, pages 319–328
© 1983 Alan R. Liss, Inc., 150 Fifth Avenue, New York, NY 10011

NEUROLOGICAL EMERGENCIES IN CANCER PATIENTS

J. Gregory Cairncross, M.D., F.R.C.P.(C)

Ontario Cancer Treatment & Research Foundation,
London Clinic,
391 South Street, London, Ontario, N6A 4G5

Central nervous system complications of systemic cancer
are common. It has been estimated that 15–20% of patients
with cancer develop neurological symptoms at some point in
their illness. Neurological complications in the cancer
patient may be sudden, devastating and irreversible.
However, most serious neurological problems begin in a subacute fashion, are heralded by warning symptoms, and are
amenable to treatment. With prompt diagnosis and
appropriate management, symptoms resolve or improve in most
patients. Moreover neurological improvement is often
maintained until the patient succumbs to systemic disease.
This is often true of patients with brain metastasis and
epidural spinal cord compression; two common and serious
neurological problems in cancer patients.

The neurological complications of systemic cancer are
protean. For a complete discussion of this topic the reader
is referred elsewhere (Posner 1979). This review emphasizes
those neurological problems which require urgent attention
and for which effective treatment is available. These
problems include cerebral herniation, seizures, epidural
spinal cord compression, and CNS infections. Encephalo-
pathies due to reversible metabolic disturbances are
discussed elsewhere.

CEREBRAL HERNIATION

Expanding intracranial mass lesions if unrecognized or
neglected lead to cerebral herniation. As intracranial mass

lesions increase in size the brain herniates in the direction of at least resistance, i.e., the brain shifts in a rostral-caudal direction through the tentorial opening and foramen magnum. There are three important and clinically distinguishable cerebral herniation syndromes (Plum, Posner 1980). The uncal and central herniation syndromes are caused by supra-tentorial mass lesions which by virtue of their expanding nature push normal brain through the narrow tentorial opening. Mass lesions in the posterior fossa push the cerebral tonsils and lower brain stem through the foramen magnum producing the clinical picture of tonsillar herniation.

Uncal herniation is characteristic of laterally placed rapidly expanding masses. The medial surface of the temporal lobe (the uncus) is displaced, medially and inferiorly, compressing the upper brain stem and the two important structures which pass between the lateral aspect of the upper brain stem and the medial edge of the tentorium, namely the posterior cerebral artery and the third cranial nerve. Rapid loss of consciousness, unilateral pupillary dilatation and ipsilateral hemiparesis from compression of the opposite cerebral peduncle against the tentorial edge are the hallmarks of uncal herniation. Central herniation is usually the result of multifocal supratentorial mass lesions, subacutely expanding unifocal mass lesions in the frontal or parietal areas, or hydrocephalus. The symptoms of the central syndrome result from slow, downward displacement of the diencephalon and distortion of the upper brain stem. The earliest signs of central herniation reflect symmetrical, diencephalic compression and are characterized by a gradual decrease in consciousness, small reactive pupils, and periodic respirations. Focal neurological signs such as hemiparesis are often absent. As the central herniation syndrome evolves more prominant neurologic signs appear such as hyperventillation, disconjugate eye movements, pupillary fixation, and abnormal motor responses. In its early stages the central herniation syndrome is often mistaken for metabolic brain disease because it evolves slowly and because the level of consciousness is often depressed out of proportion to focal neurological findings. Potentially hazardous lumbar punctures may be performed because structural intracranial disease is not considered in the differential diagnosis. In the cancer patient a history of headache or focal neurological symptoms, or the presence of focal signs, no matter how subtle, are indications for a CT scan prior to CSF examination. The symptoms and signs of tonsillar herniation result from direct

brain stem compression and from acute obstructive hydrocephalus. Decreases in consciousness accompanied or preceeded by occipital headache, vomiting, hiccoughs, and neck
stiffness suggest herniation from a posterior fossa mass
lesion. Opisthotonus, skew deviation of the eyes, hypertension, orthostatic hypotension, and syncope with cough or
sudden postural change are less common manifestations of
posterior fossa mass lesions and incipient tonsillar herniation. Respiratory changes are the most serious and life
threatening sign of this disorder. A variety of irregular
respiratory patterns occur and at times, particularly
following ill-advised lumbar puncture, sudden apnea may be
the only sign of tonsillar herniation.

The major causes of cerebral herniation in cancer
patients are brain metastasis and intracerebral hemorrhage.
Subdural hematoma, brain abscess, acute hydrocephalus, and
radiation necrosis are occasionally responsible. Brain
metastasis occurs frequently in patients with carcinomas of
the lung, breast, colon, kidney and testicle, and with
choriocarcinoma and melanoma. Intracerebral hemorrhage
occurs in two settings; thrombocytopenic patients with acute
leukemia, and patients with brain metastasis from melanoma,
hypernephroma, choriocarcinoma, and testicular carcinoma.
Subdural hematomas develop in thrombocytopenic patients
with acute leukemia and occur occasionally in patients with
other tumor types, usually in the setting of severe thrombocytopenia and dural metastases. Subdural hematomas should
always be suspected in patients on chronic anticoagulants
who develop symptoms and signs of cerebral herniation.
Brain abscess may complicate the leukemias, lymphomas, and
head and neck malignancies. Acute hydrocephalus develops
in patients with posterior fossa and pineal metastases,
leptomeningeal metastasis, and occasionally in those with
basal meningitis (e.g., cryptococcal meningitis). Radio-
necrosis of the brain is an uncommon, late complication of
radiation therapy to the head.

The management of acutely decompensating patients with
rapidly expanding intracranial mass lesions is summarized.
Maintaining a clear airway is critical. $CO_2$ retention
causes cerebral vasodilatation and further increases intracranial pressure. After securing the airway, hyperventillation lowers intracranial pressure by decreasing
$pCO_2$ which in turn decreases brain blood volume by producing
cerebral vasoconstriction. $CO_2$ tension should not be

reduced below 20-25 mm/Hg since lower levels may lead to brain acidosis and cerebral vasodilatation. Mannitol in a dose of 25-100 gm (20% solution) is given intravenously. The effect of mannitol lasts only 4-6 hours and may need to be repeated. Adrenocorticosteroids are given intravenously (e.g., dexamethasone 100 mg) to reduce the edema associated with intracranial mass lesions, especially brain metastasis and brain abscess. Steroids are not effective for several hours even after intravenous administration. The diagnosis of cerebral herniation is made on clinical grounds and treatment instituted, in many instances, before an etiologic diagnosis is established. Once treatment is underway the CT scan is the diagnostic procedure of choice. If the scan reveals an accessible lesion then surgical evacuation should be considered. In some instances, cerebral herniation can be controlled by pharmacologic measures followed by definitive treatment by means other than surgery. For example, a patient with a large brain metastasis or brain abscess may respond dramatically to mannitol and adrenocorticosteroids, stabilize, and then respond to radiation therapy or anti-biotics.

SEIZURES

Seizures are often the first sign of neurological disease in cancer patients. Seizures may be due to metastatic disorders such as intracerebral, calvarial, dural, or lepto-meningeal metastases, or a variety of non-metastatic dis-orders including metabolic-toxic disturbances, vascular problems, or infections. Effective management includes treatment of both the specific cause of the seizure and the seizure itself. The diagnostic evaluation of cancer patients with seizures includes blood tests (glucose, BUN, electro-lytes, calcium, magnesium, liver function tests, arterial blood gases, blood cultures, coagulation profile), CT scan, and lumbar puncture. Seizures in and of themselves are dangerous and must be controlled. In addition to the obvious dangers of physical injury and vomiting with aspiration seizures increase cerebral blood flow and cerebral blood volume and can cause cerebral herniation in patients with previously compensated mass lesions. Therefore seizures should be stopped as soon as possible and the patient carefully observed during the postictal period for signs of cerebral herniation. A number of medications are available to treat seizures; the drug, dose, and route of

administration will vary with the clinical situation. For
example, patients with readily correctable metabolic disturbances (e.g., hypoxia, hypoglycemia) will not require anticonvulsants. Those with a single seizure from a brain
metastasis can be treated with oral phenytoin. Patients with
repetitive generalized seizures (i.e., status epilepticus)
must be treated aggressively with parenteral anticonvulsants
and may require assisted ventilation. The seizures are
stopped with intravenous valium, the airway is secured, and
further seizures are prevented by the parenteral administration of loading doses of phenytoin or phenobarbital. For
specific suggestions regarding drugs and dosages the reader
is referred elsewhere (Cairncross, Posner 1981).


SPINAL CORD COMPRESSION

Spinal cord compression is a serious and frequent
complication of systemic cancer. Early diagnosis and prompt
treatment are essential in order to preserve neurologic
function. Once completely paralyzed the likelihood of
meaningful recovery is small. In the cancer patient spinal
cord compression may result from epidural or intramedullary
metastases, vertebral subluxation, or spinal subdural
hematoma.

The tumors which commonly cause epidural spinal cord
compression are carcinomas of the breast, lung, and prostate.
This is a reflection of both the prevalence of these tumor
types and the tendancy for these tumors to metastasize to
the spine. The interval between the diagnosis of cancer and
the development of spinal cord compression is variable.
Pain, either local or radicular, is the initial symptom in
95% of patients with epidural metastases. In general, the
location of the pain coincides with the level of the spinal
tumor. The clinical diagnosis of epidural spinal cord
compression is confirmed by radiographic procedures.
Although plain x-rays of the spine are frequently abnormal
at the level of cord compression precise localization
requires myelography. If a complete block is found from
below, a lateral C1-C2 myelogram is performed to delineate
the upper level of the lesion. The contrast material is
not removed so that at a later date fluoroscopy can be done
to establish the results of therapy, of if need be, to
rapidly assess new spinal symptoms.

Once the diagnosis has been established treatment must begin immediately since minor degrees of weakness may progress within hours to irreversible paraplegia. Radiation therapy is the mainstay of treatment for these patients. The literature does not support the widely held view that surgery and radiation therapy are more effective than radiation alone (Gilbert, Kim, Posner 1978). The importance of early diagnosis and prompt treatment is emphasized by the fact that 80% of patients ambulatory at the time of treatment remain so, while only 30-40% of patients unable to walk when treatment begins will walk again. Although patients with radio-sensitive tumors tend to fair better, good results can be anticipated following the early diagnosis and treatment of tumors generally considered to be less radio-sensitive. In general, the findings on refluoromyelogram correlate with clinical response. Surgical intervention is certainly indicated if the cause of the cord compression is in doubt or if relapse occurs in an area of prior irradiation. Adrenocortico-steroid hormones appear to be an important adjunct to radiation therapy in the treatment of cord compression and probably exert their beneficial effect by reducing spinal cord edema. Large doses of adrenocorticosteroids often dramatically improve the severe back pain associated with vertebral and epidural tumor thereby hastening early ambulation in patients who might otherwise be restricted to bed (Greenberg, Kim, Posner 1981).

Atlanto-axial subluxation is a potentially fatal complication of metastatic tumor to the upper cervical spine. Metastases to the axis (C2) lead to pathological fractures of the odontoid process and subsequent anterior dislocation of the atlas (C1) on the axis. Upper cervical spinal cord compression and respiratory arrest may result. As with epidural tumor at other spinal levels pain is the presenting complaint in the majority of patients. The diagnosis is usually established by lateral x-rays of the cervical spine, however, tommography may be useful in the detection of early non-subluxed lesions. In most instances myelography is not necessary and may in fact be hazardous. Early lesions without major subluxation can be safely treated with a soft cervical collar and radiation therapy. Management is more difficult once subluxation has occurred. Reduction by cervical traction followed by posterior cervical fusion and radiation therapy is the treatment of choice in patients whose general condition permits surgery. Those who are not surgical candidates can be managed conservatively with good results in most cases. Support of the head and neck in a Philadelphia collar followed by steroids and radiation therapy is often successful. The wide sagittal diameter of the spinal canal at this level, the splinting properties of the cervical muscles, and apparent fusion in the subluxed position after RT are factors which permit the non-surgical management of atlanto-axial subluxation in a selected group of patients (Sundaresan et al 1981).

Spinal subdural hematoma is a recognized complication of lumbar puncture in thrombocytopenic cancer patients (Edelson, Chernik, Posner 1974). Back pain and rapidly progressive paraparesis within 24 hours of a lumbar puncture in a patient with fewer than 20,000 platelets, or a rapidly falling platelet count, suggest this diagnosis. Unfortunately severe thrombocytopenia usually precludes emergency myelography and surgical decompression. Likewise, attempted drainage of the subdural hematoma by needle aspiration is likely to produce further bleeding and not relieve symptoms. In general these patient should be given platelet transfusions and started on high dose steroids. Although not of proven benefit some patients appear to be responsive to this treatment.

## CENTRAL NERVOUS SYSTEM INFECTIONS

Central nervous system infections are medical emergencies. Early, accurate diagnosis and prompt treatment are essential to prevent death or permanent disability. Patients with cancer are susceptible to CNS infections for many reasons. Steroids, chemotherapy, splenectomy, irradiation, and in some instances the underlying disease, all impair immune mechanisms. The organisms responsible for infections in the cancer patient are different from those encountered in the general population. Further, the spectrum of causative organisms varies with the underlying disease. The majority of infections occur in patients with lymphoma, leukemia, and head and neck tumors (Chernik, Armstrong, Posner 1973). The latter frequently dispose to CNS infections because surgical defects or fistuli from progressive erosion by tumor permit organisms to gain access to the para-meningeal or subarachnoid spaces.

Headache, fever, and obtundation are the hallmarks of

meningitis. Delays in diagnosis occur in cancer patients because headache is attributed to brain metastasis, fever to systemic infection, and drowsiness to medications or metabolic disturbances. A lumbar puncture is indicated in all cancer patients with fever and depressed level of consciousness. An emergency CT scan prior to lumbar puncture may be necessary for patients in whom an intracranial mass lesion is suspected. Knowledge of the underlying malignancy and the peripheral white count often permit an accurate prediction of the offending organism, and guide initial therapy. Patients with lymphoma and normal peripheral white cell counts are susceptible to infection by Listeria monocytogenes, Diplococcus pneumoniae, and Cryptococcus neoformans. Hemophilus influenzae and Neisseria meningitidis, common causes of meningitis in the general population, are rarely encountered. The gram negative organisms including Pseudomonas aeruginosa, Escherichia coli, and Proteus mirabilis are the usual causes of meningitis in lymphoma patients with depressed peripheral white counts. Patients with acute leukemia and depressed peripheral white counts are vulnerable to CNS infections by gram negative rods (esp., Pseudomonas aeruginosa), fungi other than Cryptococcus neoformans, and occasionally Listeria monocytogenes. With the exception of Cryptococcus neoformans, meningitis rarely complicates the chronic leukemias. In patients with head and neck cancers Staphylococcus aureus (coagulase positive) is the most frequent cause of meningitis. Streptococci and gram negative rods are other causes of meningitis in this group. Many of these infections are acquired in the hospital during the postoperative period. Meningitis in other cancer patients is infrequent but with a spectrum similar to that of the lymphomas; Listeria monocytogenes, Diplococcus pneumoniae, and Cryptococcus neoformans in patients with normal peripheral white counts and the gram negative organisms in those with low peripheral white counts. Specific and effective antimicrobial therapy is available to treat the majority of cancer patients with meningitis. The treatment of patients with gram negative meningitis, refactory cryptococcal meningitis, or shunt and reservoir infections may pose special problems. For a detailed discussion of these specific infections the reader is referred elsewhere (Kaiser, McGee 1975; Bennett et al 1979; Diamond, Bennett 1973).

Brain abscess and viral meningitis occur in cancer patients, but are not common problems (Chernik, Armstrong, Posner 1979). Toxoplasmosis, however, deserves special

mention. In the cancer population intracranial infections
with Toxoplasma gondii are found almost exclusively in
patients with lymphoma. It is a potentially fatal CNS
infection for which effective treatment exists. Cerebral
toxoplasmosis may present clinically as a diffuse encephalopathy with or without seizures, as a meningoencephalitis,
or as single or multiple progressive mass lesions. Because
of difficulties in serological diagnosis, brain biopsy is
frequently necessary in order to establish the diagnosis.
Marked clinical improvement or complete remission of
symptoms and signs have been reported to occur in 80% of
patients treated with the combination of sulfanomides and
pyrimethamine (Ruskin, Remington 1976).

All neurological problems in cancer patients are of
concern and require prompt attention. Cerebral herniation,
seizures, epidural spinal cord compression, and CNS
infections are especially important problems in as much as
they are eminently treatable provided undue delay has not
resulted in death or permanent disability.

Bennett JE et al (1979). A comparison of Amphotericin B
  alone and combined with Flucytosine in the treatment of
  cryptococcal meningitis. New Eng J Med 301: 126.
Cairncross JG, Posner JB (1981). Neurological complications
  of systemic cancer. In Yarbro JW, Bornstein RD (eds):
  "Oncologic Emergencies," New York: Grune and Stratton,
  p 73.
Chernik NL, Armstrong E, Posner JB (1973). Central nervous
  system infections in patients with cancer. Medicine
  52: 563.
Diamond RD, Bennett JE (1973). A subcutaneous reservoir
  for intrathecal chemotherapy of fungal meningitis. New
  Eng J Med 288: 186.
Edelson RN, Chernik NL, Posner JB (1974). Spinal subdural
  hematomas complicating lumbar puncture: Occurrence in
  thrombocytopenic patients. Arch Neurol 31: 134.
Gilbert RW, Kim J-H, Posner JB (1978). Epidural spinal
  cord compression from metastatic tumors: Diagnosis and
  treatment. Ann Neurol 3: 40.
Greenberg HS, Kim J-H, Posner JB (1980). Epidural spinal cord
  compression from metastatic tumors: Results with a new
  treatment protocol. Ann Neurol 8: 361.

Kaiser AB, McGee ZA (1975). Aminoglycoside therapy of gram negative bacillary meningitis. New Eng J Med 293: 1215.

Plum F, Posner JB (1980). "The diagnosis of stupor and coma." Philadelphia, FA Davis, p 87.

Posner JB (1979). Neurological complications of systemic cancer. Med Clin North Am 63: 783.

Ruskin J, Remington JS (1976). Toxoplasmosis in the compromised host. Ann Int Med 84: 193.

Sundaresan N et al (1981). Treatment of odontoid fractures in cancer patients. J Neurosurg 54: 187.

**13th International Cancer Congress, Part D**
**Research and Treatment, pages 329–336**
© 1983 Alan R. Liss, Inc., 150 Fifth Avenue, New York, NY 10011

NEOPLASIA ASSOCIATED SUPERIOR VENA CAVA SYNDROME

Cary A. Presant, M.D., F.A.C.P.*†; Carlos A.
Perez, M.D.‡; Marcelle Bertrand, M.D.†; Leonard
Klein, M.D.†

Wilshire Oncology Medical Group, Los Angeles, CA
91790*; City of Hope National Medical Center,
Duarte, CA 91010†; Washington Univ. School of
Medicine, St. Louis, MO 63108‡

One of the most common medical emergencies facing the
oncologist is the development of superior vena cava (SVC)
syndrome. A detailed summary of the clinical syndrome,
pathophysiology, and certain aspects of treatment has
appeared (Simpson et al, 1980). This manuscript will stress
certain aspects of the etiology of SVC syndrome, including
the identification of a new syndrome of iatrogenic etiology;
the need for prompt institution of diagnostic tests; and a
general schema for management of the syndrome.


ETIOLOGY

The superior vena cava is a short vein with high flow
rate, extending from the confluens of the right and left
innominite veins (just above the pericardium) to the juncture
with the right atrium. Because of its mediastinal location,
adjacent structures include numerous lymph nodes, mediastinal
connective tissue, and the pericardium. Rarely, substernal
thyroid tissue may also be adjacent to the SVC. In 90% of
instances, SVC syndrome is associated with neoplastic disease
(Table 1). Since most of the infections affecting the mediastinum can currently be controlled in symptomatic stages
existing prior to the occurrence of infectious lymphadenitis
or mediastinitis, it is not surprising that the incidence of
SVC syndrome due to non-neoplastic etiologies is rare. This
is usually due to bronchogenic carcinoma (most frequently

Table 1
Etiology of SVC Syndrome

Neoplasia Associated (90%)
    Bronchogenic Carcinoma
    Malignant Lymphoma
    Hodgkin's Disease
    Carcinoma
        Esophagus
        Colon
        Breast
        Testes
    Sarcoma
    Iatrogenic SVC Syndrome (ISVEC)

Non-neoplastic (10%)
    Infectious (tuberculosis, syphilis, bacterial media-
      stinitis)
    Thrombosis (traumatic, spontaneous)
    Substernal Thyroid
    Sarcoidosis
    Pericarditis

small cell carcinoma), although other carcinomas can, in
unusual circumstances, also be associated with SVC syndrome.
The most common of these is esophageal carcinoma, in which
SVC occlusion occurs secondary to direct neoplastic encroach-
ment, with extrinsic compression or invasion. Malignant
lymphoma, Hodgkin's disease, and (rarely) thymoma may also
precipitate SVC syndrome.

    Recently, the frequent use of subclavian catheters for
either short-term or long-term administration of chemotherapy
and hyperalimentation fluids has resulted in an increasing
number of patients at risk of complications of venous cathe-
terization. In four patients, two of whom had unilateral
and two of whom had sequential bilateral subclavian vein
catheterizations, subclavian and superior vena caval thrombosis occurred (Table 2). Catheters had been in place for a
considerable period of time (up to 20 months) prior to the
occurrence of SVC syndrome. The occurrence of the syndrome
was in each case associated with no evidence of recurrence
or progression of the tumor in the region of the superior
vena cava. In two cases, anticoagulation was associated
with complete or partial resolution of the SVC syndrome

Table 2
ISVEC Syndrome

| Case | Diagnosis | Subclavian Catheters | Catheter Duration until SVC Syndrome | Therapy Initial | Therapy Subsequent | Catheter | Result |
|------|-----------|---------------------|--------------------------------------|-----------------|--------------------|----------|--------|
| 1 | Ewings Sarcoma | Bilateral | 9 mo. | Heparin | Coumadin | Not Removed | Partial Resolution |
| 2 | Breast Carcinoma, Acute Un-differen-tiated Leukemia | Unilateral | 20 mo. | Heparin | Coumadin | Removed | Complete Resolution |
| 3 | Myelofi-brosis | Unilateral | 3 mo. | Strepto-kinase | None | Removed | Complete Resolution |
| 4 | Breast Carcinoma | Bilateral | 7 mo. | None | None | Removed | No change |

without additional therapy directed to any mediastinal neoplasia. In one case, fibrinolytic therapy and catheter removal was successful. Resolution was associated both with catheter removal (two cases) as well as leaving the subclavian catheter in place for continued administration of fluids and medication (one case). It is important to note that in case number 4, catheter removal without anticoagulation or fibrinolytic therapy did not relieve the SVC syndrome.

The identification of SVC syndrome in a patient with previously diagnosed malignancy in the absence of progression of mediastinal tumor is important. Prior to the recognition of this iatrogenic SVC (ISVEC) syndrome, patients may have been presumed to have progression of tumor in the region of the SVC, and may have been considered for radiation therapy or changes in chemotherapy. These patients illustrate that anticoagulation alone, with or without catheter removal, may result in resolution of the syndrome without definitive mediastinal antitumor therapy. In some patients, fibrinolytic therapy may be required to completely resolve the syndrome. However, it is imperative in patients presenting with SVC syndrome and subclavian catheters that a careful search be made for progression of tumor in the mediastinum (by use of tumor scans, mediastinal tomography, or computerized axial tomography of the chest) before concluding that the ISVEC syndrome exists.


DIAGNOSIS

An old "saw" in medicine is that the three most important aspects of patient management are "the diagnosis, the diagnosis, and the diagnosis." In previously undiagnosed patients presenting with SVC syndrome likely associated with neoplasia, rapid consideration of diagnostic tests prior to the emergent institution of therapy is extremely important in order to adequately plan subsequent therapy (Table 3). In a series of 84 patients with SVC syndrome whom we analyzed (Perez, Presant, and Van Amburg, 1978), most patients had sufficiently indolent diesase to allow bronchoscopy. Similar numbers were also able to be assessed with cytology, either obtained on sputum or bronchoscopic specimens, and/or lymph node biopsy from the supraclavicular region. All three types of evaluations were successful in producing histologic or cytologic diagnosis of the nature of the malignancy in approximately two-thirds of patients tested.

Table 3
Diagnostic Tests

| Test | % of Patients Undergoing Test | % of Tests Histo-logically Diagnostic |
|---|---|---|
| Bronchoscopy | 54 | 62 |
| Cytology | 49 | 66 |
| Lymph Node Biopsy | 48 | 63 |
| Mediastinoscopy | 13 | 81 |
| Thoracotomy | 19 | 100 |

Although the likelihood of producing a diagnostic histologic result is higher with mediastinoscopy or thoracotomy (80 to 100%), less than 20% of patients either require these procedures (since a diagnosis may have been made with less invasive tests), or have a syndrome sufficiently chronic as to allow use of these procedures.

Regardless of the type of test employed, we recommend institution of diagnostic tests within 24 hours of the appearance of SVC syndrome so that emergency definitive radiotherapy or chemotherapy may be instituted.

MANAGEMENT

Based upon our previous experience (Perez, Presant, and Van Amburg, 1978; Simpson et al., 1980), patients with neoplasia-associated SVC syndrome may be managed according to the outline described in Table 4. Patients with bronchogenic carcinoma of non-small cell undifferentiated cell type should be managed at present with emergency institution of radiation therapy. A tumor dose of at least 4000 rads is required to minimize the likelihood of recurrence of the syndrome. Comparative assessments of patients treated with 400 rads per fraction versus 200 rads per fraction for the first four fractions demonstrated equivalent results; therefore, administration of 200 rads per fraction seems satisfactory in patients with this diagnosis. The addition of chemotherapy in patients with this diagnosis results in no improvement in survival, and probably a decreased frequency of excellent or good responses to therapy (since frequently radiation therapy must be discontinued due to side effects of chemotherapy). We therefore discourage the use of simultaneous chemotherapy in this situation, at least until more effective chemothera-

Table 4
Management Outline

| Diagnosis | Primary Treatment | Secondary Treatments |
|---|---|---|
| Bronchogenic Carcinoma | | |
| Non Small-cell undifferentiated | Radiotherapy (at least 4000 R, 200 R/fraction) | Chemotherapy, anticoagulants, fibrinolytics |
| Small Cell undifferentiated | Chemotherapy (e.g. Cyclophosphamide, doxorubicin + Vincristine) | Radiotherapy |
| Malignant Lymphoma or Hodgkins Disease | | |
| Stages I,II (histologies curable by radiotherapy) | Radiotherapy | Chemotherapy |
| Stages III, IV | Chemotherapy | Radiotherapy |
| Tumor pending histologic processing | Radiotherapy for 1 to 2 days until pathology report is completed, then proceed with appropriate regimen | — |
| ISVEC* | Heparin | Catheter withdrawal Fibrinolytics |

*Iatrogenic SVC syndrome with SVC thrombosis

peutic regimens are discovered. If patients recur after radiation therapy, or fail to respond satisfactorily to radiation therapy, we recommend reevaluation of the nature of the SVC syndrome. Superior vena cavagrams are necessary to indicate whether or not intrinsic thrombosis is associated with the tumor; in such situations, anticoagulants and/or fibrinolytic therapy may be instituted with improvement in the syndrome. In most circumstances, recurrence or failure to respond are associated with persistance of the neoplasm, and in such circumstances, chemotherapy should be utilized.

In patients with small cell undifferentiated carcinoma, responses to chemotherapy are usually dramatic, both in degree and in the rapid rate of induction of the response. Therefore, we recommend that primary treatment in such patients be chemotherapy, provided an effective combination chemotherapeutic regimen is employed, such as cyclophosphamide, doxorubicin, plus vincristine; or cyclophosphamide, methotrexate plus CCNU; and provided that the patients are not refractory to prior chemotherapy. In patients who refuse chemotherapy, patients who cannot tolerate chemotherapy, or situations in which the tumor recurs after chemotherapy or fails to respond to chemotherapy, radiation therapy should be instituted at doses listed in the paragraph above.

In patients with malignant lymphoma or Hodgkin's disease, appropriate consideration should be given to the apparent stage of the disease. Although there may not be sufficient time for definitive staging evaluations, a likely stage can be presumed according to the clinical situation. In patients with limited stages of disease (Stages I or II), histologies potentially curable by radiation therapy should be initially approached with radiotherapy. Chemotherapy should be withheld until disease fails to respond to radiotherapy, or disease recurs subsequently.

In patients with more extensive stages of disease (Stages III and IV), or in patients with histologies unlikely to be cured by radiation therapy to limited stage disease, institution of chemotherapy appropriate to the histologic diagnosis should be the primary treatment. Radiation therapy in such instances can be delayed until recurrence appears, if the syndrome incompletely responds to initial therapy, or if the syndrome occurs initially following resistance to prior chemotherapy.

Frequently, the pathologist or cytologist is unwilling to make a definitive diagnosis without more complete processing of specimens already obtained. In such circumstances, we recommend institution of radiation therapy for 1 to 2 days, since such treatment is likely to result in favorable improvement of the SVC syndrome, and such therapy will not preclude the full dose chemotherapy if the patient is found to have small cell undifferentiated bronchogenic carcinoma, or malignant lymphoma of higher stage. The alternative possibility (presuming that the patient has a chemotherapy-sensitive neoplasm and initiating full-dose chemotherapy) might preclude adequate radiation therapy in a situation in which chemotherapy is unlikely to produce a satisfactory response (non-small cell undifferentiated bronchogenic carcinoma, or less chemotherapy-sensitive carcinomas of other histologic type).

The management of ISVEC syndrome has been previously discussed above. Obviously, patients should be adequately supported during the period of diagnostic evaluation and staging and preparation for treatment. Supportive measures can include head elevation, oxygen administration, maintenance of patent airway, and occasionally, use of diuretics and/or corticosteroids. Anticoagulants should be withheld until superior vena cavagrams have demonstrated thrombosis.

REFERENCES

Perez CA, Presant CA, Van Amburg AL (1978). Management of superior vena cava syndrome. Seminars Oncol 5:123.
Simpson JR, Perez CA, Presant CA, Van Amburg AL (1980). Superior vena cava syndrome. In Yarbro JW, Bornstein RS (eds): "Oncologic Emergencies," New York: Grune & Stratton, Inc., p 43.

**13th International Cancer Congress, Part D**
**Research and Treatment, pages 337–346**
© **1983 Alan R. Liss, Inc., 150 Fifth Avenue, New York, NY 10011**

ONCOLOGIC EMERGENCIES: METABOLIC DERANGEMENTS OF CLINICAL
IMPORTANCE

W. P. Laird Myers, M.D. and Marian Isaacs, M.D.

Department of Medicine
Memorial Sloan-Kettering Cancer Center
New York, New York    10021

Metabolic derangements in clinical oncology are deserv-
ing of the same concern assigned to the more dramatic oncologic emergencies such as hemorrhage and obstruction because
they have the same potential for a lethal outcome and they
can add significantly to the morbidity of the patient's
course. Awareness of their possible occurrence and early
recognition are critical to their appropriate management.

These disturbances may result from (1) tumor invasion
of an organ, (2) elaboration of physiologically active tumor
products which may cause abnormalities directly or by causing release of an endogenous product, and (3) antitumor therapy, both supportive and tumor-specific.

Tumor invasion of an organ may be directly responsible
for the failure of the normal physiologic functions of that
organ causing such disturbances as hepatic coma and hypoglycemia (liver), diabetes insipidus (pituitary), exocrine deficiency with steatorrhea (pancreas), azotemia (ureters),
and hypoxemia (lungs). Examples of physiologically active
tumor products are hormones (ectopic or natural to the tissue
of origin), growth factors, prostaglandins, catecholamines,
hydroxyindoles, and lactic acid. Many of these diverse substances have been identified only in recent years and it can
be confidently predicted many more will be identified in the
near future. The clinical manifestations of excess hormone
production are those characteristic of the hormone: hypercalcemia (parathyroid hormone), Cushing's syndrome (ACTH),
hypertension (catecholamines, renin), and erythrocytosis
(erythropoeitin). Those produced by prostaglandins are less

well defined but appear to include bone resorption and hyper-calcemia as noted below while those caused by hydroxyindoles include the long-recognized carcinoid syndrome (flushing, diarrhea, asthma). Metabolic disturbances secondary to treatment (Harrington, 1979) may soon constitute the largest of the groups since more are recognized with each new thera-peutic advance. Examples include immunosuppression (alkyla-ting agents), changes in osmolality (vincristine, cyclophos-phamide), hypocalcemia (cisplatin, mithramycin), hyper-calcemia (sex steroids), cardiac failure (doxorubicin), hypomagnesemia (aminoglycosides) and metabolic alkalosis (ticarcillin, carbenecillin). More recently prostaglandin inhibitors have been found to induce hyperkalemia and gallium nitrate hypocalcemia. These few examples will serve to ill-ustrate the point that metabolic derangements are simply ubiquitous accompaniments of cancer as seen clinically.

In order to monitor these metabolic changes in our patient population, for a number of years the Clinical Bio-chemistry Department at MSKCC has routinely notified the Clinical Physiology and Renal Service of substantial devia-tions in blood biochemical measurements. Many of the abnor-malities are of such magnitude that they are considered to be life-threatening (Table 1). On receiving this notifica-tion the Service promptly volunteers to see the patient and offers consultative advice on management. This procedure was established to minimize delays between the completion of a biochemical test and diagnosis and treatment of the abnor-mality noted. A perusal of Table 1 will reveal that a sub-stantial number of metabolic abnormalities were encountered in the twelve month period March, 1980 through February, 1981. In that period 4,277 patients had 9,427 blood biochemical abnormalities of considerable magnitude. Since patients usually had more than one abnormality, this analysis is de-rived from 2,612 individual patients. The causes of the changes observed varied considerably but, in general, they could all be classified as having been secondary to tumor invasion of an organ, or the consequence of a physiologically active tumor product, or the result of antitumor therapy, both specific and supportive. It is beyond the scope of this paper to review all of the possible consequences of the impact of various cancers on the human organism, but the following metabolic derangements will serve as examples: (1) Tumor lysis syndrome, (2) Hyper- and hypocalcemic dis-orders, and (3) Sepsis, respiratory alkalosis, and hypophos-phatemia.

1. Table 1. Substantial deviations in blood biochemical tests. March, 1980 – February, 1981

| Lower Normal | Test | Less Than | # of Pts.* | # of Tests |
|---|---|---|---|---|
| 24 | $CO_2$ | 15 | 449 | 1,012 |
| 3.8 | K | 2.8 | 398 | 842 |
| 85 | $pO_2$ | 65 | 273 | 418 |
| 9.2 | Ca | 7.0 | 227 | 637 |
| 38 | $pCO_2$ | 25 | 207 | 315 |
| 7.36 | pH | 7.30 | 197 | 337 |
| 1.4 | Mg | 1.0 | 185 | 382 |
| 136 | Na | 120 | 98 | 168 |
| 70 | Glucose | 50 | 56 | 79 |
| 2.5 | P | 1.0 | 44 | 59 |
| 95 | Cl | 70 | 17 | 20 |
| 280 | Osmolality | 275 | 16 | 22 |
| TOTALS | | | 2,167 | 4,291 |

| Test | Upper Normal | More Than | # of Pts.* | # of Tests |
|---|---|---|---|---|
| pH | 7.44 | 7.51 | 522 | 896 |
| K | 5.2 | 6.2 | 369 | 490 |
| Glucose | 110 | 400 | 290 | 896 |
| Ca | 10.8 | 12.0 | 232 | 1,261 |
| BUN | 20 | 100 | 161 | 540 |
| $pCO_2$ | 42 | 55 | 112 | 214 |
| Cl | 110 | 115 | 111 | 212 |
| $CO_2$ | 30 | 35 | 108 | 253 |
| P | 4.2 | 8.0 | 90 | 177 |
| Uric Acid | 8.5 | 15 | 64 | 129 |
| Mg | 2.2 | 3.0 | 31 | 41 |
| Na | 146 | 160 | 20 | 27 |
| TOTALS | | | 2,110 | 5,136 |

* Number of patients in descending order of frequency

Number of Tests  4,291 + 5,136 = 9,427
Number of Patients  2,167 + 2,110 = 4,277
Number of Individual Patients  = 2,612

Tumor lysis syndrome. In certain tumors, notably lymphomas and leukemias, the destruction of neoplastic cells may be marked in response to cytolytic chemotherapy or radiation therapy. This lysis of cells releases nucleic acids which are degraded metabolically to uric acid and hyperuricemia results. The solubility of uric acid varies with pH: at blood pH 7.40 it exists as the soluble monovalent urate ion, whereas at a urinary pH of 5, it exists in the much less soluble, non-ionized form. The likelihood of precipitation of uric acid crystals in the distal portions of the nephron (the region of maximal acidification of urine) is great under these conditions, and widespread intrarenal, and possibly ureteral, obstruction may occur resulting in oliguria or anuria. The full syndrome including azotemia, metabolic acidosis, hyperkalemia, hyperphosphatemia and hypocalcemia, may rapidly develop and end fatally unless treated promptly and adequately. Since prevention is more to be desired than treating the established syndrome, the following considerations must be kept in mind: (1) Be aware of its likely development in any patient with lymphoma (Cohen, Balow, Magrath, Poplack, Ziegler, 1980), especially those with bulky disease or an elevated lactic dehydrogenase, or leukemia, notably acute lymphocytic leukemia. Hyperuricemia may also be seen with certain rapidly developing carcinomas, especially in the presence of renal disease, and the syndrome might develop in these patients with cytolytic therapy. (2) In patients at risk, start treatment with allopurinol 600-900 mg orally daily at least three days before the administration of antitumor therapy. At times such a delay in treatment is not possible, but the point to be made is that prior treatment with allopurinol will be far more effective than if it is given simultaneously with the antitumor treatment. (3) Insure adequate hydration and establish an alkaline diuresis of 100-150 ml/hr prior to the administration of therapy. This can be achieved with 5% dextrose in water with added sodium bicarbonate 50 mEq/L. In patients who do not achieve appropriate urine volumes, 12.5 grams of mannitol (25% solution) should be given intravenously (IV) to induce a diuresis; 3-5 gm/hr will generally maintain a good urine output. Because mannitol is an osmotic diuretic, electrolyte excretion will increase; therefore, serum electrolytes (as well as uric acid, BUN and creatinine) should be monitored every 6 hours and losses replaced appropriately. An equivalent diuresis can usually be induced with IV furosemide: 40 mgm IV followed by 3-5 mg/kg/24 hrs in an IV infusion (Isaacs, 1979).

In some patients, particularly those who present with azotemia, hyperuricemia or hyperphosphatemia, dialysis either prior to therapy or on an emergency basis may have to be done because of the rapidity with which uremia can develop. This is most likely to occur in patients with marked hyperphosphatemia, since intrarenal precipitation of calcium phosphate salts may contribute to the development of renal failure. Acutely ill patients may have to be dialyzed daily and therapy instituted to reduce hypercatabolism, if present (adequate calories and protein via parenteral nutrition, antibiotics for sepsis, and other supportive measures as indicated). Anemia, disseminated intravascular coagulation, and thrombocytopenia are not contraindications to dialysis in our experience. Peritoneal dialysis is useful primarily for fluid overload syndromes, in those who are hemodynamically unstable, and in small children. It is not as useful as hemodialysis for clearing uric acid from the blood. As part of the overall management of these patients drug dosages must be monitored and reduced as indicated in the presence of renal failure. In summary, the syndrome is a dramatic one, should usually be preventable, and is readily managed by the measures noted.

Hypercalcemia, hypocalcemia. Abnormalities of serum calcium concentration constitute a common metabolic derangement in cancer - one which may very well be life threatening. Hypercalcemia has received considerable attention in recent years but hypocalcemia in our experience is becoming increasingly common. Thus, in the twelve month review referred to above (Table 1), there were 232 patients who had serum calcium levels above 12 mg/dl, but there were also 227 patients whose serum calciums were less than 7 mg/dl. There are numerous and fascinating reasons behind these changes. Although most patients with hypercalcemia have bone metastases, many do not. Originally thought to be the consequence of tumor invasion of bone causing calcium release into the extracellular compartment faster than the kidneys could remove it, hypercalcemia is now considered more in humoral terms. That is, tumor products are thought to be largely responsible for osteolysis whether they are elaborated locally in bone or systemically. The three products which have been most often cited include parathyroid hormone (PTH) or a PTH-like substance, prostaglandins - notably $PGE_2$, and a lymphokine, osteoclast activating factor - OAF. More recently other biological substances have been demonstrated to have bone-resorbing actions in vitro. These include vaso-

active intestinal peptide, epidermal growth factor and platelet derived growth factor.  In addition, evidence for a tumor-
derived growth factor with prostaglandin-independent bone
resorbing activity has been reported in an animal tumor which
causes hypercalcemia (Ibbotson, D'Souza, Osborne, Niall, Wah,
Martin, Mundy, 1982).

In recent years it has been shown that resorbing bone
is chemotactic for tumor cells and that tumor cells can resorb bone directly without the cellular intermediation of
osteoclasts or osteocytes.  The sequence of events in bone
break-down has been considered to be a two-step event in
which initially tumor products cause bone to resorb either
directly or through the intermediation of osteoclasts (stimulated, for example, by OAF, with $PGE_2$ serving as a necessary
intermediary).  The resorbing bone in turn attracts tumor
cells which in the second step join the osteoclasts on the
bone surface to further bone lysis.  In instances where the
skeleton is not invaded only the first of these two steps
would be operative.  In clinical terms virtually every known
tumor may be attended by hypercalcemia at one time or another
in the patient's course.  The exact incidence varies with the
tumor, being most common in breast cancer in our experience,
followed in decreasing order of frequency by hematological
neoplasms and by cancers of the lung, kidney, head and neck,
cervix, prostate and a variety of miscellaneous tumors.
Patients with cancer who have hypercalcemia, hypophosphatemia
and hypercalciuria have the typical biochemical parameters of
hyperparathyroidism solely on the basis of their tumors (so-
called ectopic hyperparathyroidism) or on the basis of co-
existing primary hyperparathyroidism.  With regard to the
latter, several reports have called attention to the concurr-
ence of primary hyperparathyroidism and cancer, notably
breast cancer.  Thus, a patient with breast cancer who has
hypercalcemia and hypophosphatemia (rare in breast cancer in
contrast to lung or renal cancer) should be strongly suspected of having co-existent primary hyperparathyroidism.

Treatment can be considered in four categories: (1) General measures:  These are directed against dehydration and
toward fostering renal excretion of calcium by infusions of
5% dextrose in normal saline initially and 0.45% saline subsequently.  Diuretics may be used - that is furosemide, not
thiazides which reduce calcium excretion.  (2)  Non-specific
measures:  Inhibition of the basic lesion of cancer hypercalcemia - increased bone resorption - can be accomplished

with oral phosphates (caution: avoid using in the azotemic patient), mithramycin (caution: injudicious use can cause fatal hypocalcemia), calcitonin (perhaps more effective if given in conjunction with phosphate), and diphosphonates (oral ethane hydroxydiphosphonate - EHDP). Corticosteroids are useful primarily in the hypercalcemia of myeloma, lymphoma and breast cancer and presumably work via tumor inhibition and by suppressing prostaglandins needed at the bone surface to mediate OAF resorption. Prostaglandin inhibitors, notably aspirin and indomethacin, have been reported to correct hypercalcemia in those patients whose bone resorption is primarily caused by prostaglandins. For the most part they have not proved very effective clinically. (3) Specific measures: The most important way to control cancer-induced hypercalcemia is to control the cancer whether by surgery, chemotherapy or radiation therapy. Sex steroid treatment of breast cancer (estrogens, anti-estrogens, androgens, and progestins) may at times cause hypercalcemia and should be discontinued in such instances. (4) Associated problems: Avoidance of protracted immobilization is at times difficult to achieve, but worthy of doing whenever possible. Patients with hypercalcemia may also have associated hypokalemia, alkalosis, and hypomagnesemia and these should be looked for and treated as necessary (Myers, 1973).

Hypocalcemia has been reported in a **variety** of clinical situations: (1) In the "hungry bones" syndrome, in which intense osteoblastic activity causes marked skeletal uptake of calcium; (2) In hypomagnesemia, the result of renal losses, induced by chemotherapy (cisplatin) and antibiotics (amphotericin B and gentamicin), or gastrointestinal losses; (3) In hypoalbuminemia; (4) In malabsorption secondary to tumor involvement of the intestine or pancreas, to massive resection of the small bowel, or to avitaminosis D; (5) In hyperphosphatemia secondary to the tumor lysis syndrome; (6) In surgical removal of the parathyroid glands with radical neck dissections for cancer; (7) In metastatic destruction of the parathyroid glands; (8) In patients with hypophosphatemia and osteomalacia secondary to mesenchymal tumors; and (9) In antitumor treatment, or treatment for hypercalcemia, such as with mithramycin or phosphate. Symptomatology is variable from none to weakness, confusion, paresthesias, carpal pedal spasm and tetany. Treatment should be directed at the cause, but acute symptomatic hypocalcemia must be treated with intravenous calcium gluconate. Long term management may call for the use of oral calcium supplements and vitamin D.

  Sepsis, respiratory alkalosis and hypophosphatemia.
There are a number of disorders in patients with cancer that
can lead to respiratory alkalosis, that is a primary decrease
in $pCO_2$ caused by increased depth or frequency of respirations.
Thus, respiratory alkalosis has been described in patients
with pulmonary metastases, mechanical and voluntary overven-
tilation, hypoxia, hepatic coma and central nervous system
afflictions. Although these causes must be considered in
any differential diagnosis, we have become particularly
impressed by the frequent occurrence of sepsis (gram-negative
and gram-positive sepsis) in our patient population as a
cause of respiratory alkalosis. In one review of our patient
population 54% of 47 patients with positive blood cultures
had respiratory alkalosis (Scheiner, Isaacs, Vanamee, 1966).
Hyperventilation and respiratory alkalosis may precede the
fever and shock of sepsis so that all patients who are found
clinically to be hyperventilating now routinely have blood
cultures. Patients with respiratory alkalosis have hyperchloremia and this must be remembered to avoid the snap conclusion that a patient with hyperchloremia and a low serum
bicarbonate has hyperchloremic acidosis. In fact, in our
experience, 60% of low serum bicarbonate determinations are
caused by respiratory alkalosis. An additional finding in
these patients has been hypophosphatemia. Hypophosphatemia
less than 2 mg/dl has been reported to be associated with
41% of patients with gram-negative sepsis and only 14% of
those with gram-positive sepsis (Riedler, Scheitlin, 1969).
Hypophosphatemia apparently is secondary to the respiratory
alkalosis, which causes an increased cellular uptake of phosphate. Of interest is the observation that alkalosis of
metabolic origin does not induce hypophosphatemia as frequently or to the same extent as respiratory alkalosis of similar
magnitude. Cancer patients may also have other disorders,
existing concurrently with respiratory alkalosis and sepsis,
that can aggravate the phosphate abnormality. For example,
phosphate depletion may result from malabsorption following
gastrectomy or with renal phosphate wasting as seen in leukemia and in the Fanconi syndrome associated with multiple
myeloma. Medical interventions such as glucose infusions,
hyperalimentation, diuretics and phosphate-binding antacids
also may be contributory factors.

  The physiological consequences of hypophosphatemia
(Knochel, 1977) include a variety of disturbances best

remembered by the target tissues affected: red cells, leucocytes, platelets, the central nervous system, muscle, bones and kidneys. A decrease in red cell 2,3-diphosphoglycerate (DPG) and adenosine triphosphate (ATP) results in a shift to the left of the oxyhemoglobin dissociation curve with a reduction in P50 (oxygen tension at which hemoglobin is 50% saturated), an increased affinity of hemoglobin for oxygen, and tissue hypoxia. In severe hypophosphatemia hemolytic anemia may be seen. A decrease in leukocyte ATP is accompanied by abnormalities in chemotaxis and phagocytosis. Thrombocytopenia, accelerated rate of disappearance of platelets from the blood, diminished platelet aggregation and poor clot retraction may occur, as well as tissue hypoxia of the central nervous system which may lead to ataxia, seizures and coma. Muscle cell membrane functional changes occur with the reduction in muscle ATP and may ultimately be attended by rhabdomyolysis with release of creatine phosphokinase and heme pigment. Osteomalacia has been described in severe phosphate depletion. The kidney responds to hypophosphatemia with a decrease in urinary phosphate (to less than 4 mg/dl when the serum phosphorus is below 2 mg/dl) and an increase in the excretion of calcium, bicarbonate and glucose. Treatment includes careful monitoring of the serum phosphate in patients whose clinical settings are likely to be associated with the disorder with addition of phosphate supplements as indicated. Skim milk is a good source of phosphorus (0.9 mg/ml) for those who can take nourishment orally. Phosphate salts may be given orally but often cause diarrhea. In some patients the intravenous route must be used and the administration of 10-20 mM per 24 hours, depending on the severity of the losses and the hypophosphatemia, is usually recommended. It may be given as potassium phosphate to treat hypokalemia which frequently coexists, but usually potassium deficits have to be met independently.

In conclusion, some general aspects of metabolic derangements in cancer have been cited and three (the tumor lysis syndrome, hyper- and hypocalcemia, and sepsis with respiratory alkalosis and hypophosphatemia) have been reviewed from the standpoint of their pathogenesis and treatment. When fully developed these derangements constitute true oncologic emergencies which must be recognized and treated appropriately to avoid unnecessary fatalities.

Cohen LF, Balow JE, Magrath IT, Poplack DG, Ziegler JL (1980). Acute Tumor Lysis Syndrome. A review of 37 patients with Burkitt's lymphoma. Amer J Med 68:486.

Harrington WJ (1979). Iatrogenic Disorders from Cancer Treatment. Advances Int Med 24:141.

Ibbotson K, D'Souza SM, Osborne CK, Niall M, Wah K, Martin TJ, Mundy GR (1982). Evidence that a tumor-derived growth factor is responsible for the humoral hypercalcemia of malignancy. Amer Soc Bone Min Res Abstr 4th Annual Meeting p531.

Isaacs M (1979) Life-threatening fluid and electrolyte abnormalities in patients with cancer. Current Problems in Cancer 4:6.

Knochel JP (1977). The pathophysiology and clinical characteristics of severe hypophosphatemia. Arch Int Med 137:203.

Myers WPL(1973). Hypercalcemia associated with malignant diseases. In Samaan NA (ed) "Endocrine and Non-Endocrine Hormone-Producing Tumors". Chicago: Year Book Medical Publishers, Inc. p 147.

Riedler GF, Scheitlin WA (1969). Hypophosphataemia in Septicaemia: Higher incidence in gram-negative than in gram-positive infections. Brit Med J 1:753.

Scheiner E, Isaacs M, Vanamee P (1966). Water and electrolyte disturbances in cancer patients. Med Clin North Amer 50:711.

13th International Cancer Congress, Part D
Research and Treatment, pages 347–360
© 1983 Alan R. Liss, Inc., 150 Fifth Avenue, New York, NY 10011

# MALIGNANT EFFUSIONS AS ONCOLOGIC EMERGENCIES

Frederick Hausheer, M.D.
J.W. Yarbro, M.D., Ph.D.
Department of Medicine
University of Missouri
Columbia, MO  65212

Malignant pleural, pericardial, and ascitic effusions often develop as chronic recurrent complications of cancer. It is still generally true that the development of a malignant effusion is a signal that the cancer has become incurable and therapy can, at best, improve the quality of life for a few months.

On the other hand the number of exceptions to this generally pessimistic analysis is increasing each year. Increasingly with modern multimodal therapy, cures are possible of cancers disseminated to the point of producing effusions. Improved palliative treatment may add years to life, the quality of which will be determined by our ability to control a recurrent effusion. Finally, not infrequently malignant effusions may present as oncologic emergencies requiring rapid diagnosis and appropriate therapy if the patient is to have an opportunity to receive the benefits of our much improved therapeutic armamentarium against cancer.

## PATHOPHYSIOLOGY

The pleural, pericardial and peritoneal spaces normally contain a small quantity ($<$ 35 ml) of serous fluid with a protein content $<$ 2 gm/dl and a pH and glucose equilibrated with plasma. This fluid has a rapid turnover, for pleura 35-75% per hour, in accordance with the Starling equation:

$$F = K \left[ (P_{cap} - P_{if}) - (O_{cap} - O_{if}) \right]$$

## MALIGNANT EFFUSIONS

where F = fluid movement, K = permeability constant in ml/sec/cm$^2$/cmH$_2$O, Pcap = capillary hydrostatic pressure, Pif = pericapillary interstitial fluid hydrostatic pressure (or effusion hydrostatic pressure), Ocap = plasma osmotic pressure, and Oif = interstitial fluid osmotic pressure (or effusion osmotic pressure).  At equilibrium, fluid entering the space is equal to fluid leaving.  The K for the entry point is not necessarily the same as the K for the exit point as is illustrated by the increased number of microvilli of visceral pleura mesothelial cells compared to parietal.  Any factor that alters any of the four pressure functions or the permeability constant may lead to fluid accumulation.  Such factors may be systemic or local.

The most common systemic cause of effusion is congestive heart failure which increases Pcap leading to accumulation of sufficient fluid to produce a compensating rise in Pif in the space.  Constrictive pericarditis produces ascites and pleural effusion in a similar fashion.  A fall in serum protein will lower Ocap and fluid will accumulate until the Pif of the effusion raises fluid outflow to equal inflow.  Myxedema represents a rare cause of high protein effusion, presumably due to altered membrane permeability, that may present diagnostic difficulties.

Local factors may alter the elements of the Starling equation.  A local or regional increase in Pcap may result from venous obstruction of portal veins, hepatic veins (Budd Chiari syndrome), inferior vena cava, and pulmonary veins, with or without concomitant lymphatic obstruction.  These relationships may become quite complex; the exact pathophysiology is in many cases still controversial (Witte et al, 1980).  Infection within a space, or tumor cell invasion may increase the protein content ($\uparrow$ Oif) and inflammation may alter the permeability of the serous lining ($\Delta$ K).

It is traditional to classify effusions as exudates or transudates, based on high or low protein content.  Light et al (1972) defined an exudate based on the content of protein and LDH relative to serum: the effusion was considered an exudate if the effusion/serum protein ratio was > 0.5, the LDH ratio > 0.6, or if the absolute LDH content of the effusion was > 200 I.U.  This is a useful, but by no means infallible, aid in diagnosis.

The pathophysiology of malignant effusion is complicated by the multiplicity of mechanisms by which cancer may alter fluid balance in the space:

1. Tumor cells and inflammation within the space may alter permeability ($\Delta$ K).
2. Some tumors secrete protein in the space ($\uparrow$ Oif).
3. Regional lymphatics and/or venous drainage may be compromised ($\uparrow$ Pcap).
4. Malnutrition secondary to cancer may lower serum protein ($\uparrow$ Ocap).
5. Complications such as congestive heart failure ($\uparrow$ Pcap), post obstructive pneumonitis ($\uparrow$ Oif) etc., may produce effusions.

It is a virtual certainty that these mechanisms operate in various combinations for different tumors in different spaces. For example, lung cancer may produce an exudative pleural effusion by invasion of the pleura or a transudative effusion by vascular compromise within the lung, or a combination of both. Exudative ascites may follow peritoneal implantation of mucin secreting ovarian or gastric tumors or transudative ascites may result from hepatic metastases. In general, of course, malignant effusions are exudates.

Once the equilibrium of the Starling equation is shifted toward fluid accumulation it may progress to some stable point where the increase in Pif balances the equation at an asymptomatic or mildly symptomatic clinical stage; alternately, the effusion may continue to accumulate at a variable rate producing an emergency, hypoventilation in the case of pleural or peritoneal effusion and cardiac tamponade in the case of pericardial effusion.

Pleural effusion acts as a plombage, that is it occupies space in the chest compromising the ability of both lungs to expand by reducing compliance, and causing mild symptoms, usually not requiring therapy. Chernow and Sahn (1977) reviewed 96 cases of malignant pleural effusion: 23% were asymptomatic, 57% had dyspnea; the effusion was bilateral in 31% and massive in 13%; the mean $pO_2$ of these patients was 55.6 $\pm$ 2.2 (range 26-77) normal = 70 $\pm$ 5, and the mean $pCO_2$ was normal; 56% did not require treatment for the effusion. It is likely that patients who develop respiratory compromise from pleural effusion had marginal pulmonary function before the effusion developed.

Pericardial effusion produces its pathophysiological effects by initiating a chain of events in which compensation is effective in the majority of cases; in a minority, however, continued increase in the effusion leads to a catastrophic decompensation (tamponade). As the accumulating effusion raises pericardial pressure there is an increase in ventricular diastolic pressure and mean atrial pressure, the latter initiating tachycardia via the Bainbridge reflex; decreased ventricular filling leads to decreased stroke volume with fall in cardiac output and resultant vasocontriction. Central venous pressure rises to allow blood to continue to enter the heart against the pressure gradient induced by the effusion, and renal salt and water retention further elevate the volume in the venous pool. Cardiac output is maintained by vasoconstriction, tachycardia, increased blood volume, and increased venous pressure. Vasoconstriction maintains, or may even increase, diastolic pressure. Pulmonary venous pressure is also elevated, but pulmonary edema is quite rare because the output of the right heart is also reduced and, as Spodick (1967) has pointed out, "signs of left heart failure cannot occur without right heart success".

If the effusion continues to accumulate, the stroke volume may fall below the level that allows cardiac output to maintain systolic pressure and collapse is catastrophic over a few hours with no further compensation possible.

Interruption of this chain of events requires that one first address the altered pressure relationships in the pleural, peritoneal, or pericardial space and, if necessary, remove sufficient fluid to alleviate any emergency. This will only occasionally be necessary for pleural and peritoneal effusions, but will be required more often for pericardial effusions. Once pressure relationships are temporarily restored the question of restoring balance between ingress and egress of fluid into the space must be considered. This is obviously best achieved by addressing the primary cause. When a curable or highly responsive cancer is present, systemic treatment is always to be preferred (except for relief of acute manifestations). But all too often, a reversal of the primary pathology may not be possible. Under these circumstances, local control of the effusion is attempted either by obliterating the space by fusion of the surfaces as in the case of the pleura, by eliminating the space as in the case of pericardiectomy, or by draining the space as by LeVeen shunt for ascites or pleuropericardial window for pericardial effusion. In some tumors there may be a role for local tumor control (by drugs or radiation) even when systemic control is not possible. In any event, as the therapeutic modalities escalate in complexity, morbidity, and mortality, careful judgment must be exercised. Drastic local measures are not indicated in a patient who will soon die from systemic cancer.

## DIAGNOSIS

In most patients, the diagnosis of cancer will have been established long before the patient presents with an effusion. It is still necessary to establish that the effusion is malignant in origin and signals cancer progression. Patients whose cancer has been cured or has entered prolonged remission may develop benign effusions. Posner et al (1981) reviewed the records of 31 cancer patients with an antemortem diagnosis of pericardial disease: In 13 (42%) the involvement was considered benign.

In a few patients the effusion may be the initial manifestation of malignancy. Of 106 patients with malignant pleural effusions studied by Martini et al (1975), the effusion was the only clinical and radiologic finding initially in 68 (64%). Such presentations are rather common in lung cancer but far less common is breast cancer: only 2/33 breast cancer patients in this series presented initially with pleural effusion. Pericardial effusion with tamponade may be the presenting sign on rare occasions in acute myelogenous leukemia (Saha et al, 1977), lymphoma (Levitt et al, 1979), Hodgkin's disease, melanoma, thymoma, and breast cancer (Anderes et al, 1979); but, most of the reported cases in which a malignancy presents with tamponade are due to lung cancer (Brown et al, 1976, Damuth et al, 1979, Strauss et al, 1977). Adenocarcinoma of the lung may be of particular importance in this regard. Of 23 cases of malignant tamponade studied by Anderes et al (1979), tamponade was the presenting sign in nine (39%), and lung cancer was the cause in six of these nine.

Dyspnea is by far the most common complaint in both pleural and pericardial effusion and dyspnea will be the chief complaint in most patients who require immediate therapy for malignant ascites. Fluid produces a flat percussion note commonly seen in pleural effusion but present as substernal flatness in pericardial effusion, and as the "puddle sign" when patients with ascites are positioned on hands and knees with abdomen dependent. The upright chest x-ray will detect as little as 300 ml of effusion and the lateral decubitus 100 ml. The echocardiogram allows detection of very small quantities of pericardial effusion, less than 50 ml. The classic shifting dullness of ascites is not seen until two liters of fluid are present but the "puddle sign" sign may be elicited with 300-400 ml.

The evaluation of a patient with pleural effusion of unknown etiology should begin with thoracocentesis to obtain at least 250 ml for study of cytology, protein content, pH, LDH, and culture. A diagnosis of cancer will be made in 50-60% of malignant effusions in this manner. Needle biopsy of the pleura and cytogenetic studies will increase the diagnostic yield to 80-90%, and when two centeses have failed, pleuroscopically directed biopsy will permit diagnosis of 90-95% of patients (Weissburg et al, 1980). Exploratory thoracotomy is the final diagnostic step and even this procedure may sometimes fail to provide a diagnosis; two-thirds of such patients never have a recurrence of fluid and one-fourth are later found to have cancer (Ryan et al, 1981).

Diagnosis of pericardial effusion should be based on the echocardiogram which has largely replaced the other techniques once used in this diagnosis. Not all effusions, of course, produce tamponade. A compromise of cardiac function is suggested by elevated venous pressure with exaggerated pulsations, tachycardia with narrowed pulse pressure, and pulsus paradoxus which probably results from "internal tamponade" of the left ventricle by a right ventricle enlarged by the influx of blood induced by inspiration (Spodick, 1967). Cytology of pericardial fluid is accurate in establishing the diagnosis of malignant effusion in 57% to 80% of cases (Yazdi et al, 1980, Zipf and Johnson, 1972).

The proportion of all effusions that ultimately turn out to be malignant is difficult to determine from a study of the literature. Congestive heart failure is clearly the leading cause of effusions but these cases are often not reported (as for pleural effusion) or not diagnosed (as for pericardial effusion) so that reported "incidence" data relate to selected effusions. About half of all reported effusions of sufficient clinical significance to be tapped for diagnostic and/or therapeutic purposes are malignant (Table 1). There is wide variation in the criteria for inclusion in reported series but the data are surprisingly consistent. Not all investigators distinguish between effusions seen in patients with cancer and effusions with cancer cells in the fluid. This is an important distinction particularly in pericardial effusion where cured Hodgkin's disease patients may present with radiation pericarditis (Krikorian and Hancock, 1978).

Table 1. Causes of pleural, pericardial, and ascitic effusions classified as malignant. Data are expressed as number of malignant effusions/total effusions studied and percent malignant. Data are from Leuallen and Carr (1955), Storey et al (1976), Cardazo (1966), Hirsch et al (1979), Anderes et al (1979), Lajos et al (1975), Williams and Soutter (1954), Krikorian and Hancock (1978), Hyman et al (1963), Berner et al (1964) and Tavel (1959).

| PLEURAL | | PERICARDIAL | | ASCITIC | |
|---|---|---|---|---|---|
| 229/436 | 53% | 23/40 | 58% | 199/344 | 58% |
| 64/133 | 48% | 15/32 | 47% | 53/142 | 38% |
| 546/1248 | 44% | 50/120 | 42% | 37/100 | 37% |
| 117/300 | 39% | 7/17 | 41% | 34/100 | 34% |

Only a relatively few cancers tend to produce malignant effusions with a high degree of frequency presumably because they combine a naturally high incidence with a tendency to invade serosal surfaces or to occupy strategic regional locations. Table 2 lists the tumors most commonly associated with malignant effusions. About half of the significant pleural and pericardial effusions are produced by cancers of the lung and breast (about equally). Lymphoma is the third most common cause. Any large series of pericardial effusions will include several cases of melanoma, which metastasizes to the heart with a very high frequency, as high as 64% in one study (Glancy and Roberts, 1968), but because it is less common that the other cancers (and because cancers metastatic to the heart do not usually cause symptoms) it represents only a small fraction of cases presenting with symptomatic pericardial effusion. Consistent data on the incidence of various types of cancer in patients with malignant ascites is surprising difficult to obtain. A special variant of malignant ascites, chronic chylous ascites, is malignant 80% of the time and usually due to lymphoma.

Table 2.   Tumors most commonly associated with malignant effusions listed in approximate order of frequency.

| Pleural | Pericardial | Ascitic |
|---------|-------------|---------|
| Lung | Lung | Ovary |
| Breast | Breast | Hepatoma |
| Lymphoma/Leukemia | Lymphoma/Leukemia | Lymphoma |
| Ovary | Melanoma | Other G.I. |
| Mesothelioma | Mesothelioma | Mesothelioma |

## THERAPY OF MALIGNANT EFFUSIONS

Therapeutic strategy for management of malignant effusions should be considered in three phases:  emergency, curative, and palliative.  Emergency therapy may be required to correct the acute compromise of function produced by the pressure of the accumulating fluid.   Curative therapy is still possible in some cancers even after effusion develops; surgical cure is almost never possible and the theoretical possibility of curing a lung cancer in which the effusion is a transudate due to intrapulmonary obstruction is sufficiently rare that data are limited to isolated case reports.  Palliative therapy, which is what most patients with malignant effusion require, may be subdivided into antitumor therapy, space obliteration therapy, and long-term space drainage.  Where possible, local palliation should be combined with attempts to control the systemic or regional cancer and the extent of the local therapy should be calibrated to the overall prognosis of the patient.

### Emergency Therapy

Emergency therapy for malignant pleural effusion will occasionally be required and this decision is best made on the basis of the clinical picture of respiratory distress and blood gas studies indicating anoxia.  The initial thoracocentesis may be both diagnostic and therapeutic.  Most patients who require therapeutic thoracocentesis probably should have either a catheter or chest tube inserted initially to prevent recurrence of the effusion.

Emergency centesis for ascites is rarely necessary but when required may dramatically relieve respiratory distress.

Unlike either pleural or pericardial effusion, placement of catheter or tube drainage is not ordinarily recommended. In the past, removal of massive quantities of ascitic fluid was commonplace; but, because this is occasionally followed by rapidly reaccumulating fluid reducing blood volume and producing shock, most investigators now recommend that no more than one or two liters be removed.

Pericardial effusion with tamponade is the prototype oncologic emergency produced by malignant effusion. When tamponade is diagnosed on the basis of echocardiogram, narrowing pulse pressure, pulsus paradoxus, elevated venous pressure and other less common signs, immediate decompression is required. While preparations for this decompression are underway, fluids should be used to increase the filling pressure of the heart, and isoproterenol should be administered. Isoproterenol stimulates contraction, reduces heart size (diminishing tamponade), and increases cardiac output. When shock is present, norepinephrine should be added to isoproterenol (Fowler and Holmes, 1969). Vasodilators such as nitroprusside are contraindicated because they reduce filling pressure. Positive pressure respiratory therapy is also contraindicated because it raises pericardial pressure and reduces filling. Digitalis is often said to be contraindicated because of an older study (McMichael and Sharpey-Schafer, 1944) indicating it reduced atrial pressure (this might reduce filling) but this is open to debate when the full implications of this original study are evaluated. Furthermore, severe congestive failure sometimes follows decompression of tamponade. Thus the use of digitalis is probably justified when clinical judgment dictates.

Decompression of tamponade may be effected by pericardiocentesis or by a surgical procedure and the decision as to which alternative is preferred is based on the nature of the tamponade and the clinical expertise available. In general surgical decompression is indicated when the effusion is purulent (and thus too thick to drain by catheter), traumatic and bloody (in which case repair may be required), effusive-constrictive (in which removal of the visceral pericardium is required for decompression), when pericardiocentesis fails or fluid reaccumulates rapidly, or in the absence of a cardiologist skilled in centesis. When removal of the visceral pericardium is likely to be necessary, a sternal splitting approach is mandatory; otherwise, a left thoracotomy may be used. For reversible tamponade a subxiphoid pericardiostomy under local is preferred by some (Lajos et al, 1975) whereas others prefer pericardiocentesis using a #14 needle often with insertion of a catheter (which should not be left in beyond 48 hours). Insertion of the large needle should be preceeded by local anesthetic injected through a long #20 needle inserted by a subxiphoid subcostal route aiming at the left shoulder and keeping the needle tip as close to the ribcage as possible until fluid can be withdrawn from the pericardium. Some operators prefer to attach a V-lead EKG to the hub of the needle to signal if the myocardium is touched.

## Curative Therapy

Some tumors may be curable even though sufficiently advanced to produce malignant effusions. Of the tumors commonly associated with malignant effusions, curable tumors include Hodgkin's and some non-Hodgkin's lymphoma, small cell lung cancer, and ovarian cancer. Less commonly germ cell neoplasms or another curable cancer may be encountered. Under such circumstances, after any emergency situation is dealt with by decompression, appropriate potentially curative therapeutic regimens should be initiated.

## Palliative Therapy

Most malignant effusions are associated with neoplasms that are incurable in the stages in which effusions develop. However, some of these - notably breast cancer - may be controlled by palliative systemic therapy for long periods of time and adequate control of the effusion may markedly improve the quality of the patient's remaining life. Three basic therapeutic strategies are available: 1) control of the tumor within the space by radiation or anti-tumor drugs; 2) obliteration of the space by sclerotic drugs (anti-tumor or other sclerosing drug), by talc, or by surgical pleurectomy; and 3) long-term drainage by parietal pericardiectomy or LeVeen shunt. The appropriate strategy depends on the nature of the tumor, the pathophysiology of the effusion, and the overall prognosis of the patient.

For radiosensitive tumors, especially of the pericardium, radiation therapy has produced excellent results.

For tumor sensitive to non-sclerotic antineoplastic drugs, especially ovarian cancer with ascites, agents such as thiotepa have value. For the most part, however, in the pleural space where sclerosis is particularly effective, sclerotic agents (whether or not they are antineoplastic) are the agents of choice. It is clear that thoracocentesis alone is followed by recurrence over 95% of the time unless the systemic treatment of the cancer is successful. Tube drainage alone is better but a sclerotic agent administered through a tube (under water seal after full lung expansion is documented) is the treatment of choice. Table 3 shows results reported by numerous investigators using various drugs. Data are far from clear as to the agent of choice and although tetracycline is recommended widely a close study of the data do not indicate it to be clearly superior. Several studies show Bleomycin to be quite effective (though it is costly) and early data on Adriamycin are encouraging. When sclerosing drugs fail, talc is often effective and the procedure of final recourse is pleurectomy which is virtually 100% effective but carries on operative (30 day) mortality rate of 10-18% (Martini et al, 1975, Jensik et al, 1963).

Table 3. A summary of numerous reports of the rate of control of pleural effusion using a variety of agents and not always using tube drainage. Only those reports were selected in which follow-up data were given and control was defined as at least one month free of recurrence. The numerous references reviewed will be cited in a subsequent more detailed report. The reader should consult the following sources: for adriamycin Kefford et al, 1980; for Bleomycin Bitran et al, 1981 and Paladine et al, 1976; for talc Weissburg and Kaufmann, 1980, Harley, 1979, Adler and Sayek, 1976, and Prorok and Nealon, 1968.

| AGENT | RANGE OF REPORTED RESPONSES | MEDIAN |
|---|---|---|
| Nitrogen Mustard | 28 - 88% | 52% |
| 5-FU and ThioTEPA | 30 - 63% | 55% |
| Tetracycline | 55 - 75% | 67% |
| Adriamycin | 73% | 73% |
| Quinacrine | 72 - 86% | 80% |
| Bleomycin | 85 - 89% | 87% |
| Talc | 90 - 100% | 95% |

Adler RH, Sayek I (1976). Treatment of malignant pleural effusion: A method using tube thoracostomy and talc. Ann Thorac Surg 22:8-15.

Anderes U, Heierli B, Follath HF (1979). Herztamponade bei malignen Tumoren. Schweiz Med Wsch 109:791-793.

Berner C, Herbert FL, Riggs S, and Davis JS (1964). Diagnostic probabilities in patients with conspicuous ascites. Arch Int Med 113:687-690.

Bitran JD, Brown C, Desser RK, Kozloff MF, Shapiro C, and Billings AA (1981). Intracavitary Bleomycin for the control of malignant effusions. J Surg Oncol 16:273-277.

Brown SE, Harder HI, Brown AF (1976). Bronchioalveolar carcinoma presenting as pericardial effusion with tamponade. West J Med 124:500-502.

Cardoza PL (1966). A critical evaluation of 3000 cytologic analyses of pleural fluid, ascitic fluid, and pericardial fluid. Acta Cytol 10:455-460.

Chernow B and Sahn SA (1977). Carcinomatous involvement of the pleura. Am J Med 63:695-702.

Damuth TE, Bush CA, Leier CV (1979). Adenocarcinoma of the lung: pericardial tamponade as the major presenting feature. Ohio State Med J 75:25-27.

Fowler NO, Holmes JC (1969). Hemodynamic effects of isoproterenal and norepinephrine in acute tamponade. J Clin Invest 48:502-507.

Glancy DL, Roberts WC (1968). The heart in malignant melanoma. A study of 70 autopsy cases. Amer J Cardiol 21:555-571.

Harley HR (1979). Malignant pleural effusions and their treatment by intercostal talc pleurodesis. Br J Dis Chest 73:173-177.

Hirsch A, Ruffie P, Nebut M, Bignon J, Chretien J (1979). Pleural effusion: laboratory tests in 300 cases. Thorax 34:106-112.

Hyman S, Villa F, Steigman F (1963). Mimetic aspects of ascites. JAMA 183:651-658.

Jensik R, Cagle JE Jr, Milloy F et al (1963). Pleurectomy in the treatment of pleural effusion due to metastatic malignancy. J Thorac Cardiovasc Surg 46:322-330.

Kefford RF, Woods RL, Fox RM, Tatterall MH (1980). Intracavitary adriamycin, nitrogen mustard, and tetracycline in the control of malignant effusions: a randomized study. Med J Aust 2:447-448.

Krikorian JG, Hancock EW (1978). Pericardiocentesis. Am J Med 65:808-814.

Lajos TZ, Black HE, Cooper R et al (1975). Pericardial

decompression. Ann Thorac Surg 19:47-53.

Leuallen EC, Carr DT (1955). Pleural effusion - a statistical study of 436 patients. N Eng J Med 252:79-83.

Levitt LJ, Ault KA, Pincus GS, Sloss LJ and McManus BM (1979). Pericarditis and early cardiac tamponade as a primary manifestation of lymphosarcoma cell leukemia. Am J Med 67:719-723.

Light RW, MacGregor MI, Luchsinger PC (1972). Pleural effusions: The diagnostic separation of transudates and exudates. Ann Int Med 77:507-513.

Martini N, Bains MS, Beattie EJ Jr (1975). Indications for pleurectomy in malignant effusion. Cancer 35:734-738.

Martini N, Freiman AH, Watson RC, and Hilaris BS (1977). Intrapericardial instillation of radioactive chromic phosphate for malignant pericardial effusion. Am J Roentgenol 128:639-641.

McMichael J, Sharpey-Schafer EP (1944). Action of intravenous digoxin in man. Quart J Med 37:123-135.

Paladine W, Cunningham TJ, Sponzo R, Donovan M, Olson K, Horton J (1976). Intracavitary bleomycin in the management of malignant effusions. Cancer 38:1903-1908.

Petersen CD, Robenson WA, Kurnick JE (1976). Involvement of the heart and pericardium in the malignant lymphomas. Am J Med Sci 272:161-165.

Posner MR, Cohen GI, Skarin AT (1981). Pericardial disease in patients with cancer: The differentiation of malignant from idiopathic and radiation-induced pericarditis. Am J Med 71:407-413.

Prorok J, Nealon TF (1968). Pleural symphysis by talc poudrage in the treatment of malignant pleural effusion. Bull de la Societe Internat de Chir 6:630-636.

Ryan CJ, Rodgers RF, Unni KK, Hepper NG (1981). The outcome of patients with pleural effusion of indeterminate cause at thoracotomy. Mayo Clin Proc 56:145-149.

Saha PK, Agrawal BC, Mishra SK et al (1977). Pleuropericardial effusion: A presenting feature of acute myelogenous leukemia. Ind Heart J 29:165-168.

Spokick DH (1967). Acute cardiac tamponade: Pathologic physiology, diagnosis, and mangement. Prog Cardiovasc Dis 10:64-96.

Storey DD, Dines DE, Coles DT (1976). Pleural effusion: a diagnostic dilemma. JAMA 236:2183-2189.

Strauss BL, Mathews MJ, Cohen MH, Simon R, Tejada F (1977). Cardiac metastases in lung cancer. Chest 71:607-611.

Tavel ME (1959). Ascites: Etiological considerations with emphasis on the value of several laboratory findings in diagnosis.  Am J Med Sci 237:727-743.

Weissburg D, Kaufmann M (1980).  Diagnostic and therapeutic pleuroscopy:  Experience with 127 patients.  Chest 78:732-735.

Williams C, Soutter L (1954).  Pericardial tamponade:  Diagnosis and treatment.  Arch Int Med 94:571-579.

Witte CL, Witte MH, Dumont AE (1980).  Lymph imbalance in the genesis and perpetuation of the ascites syndrome in hepatic cirrhosis.  Gastroenterol 78:1059-1068.

Yazdi HM, Hadju SI, Melamed MR (1980).  Cytopathology of pericardial effusions.  Acta Cytol 24:401-412.

Zipf RE Jr, Johnston WW (1972).  The role of cytology in the evaluation of pericardial effusions.  Chest 62:593-596.

CONGRESS SYMPOSIA


IMAGING TECHNIQUES FOR DETECTION AND EXTENT
DETERMINATION OF CANCER Boijsen, E., Sweden,
Chairman; Bragg, D., USA, Co-Chairman; Arena

Imaging Techniques for Detection and Extent
Determination of Cancer of the Esophagus,
Stomach and Colon. *Op-den-Orth, J. O.,
Haarlem, The Netherlands.

Imaging Techniques for Detection and Determining
the Extent of Biliary Tract Cancer.
*Bernardino, M. E., Houston, TX USA. (By Title
Only)

Imaging Techniques for Extent Determination of
Hodgkin's Disease and Non-Hodgkin's Lymphoma.
*Castellino, R. A., Palo Alto, CA USA.

CT of the Head and Neck. *Reede, D., USA. (By
Title Only)

Imaging Techniques for Detection and Extent
Determination of Genitourinary Cancer.
*Boijsne, E., Lund, Sweden.

Please note: Papers that are listed as "By Title
Only" were presented at the 13th International
Cancer Congress, but are not included in these
volumes.

13th International Cancer Congress, Part D
Research and Treatment, pages 363–364
© 1983 Alan R. Liss, Inc., 150 Fifth Avenue, New York, NY 10011

IMAGING TECHNIQUES FOR DETECTION AND EXTENT DETERMINATION
OF CANCER OF THE ESOPHAGUS, STOMACH AND COLON.

J.Odo Op den Orth M.D.

Department of Radiology
St.Elisabeth's of Groote Gasthuis
Boerhaavelaan 22, 2035 RC Haarlem, Holland.

Double-contrast radiography provides accurate visualisation
of even small esophageal tumors; it is very useful for the
detection of esophageal cancer. It also shows the
macroscopic extent of a tumor in the longitudinal direction.
CT scanning gives information on wall thickening, para-
esophageal extension and metastatic disease.

Radiographic techniques for the detection of gastric
carcinoma have greatly improved during the last decade.
Inspired by the Japanese, many Western institutions have
adopted double-contrast techniques. The anterior wall of
the gastric corpus and the gastric antrum can not be
completely explored in a routine double-contrast examination.
Therefore we advocate a biphasic examination, that combines
the advantages of double-contrast and positive-contrast
graded compression studies. To induce hypotony a pre-
medication of glucagon is routinely administered.
A biphasic examination of the stomach that has been rendered
hypotonic by an i.v. injection of glucagon has been proven
to be an accurate detector of gastric carcinoma, not only
in the advanced but also in the early stage. Early gastric
carcinoma has been defined as a carcinoma that does not
infiltrate beyond the submucosa. Such a carcinoma has a
good prognosis after treatment; the 5 year survival rate
is far over 90%. Early gastric carcinoma often barely
thickens the gastric wall. Although CT can be used to
demonstrate metastatic disease in early gastric carcinoma,
it is not the appropiate tool to detect and to stage this
kind of lesion. CT is useful however for the staging and

therapy planning of advanced gastric carcinoma and gastric
lymphoma.

Double-contrast examination of the colon is usually the
primary imaging technique in the evaluation of colonic
cancer. If there is diverticular disease in the sigmoid
colon, polypoid lesions are often difficult to detect.
We have found it therefore useful to make additional
positive-contrast films of this part of the bowel.
Extracolonic extension of a carcinoma of the colon and
metastatic disease can be detected by CT scanning.
Furthermore CT scanning is especially important in the
evaluation of recurrent carcinoma of the rectum.
Ultrasonography may detect mass lesions of the stomach
and colon before any bariumexamination has been performed;
it also gives information on tumor extent and the presence
of metastases.

13th International Cancer Congress, Part D
Research and Treatment, pages 365-372
© 1983 Alan R. Liss, Inc., 150 Fifth Avenue, New York, NY 10011

IMAGING TECHNIQUES FOR EXTENT DETERMINATION OF HODGKIN'S
DISEASE AND NON-HODGKIN'S LYMPHOMA

Ronald A. Castellino, M.D.

Division of Diagnostic Radiology
Stanford University School of Medicine
Palo Alto, California 94305, U.S.A.

Hodgkin's disease (HD) and the heterogeneous group of
disorders which comprise the non-Hodgkin's lymphomas (NHL)
are distinct entities which manifest differing modes of
presentation, patterns of involvement, and responses to
varying treatment regimens.  These malignancies usually
arise within lymph nodes or in the thymus; furthermore, the
NHLs frequently arise in extranodal lymphatic tissues such
as Waldeyer's ring and Peyer's patches, or in extralymphatic
sites such as the gastrointestinal tract.  Staging criteria
developed for HD at the Ann Arbor Conference has been
generally applied to patients with NHL, with some modification in children or in unusual histologic subtypes at
certain centers.

Careful anatomic staging of extent of disease has been
considered extremely important to determine subsequent treatment and prognosis.  High energy external beam radiation
therapy employing innovative treatment planning relies
heavily upon precise anatomic staging.  The emergence of
increasingly effective chemotherapeutic regimens, often
coupled with radiation therapy, still requires accurate
anatomic delineation of disease extent, but perhaps to a
lesser degree than previously due to the systemic effects
of drug therapy.

Table 1 shows the incidence of disease involvement at
specific anatomic sites based upon data derived from patients with newly diagnosed, previously untreated HD and NHL
who were enrolled in a prospective, nonselected manner into
the treatment protocols of Kaplan, Rosenberg and associates

at Stanford Medical Center (Goffinet et al 1977; Kaplan 1979; Filly et al 1976. Data for intra-abdominal disease is based upon histologic material obtained at staging laparotomy, whereas data for supradiaphragmatic disease is derived from analysis of standard frontal and lateral radiographs and full lung tomography.

Table 1. ANATOMIC SITES INVOLVED AT PRESENTATION

| | HODGKIN'S DISEASE | | NON-HODGKIN'S LYMPHOMA | |
|---|---|---|---|---|
| | Adult | Child | Adult | Child |
| Thoracic nodes | ——— 65% ——— | | ——— 25% ——— | |
| Lung parenchyma | ——— 10% ——— | | ——— 4% ——— | |
| Pleural effusion | 10% | 4% | 7% | 14% |
| Para-aortic nodes | 34% | 19% | 55% | 30% |
| Mesenteric nodes | ——— <5% ——— | | ——— 51% ——— | |
| Spleen | ——— 34% ——— | | ——— 33% ——— | |
| Liver | ——— 6% ——— | | ——— 14% ——— | |
| GI tract | ——— 0% ——— | | 8% | 18% |
| Urinary tract | ——— 0% ——— | | ——— 3% ——— | |

The choice of which imaging technique to use to evaluate these various sites should be based upon knowledge of the incidence of involvement; the sensitivity, specificity and accuracy of the available imaging studies (McNeil et al 1975); and the type of information required to make therapeutic and prognostic decisions. The routine evaluation of sites frequently involved by tumor is reasonable, whereas routine screening of sites with a low incidence of disease appears fruitless. However, appropriate signs or symptoms should prompt further imaging studies irrespective of the incidence of disease at that site.

## SUPRADIAPHRAGMATIC DISEASE

Whereas evaluation of extrathoracic sites is best accomplished by physical examination, intrathoracic involvement for staging purposes is determined by imaging techniques (rarely is a surgical procedure performed to clarify staging). The conventional posterior-anterior and lateral chest radiographs demonstrate the vast majority of intrathoracic abnormalities. Supplementary full lung tomography will demonstrate additional extent of disease in some 20% of cases, but this additional knowledge affects staging and/or treatment in very few patients (Castellino et al 1976). Its use is therefore optimized in patients with suspicious findings on conventional radiographs or in those where the lung parenchyma is at high risk for involvement.

Thoracic computed tomographic (CT) scanning unquestionably demonstrates enlarged mediastinal lymph nodes in patients whose chest radiographs and full lung tomograms appear unremarkable. However, to date no rigorous study has emerged which determines how frequently this occurs and how often this additional information affects patient management. Likewise, CT scanning has been shown to demonstrate pulmonary lesions in addition to those seen on conventional radiographs or tomograms. At times, however, these lesions do not represent manifestations of the underlying disease and such falsely positive information contributes to staging errors. Once again, no rigorous studies in the lymphomas have addressed this point.

CT does appear, however, to provide greater appreciation for the local extent of disease, as well as evidence of infiltration into adjacent structures, by virtue of its cross-sectional display. Such information can be important in radiotherapy treatment planning. Because of this, and our belief that CT is the preferred method to evaluate the mediastinum, we frequently employ CT scans of the thorax in staging these patients.

## SUBDIAPHRAGMATIC DISEASE

Staging laparotomy has provided information with which to determine the sensitivity, specificity, and accuracy (NcNeil et al 1975) of various imaging tests in assessing intra-abdominal disease. (Similar histologic correlative material is not available for assessing intrathoracic sites.) Prior studies have shown the relative lack of accuracy of such studies as excretory urography and inferior venacavagraphy to evaluate the retroperitoneal lymph nodes; routinely performed gastrointestinal tract barium studies to detect asymptomatic gastrointestinal tract involvement; technetium sulfur colloid radioisotope liver-spleen scans and splenic arteriography to detect involvement of these organs; and routinely performed radiographic skeletal surveys and radioisotope bone scans to detect unsuspected bone lesions.

Lymphangiography (LAG) has thus emerged as the key imaging technique to evaluate subdiaphragmatic disease, and its use is supported by a wealth of published experience documenting its sensitivity, specificity and accuracy (Kademian and Wirtanen 1977; Marglin and Castellino 1981). In the past 5 years, body CT scanning with high resolution images has emerged as a powerful imaging technique which evaluates not only the same retroperitoneal nodes opacified by lymphography, but many other potential sites of disease involvement within the abdominal cavity, retroperitoneum and pelvis. There is, however, limited data on the sensitivity, specificity and accuracy of CT scanning based upon histologic corroboration in these diseases (Best et al 1978; Breiman et al 1978). The data provided in Table 2 represent the results of an ongoing prospective study of unselected patients with previously untreated HD and NHL who underwent lymphography, CT scanning of the abdomen and pelvis, and staging laparotomy.

Para-aortic/paracaval ("retropertitoneal") lymph nodes. The majority of these lymph nodes are opacified by lymphography (LAG). A consecutive series of 632 patients (416 with HD and 216 with NHL) yielded a sensitivity, specificity, and overall accuracy in HD of 93%, 92%, and 92%, and in NHL of 89%, 86%, and 88%, respectively (Marglin and Castellino 1981). In the smaller group of patients who have also had CT scans, the LAG proved to be a better indicator of the absence or presence of disease than did CT (Table 2). This can be explained by the ability of the LAG to detect tumor deposits in nodes that are normal in size or only slightly enlarged, whereas CT requires lymph node enlargement before a positive diagnostic interpretation can be given. CT does define the extent of bulky disease more precisely than the LAG and is a less invasive diagnostic technique. Thus, CT could be employed as the initial imaging study in patients whose disease tends to be bulky, such as those with NHL. The convenience of following the residually opacified lymph nodes with surveillance abdominal films will of course be lost when lymphography is not performed.

TABLE 2.    LAG/CT/LAPAROTOMY CORRELATIONS

HODGKIN'S DISEASE (n = 87)

| | RETROPERITONEAL NODES | | MESENTERIC NODES | SPLEEN | LIVER |
|---|---|---|---|---|---|
| | LAG | CT | CT | CT | CT |
| SENSITIVITY | $\frac{14}{17}$ = 82% | $\frac{13}{17}$ - 76% | Only 1 positive biopsy in 66 patients – and that was missed by CT | $\frac{23}{38}$ = 61% | $\frac{1}{6}$ = 17% |
| SPECIFICITY | $\frac{60}{60}$ = 100% | $\frac{57}{63}$ = 90% | | $\frac{36}{49}$ = 73% | $\frac{80}{80}$ = 100% |
| ACCURACY | $\frac{74}{77}$ = 96% | $\frac{70}{80}$ = 88% | | $\frac{59}{87}$ = 68% | $\frac{81}{86}$ = 94% |

NON-HODGKIN'S LYMPHOMA (n = 24)

| | LAG | CT | MESENTERIC CT | SPLEEN CT | LIVER CT |
|---|---|---|---|---|---|
| SENSITIVITY | $\frac{14}{14}$ = 100% | $\frac{12}{14}$ = 86% | $\frac{10}{15}$ = 67% | $\frac{5}{11}$ = 45% | $\frac{2}{3}$ = 67% |
| SPECIFICITY | $\frac{6}{8}$ = 75% | $\frac{6}{8}$ = 75% | $\frac{6}{8}$ = 75% | $\frac{10}{12}$ = 83% | $\frac{21}{21}$ = 100% |
| ACCURACY | $\frac{20}{22}$ = 91% | $\frac{18}{22}$ = 82% | $\frac{16}{23}$ = 70% | $\frac{15}{23}$ = 65% | $\frac{23}{24}$ = 96% |

Mesenteric lymph nodes are rarely involved at presentation in HD and, when involved, are usually normal in size.
On the other hand, this lymph node group is frequently
involved in NHL and not uncommonly such involvement is accompanied by bulky masses. Thus, CT scanning is of no use
to evaluate this site in HD but is relatively productive in
NHL (Table 2). Whether such information in patients with NHL
is of clinical value regarding patient management is unclear,
but if desired it should be evaluated with CT scanning.

Splenic involvement is frequently noted histologically
in spleens of normal size; and conversely, enlarged spleens
do not necessarily contain histologic evidence of tumor.
When disease is present, it usually occurs as foci of tumor
deposits, often less than 1 cm in diameter. Larger lesions
can be detected by CT scanning, particularly when intravenous contrast material is used. However, CT interpretation
of involvement is usually based upon demonstration of an
enlarged spleen without focal defects. Not surprisingly, the
sensitivity (ability to detect existent disease) is not very
good (Table 2); however, this technique is as, or more,
accurate than other imaging techniques used to evaluate
this organ.

Hepatic involvement occurs relatively infrequently and
presents problems similar to those encountered with the
spleen. Tumor deposits are frequently less than 1 cm in
size and enlarged livers may not contain biopsy evidence
of tumor. Furthermore, CT evaluation of liver size is more
difficult than it is for spleen size. Due to the low
incidence of histologic liver involvement, overall accuracy
has little meaning; the important parameter is sensitivity,
which is quite low (Table 2).

Intrinsic gastrointestinal and genitourinary involvement
occurs very rarely in patients presenting with HD. However,
in NHL these organ systems are occasionally involved,
particularly in children. Intrinsic involvement is most
frequently accompanied by suggestive signs or symptoms which
should prompt appropriate imaging techniques. Conventional
barium studies of the gastrointestinal tract readily demonstrate these lesions. Renal involvement can be shown with
excretory urography, ultrasound, and CT studies.

Miscellaneous. If hydronephrosis is suspected because of bulky lymphadenopathy, ultrasound scanning provides a rapid, accurate, and noninvasive imaging test. Unsuspected bone involvement at times is noted on the chest radiographs and abdominal films taken during lymphography, as well as on CT scans. Suspected bone involvement is evaluated with radioisotope bone scanning followed by detailed radiographs of the positive sites. Evidence for extradural involvement is conventionally evaluated by myelography, but at times can be successfully evaluated in the lumbar area by CT scanning.

## IMAGING STRATEGIES

An approach to evaluating patients with HD and NHL at presentation with imaging techniques can be based upon the following assumptions: (1) routine screening is valuable for sites frequently involved with tumor if the imaging test is sufficiently accurate; however, in frequently involved sites associated with low sensitivity imaging tests, routine screening is nonproductive; and (2) routine screening (even with tests of high accuracy) has little value for sites infrequently involved with tumor; however, suggestive symptoms and/or signs at any site should prompt the performance of appropriate imaging examinations.

Our current utilization of radiologic imaging studies for staging these tumors is as follows.

1. Intrathoracic disease is usually adequately evaluated with standard posterior-anterior and lateral chest radiographs. Further evaluation is best performed by CT scanning, if available; if not, then by full lung tomography.

2. Lymphography remains the best imaging study to evaluate the "retroperitoneal" lymph nodes. This study also provides a convenient means for follow-up.

3. Abdominal and pelvic CT scanning more precisely defines the extent of bulky lymph node disease and evaluates other lymph node sites not opacified by LAG. Mesenteric lymphadenopathy is often shown by CT in NHL; however, disease at this site is not sufficiently frequent in HD to justify CT

scanning to evaluate this site in HD. To date, CT has not been particularly rewarding in evaluating the liver and spleen, unless focal defects are noted.

4. The possibility of hydronephrosis is readily studied with ultrasound, unless already evaluated as part of a prior CT scan.

5. Selective imaging studies should be used to evaluate signs and/or symptoms suggesting involvement of specific sites.

Castellino RA, Filly R, Blank N (1976). Routine full-lung tomography in the initial staging and treatment planning of patients with Hodgkin's disease and non-Hodgkin's lymphoma. Cancer 38:1130.

Best JJK, Blackledge G, Forbes WS, Todd IDH, Eddleston B, Crowther D, Isherwood I (1978). Computed tomography of abdomen in staging and clinical management of lymphoma. Br Med J 2:1675.

Breiman RS, Castellino RA, Harell GS, Marshall WH, Glatstein E, Kaplan HS (1978). CT-pathologic correlations in Hodgkin's disease and non-Hodgkin's lymphoma. Radiology 126:159.

Filly R, Blank N, Castellino RA (1976). Radiographic distribution of intrathoracic disease in previously untreated patients with Hodgkin's disease and non-Hodgkin's lymphoma. Radiology 120:277.

Goffinet DR, Warnke R, Dunnick NR, Castellino R, Glatsetin E, Nelsen TS, Dorfman RF, Rosenberg SA, Kaplan HS (1977). Clinical and surgical (laparotomy) evaluation of patients with non-Hodgkin's lymphomas. Cancer Treat Rep 61:981.

Kademian MT, Wirtanen GW (1977). Accuracy of bipedal lymphography in Hodgkin's disease. AJR 129:1041.

Kaplan HS (1979). "Hodgkin's Disease." Cambridge: Harvard University Press.

Marglin S, Castellino RA (1981). Lymphographic accuracy in 632 consecutive, previously untreated cases of Hodgkin's disease and non-Hodgkin's lymphoma. Radiology 140:351.

McNeil BJ, Keeler E, Adelstein SJ (1975). Primer in certain elements of medical decision making. N Engl J Med 293:211.

(Supported in part by CA-05838, NCI, NIH, and the T. Eckstrom Fund)

13th International Cancer Congress, Part D
Research and Treatment, pages 373–383
© 1983 Alan R. Liss, Inc., 150 Fifth Avenue, New York, NY 10011

# IMAGING TECHNIQUES FOR DETECTION AND EXTENT DETERMINATION OF GENITOURINARY CANCER

Erik Boijsen, M.D.

Department of Diagnostic Radiology
University Hospital
S-221 85 LUND
Sweden

With the advent of non-invasive imaging techniques a completely new approach to diagnosing and staging of genitourinary cancers has appeared. Over the past 20 years radiologists have largely relied upon angiography and lymphangiography to define type and extension of urogenital tumors. Today angiography is required only in selected cases and the number of lymphangiographies has reduced remarkably, being replaced by ultrasonography (US) and computed tomography (CT).

In every detected genitourinary tumor, a chest radiogram is taken for the search of metastases. For the same reason radionuclide imaging of the liver and skeleton are commonly performed. These methods have become routine procedures and will therefore not be discussed further.

## RENAL CARCINOMA

The detection of a renal carcinoma is still mainly made by urography. With adequate technique, i.e. large bolus injection and tomography, most cancers will be defined by urography. Thus, of a total of 32 cancers examined with this technique there were only two regarded as doubtful and no false negative; and of 19 cysts 4 were indeterminate because of their central position in the kidney (Dardenne, Bodart 1981).

Therefore the next step in most cases of renal cancer defined at urography, is to decide local extension of the tumor. US is a simple and reliable method to show venous invasion, but if the diagnosis of the renal carcinoma is already available, CT will give this information to an advantage, particularly with the use of contrast enhancement (Figure 1).

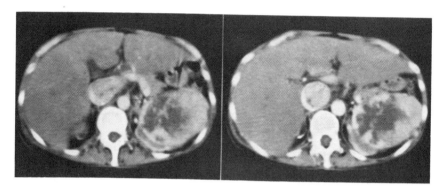

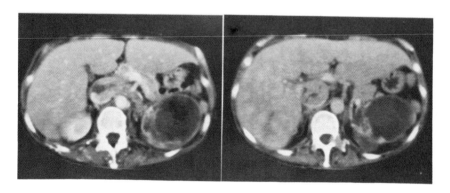

Fig. 1 a, b: Invasion of renal vein and inferior vena cava by left renal carcinoma.
c, d: 40 days after ethanol ablation of renal artery. Marked regression of tumor with gas formation both in renal tumor and in tumor thrombus.

With CT we will also better define perirenal
extension as well as nodal enlargement (Karp et al.
1981; Weyman et al. 1980). In a series of 27
patients with adenocarcinoma correct staging was
obtained in 70 %. In 3 patients overstaging occurred
because enlarged nodes observed at CT did not
represent metastases. Distant metastases to the
liver or spine will also become obvious with CT,
particularly if contrast enhancement is utilized.
In patients with indeterminate findings at urography, US could again be an appropriate method
but if a solid tumor is small a false negative
result is bound to occur (Fig. 2).

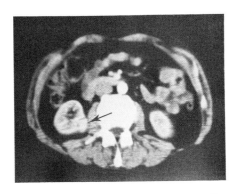

Fig. 2.   At CT a 2 cm renal carcinoma (arrow) is
present. The tumor was not found at US.

According to our experience, and others, CT
therefore is the first choice in patients where
a carcinoma or a questionable expansive lesion is
present at urography (Fig. 3).

Angiography is, with few exceptions not
necessary to perform today. US has still a position
in renal tumors, one is where nephrotomography has
revealed a cyst which always needs confirmation.
Most of these cases are unequivocal and no cyst
puncture necessary to be performed. US and cystography should, however, be performed in cases

where CT or US for some reason has not given
clearcut diagnosis of the cyst. Thus, in cases
with indeterminate lesions at CT, it was found
that US combined with cystography was diagnostic
in 84 % while angiography was useful only in 16 %
(Balfe et al. 1982).

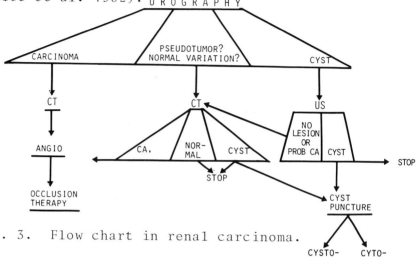

Fig. 3.   Flow chart in renal carcinoma.

For diagnostic reasons the role of angiography is limited to few indications. One is when
at urography there is a suspected vascular
abnormality (Fig. 4), another is in cases where
both CT and US are indeterminate. It is also
recommended to use angiography as a differential
diagnostic method for onkocytoma, and when adjacent tumors such as adrenal tumors, infiltrate
the kidney (Ambos et al. 1977; Weyman et al. 1980;
Bosniak 1981).

For extent determination of the renal carcinoma, angiography is rarely necessary to
demonstrate patency of inferior vena cava or renal
vein. Angiography is the best method to show
small metastases in the opposite kidney and in
the liver. Finally, renal angiography is important
for the management of tumors, i.e. in patients
where partial nephrectomy is necessary to perform,
in excessively large tumors, and in cases where
ablation is preferred (Fig. 1).

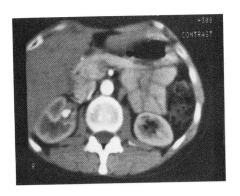 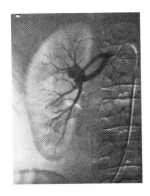

Fig. 4 a, b.  Aneurysm of right renal artery
defined at CT (a), as well as angiography (b).


NMR will add very little to the diagnosis
and extent determination of renal tumors. Phlebography, digital subtraction angiography (DSA),
lymphangiography, and biopsy are rarely of any
value in renal tumors for the diagnosis or extent
determination. Many differential diagnostic
problems still exist, but with the advent of CT
the differentiation between tumor and cyst rarely
is a problem. Thus, today urography and CT are
the methods we need for diagnosis and extent
determination in renal carcinoma, and angiography
in selected cases.


## RENAL PELVIC AND URETERIC CARCINOMA

As in renal carcinoma, renal pelvic and
ureteric carcinoma are in most cases diagnosed by
urography. Cytology is of prime importance particularly in ureteric carcinoma which is otherwise
frequently overlooked in early stages. Uretero-
pyelography is an important complementary study in
silent kidneys or in small ureteric cancers overlooked at urography. CT plays an important role
in defining transitional cell carcinoma of the
urinary tract, particularly to evaluate non-

functioning kidneys, where angiography once was
the method of choice. Because of the multicentric
origin of these tumors it is important to preserve
renal function in the event that a new lesion
develops on the opposite side. Recent studies
have recommended limited resections in stages I
and II and therefore a non-invasive staging of
this tumor is important. CT can be used to show
pelviureteral and intrarenal extension with high
degree of accuracy (Baron et al. 1982).

Thus, urography with or without ureteropyelo-
graphy and CT will cover the required information
in transitional cell carcinoma of the renal pelvis
and ureter.


BLADDER TUMORS

The diagnosis of bladder tumors is rarely
radiographic. With modern cystoscopic technique
no radiographic examination is of importance for
diagnosis.

The clinical staging of bladder tumor is
based on palpation, which obviously is a rather
crude method. Since the prognosis and management
of these tumors largely depends on the local and
distant extent, a variety of methods have been
used over the years. Urography is of prime importance to show the presence of any further transitional cell tumor in the upper urinary tract and
also the presence of local periureteral extension.
Antegrade pyeloureterography with nephrostomy
should be used if the kidney is silent at urography. Angiography was until recently the next
method which gave an accuracy of defining stage
III and IV lesions to 80 % and 85 %, respectively.
Adding lymphangiography to angiography improved
accuracy of stage IV to 95 % (Winterberger et al.
1978).

However, during the last 4-5 years it has
become obvious that both US and CT are more reliable than the invasive techniques (McLaughlin
et al. 1975; Colleen et al. 1981). Therefore the

present staging technique in most places is with CT because reproducibility and morphologic identification is simpler. It should, however, be clear that there are regions difficult to interpret and biopsy or transurethral resection may change the CT finding as can be observed in Fig. 5.

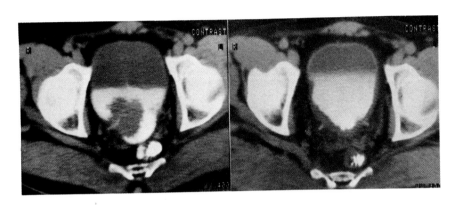

Fig. 5. Bladder carcinoma stage T2 preoperatively defined by CT (a) and verified at transurethral resection. Repeat CT three days after resection reveals extensive edema in bladder wall and the perivesical fat (b).

## PROSTATIC CARCINOMA

The diagnosis of prostatic carcinoma is not radiologic, but US/CT have potentialities to detect lesions previously only observed at autopsy. The prognosis of prostatic carcinoma is related to extent of disease and tumor grade. Thus, if the carcinoma is located to the prostate and the gland is removed the man has the same prognosis quoad vitam as the aged-matched person without prostatic carcinoma, but has the tumor been proven by histology to pass outside the gland, the survival is markedly reduced. Therefore, an accurate clinical staging is required for correct therapy.

The common clinical staging by means of rectal palpation, multiple biopsies, skeletal radionuclide imaging, and radiology of the skeleton, will not give complete information about local and distant extent of the tumors. Thus, in one quarter of the cases the local extent is underestimated when based on palpation and biopsy. Lymph node metastases occur in about 30 % of the patients that undergo lymphadenectomy despite clinical staging of A2 or B (Catalona and Stein 1982). 40-50 % of patients with stage C1-lesions (i.e. extracapsular extension without seminalvesical involvement) and 60-90 % with stage C2-lesions (i.e. seminal-vesical involvement) have lymph node metastases. Tumor grade also influences metastatic spread. Thus, additional examination to palpation per rectum, multiple biopsy of both lobes and skeletal studies should be utilized. Transrectal US or suprapubic transabdominal US improves the early detection of prostatic cancer. US is better for evaluation of bladder base than CT and more accurate than rectal palpation (Greenberg et al. 1981; Denkhaus et al. 1981). Suprapubic transverse US is suitable for monitoring progress of therapy. Lymphangiography has been advocated for lymph node involvement but it should be clear that, as in bladder tumors, lymphangiography will only pick up metastases when they have reached the iliac nodes or when they pass beyond them to the paraaortic region. With an incidence rate of 51 %, accuracy rates have been reported to be between 70-80 %, or even higher. Therefore, lymphangiography is of value in planning treatment, particularly of those with no other evidence of distant metastases. Lymphangiography can serve as an indication for radical surgery.

## TESTICULAR TUMORS

Testicular tumors are mainly diagnosed by palpation, but occasionally US of testis is of great value. The point of origin of the mass can always be determined in inconclusive cases on physical examination. Tumors more than 5 mm in size are easily detected. US is therefore of particular value to exclude testicular neoplasms. This may occur: 1/ if there is a palpable scrotal mass which is thought to be extratesticular, but could possibly be a protrusion of an intratesticular mass; 2/ if there is a hydrocele present and the testis cannot be adequately palpated; and 3/ if metastatic disease is present which could be of testicular origin with a clinically normal scrotum (Wilson et al. 1982).

US is also of value to determine local and distant extent. Local invasion of the mediastinum testis can be recognized, which is significant and indicates poor prognosis. Distant metastases are important to find because the management varies depending on whether metastases are present or not and whether the tumor is seminomatous or non-seminomatous. Previously, urography and phlebography were common procedures to detect large retroperitoneal nodes but today US or CT have replaced these methods. US has a high accuracy rate of about 80 % and the same goes for CT (73 - 87 %). Since CT is easier to handle, particularly to follow the effect of therapy, this method has been most often used. It should, however, be observed that there is a false negative rate of 30-40 % (Richie et al. 1982). Therefore, in seminoma additional examinations with lymphangiography would be indicated with negative CT.

In the non-seminoma metastases the policy at present is combination of retroperitoneal node dissection and chemotherapy. In nodes less than 2 cm, a negative CT does not need to be complemented with lymphangiography because operation is to be performed anyhow.

In summary, diagnosis and extension of genitourinary tumors have been greatly improved by the non-invasive imaging techniques. It is true that angiography and lymphangiography still should be performed in selected cases, angiography in renal carcinoma, and lymphangiography in bladder tumors, prostatic carcinoma, and testicular malignancy. The number of lymphangiographies and angiographies have been reduced remarkably owing to these non-invasive techniques. Probably, DSA and NMR will add very little to the presently used methods. Improvements in ultrasonography, as well as CT may remove most of the remaining indications for the invasive techniques. Probably, however, angiography will return and be more used as a method for therapy in many of the presented malignant tumors and their recurrencies.

## REFERENCES

Ambos MA, Bosniak MA, Madayag MA, Lefleur RS (1977) Infiltrating neoplasms of the kidney. AJR 129:859.

Balfe DM, McClennan BL, Stanley RJ, Weyman PJ, Sagel SS (1982) Evaluation of renal masses considered indeterminate on computed tomography. Radiology 142:421.

Baron RL, McClennan BL, Lee JKT, Lawson TL (1982) Computed tomography of transitional-cell carcinoma of the renal pelvis and ureter. Radiology 144:125.

Bosniak MA (1981) The role of angiography in the study of renal neoplasms in the age of computed tomography. 6th Ann. Course on Diagnostic and Therapeutic Angiography and Interventional Radiology. Book of Abstracts, p. 129.

Catalona WJ, Stein AJ (1982) Staging errors in clinically localized prostatic cancer. J Urol 127:452.

Colleen S, Ekelund L, Henrikson H, Karp W, Månsson V (1981) Staging of bladder carcinoma with computed tomography. Scand J Urol Nephrol 15:109.

Dardenne AN, Bodart P (1981) La nefro-tomografia nei processi espansivi renali. In: Pistolesi GF (ed) "La Radiologia del Rene". Ed. Libraria Cortina Verona, p. 469.

Denkhaus H, Becker H, Bücheler E (1981) Befunde bei Prostatakarzinomen und -adenomen in der suprapubischen Prostatasonographie. RöFo 135: 285.

Greenberg M, Neiman HL, Brandt TD, Falkowski W, Carter M (1981) Ultrasound of the prostate. Radiology 141:757.

Karp W, Ekelund L, Olafsson G, Olsson A (1981) Computed tomography, angiography and ultrasound in staging of renal carcinoma. Acta Radiol (Diagn) 22:625.

McLaughlin JS, Morley P, Deane RF, Barnett E, Graham AG, Kyle KF (1975) Ultrasound in the staging of bladder tumors. Brit J Urol 47:51.

Richie JP, Garnick MB, Finberg H (1982) Computerized tomography: How accurate for abdominal staging of testis tumours? J Urol 127:715.

Weyman P, McClennan B, Stanley R, Levitt R, Sagel S (1980) Comparison of computed tomography and angiography in the evaluation of renal cell carcinoma. Radiology 137:417.

Wilson PC, Day DL, Valvo JR, Gramiak R (1982) Scrotal ultrasound with an Octoson-TM. Radiographics 2:24.

Winterberger AR, Wajsman Z, Merrin C, Murphy GP (1978) Eight years of experience with preoperative angiographic and lymphographic staging of bladder cancer. J Urol 119:208.

CONGRESS SYMPOSIA


MICROSURGERY AND MYOCUTANEOUS FLAPS IN TUMOR
SURGERY Millesi, H., Australia, Chairman;
Larson, D., USA, Co-Chairman; Flag Pavilion A

Microsurgery and Mycocutaneous Flaps in Tumor
Surgery-Nerve Grafting. *Millesi, H., Vienna,
Austria.

Skeletal Reconstruction Following Tumor Surgery:
Vascularized Bone Grafts. *Buckwalter, J. A.,
Iowa City, IA USA.

Free Skin Flaps. *Melissinos, E., Houston, TX
USA. (By Title Only)

Mycocutaneous Flaps Tumor Surgery of the Head
and Neck. *Cummings, C. W., Seattle, WA USA.

Mycocutaneous Flap Reconstruction of the
Trunk and Extremities in Cancer Surgery.
*Larson, D. L., Houston, TX USA.


Please note: Papers that are listed as "By Title
Only" were presented at the 13th International
Cancer Congress, but are not included in these
volumes.

385

13th International Cancer Congress, Part D
Research and Treatment, pages 387–397
© 1983 Alan R. Liss, Inc., 150 Fifth Avenue, New York, NY 10011

MICROSURGERY AND MYOCUTANEOUS FLAPS IN TUMOR SURGERY-
NERVE GRAFTING

Hanno MILLESI, Professor, Dr.

Director Department of Plastic and Reconstructive
Surgery, 1st Surgical University Clinic and Direc-
tor of Ludwig-Boltzmann-Institute for Experimental
Plastic Surgery, A-1090 Vienna, Austria

GENERAL REMARKS ON NERVE GRAFTING

The first experimental nerve graft has been performed by
Philipeaux and Vulpian in 1870. In clinical praxis nerve
grafting was introduced by Albert in the seventies of the
last century ( Albert 1876, 1878 ). He used auto- and
allografts.

Considerable success has been reported ( Bunnell, 1927 ,
Ballance and Duel, 1932; Bunnell and Boyes ( 1980 ); Seddon,
1947; Brooks, 1955 ). In spite of these reports, nerve grafting did not become popular. It was always regarded significantly inferior to an end-to-end neurorrhaphy. Bunnell (1927),
Ballance and Duel ( 1932 ) and others bridged successfully
defects of the facial nerve after tumor surgery, but the
majority of surgeons preferred re-neurotization of the
peripheral stump of the facial nerve by hypoglossus nerve
transfer or other nerve transfers.

What Do We Expect From Successful Nerve Grafts?

The nerve graft has to survive completely and it should
behave like a peripheral stump after nerve transsection.
This means that no fibrosis must develop and the Schwann
cells have to survive. The axon sprouts from the proximal
stump must be able to cross into the graft and from the graft
to the distal stump without being blocked by scar tissue.
The axon sprouts which enter the nerve graft at its proximal
end and leave the nerve graft at its distal end should do
this in an area of the cross-section of the distal stump

where the functionally corresponding peripheral cndoneurial tubes are located.

Trunk Grafts

Free grafting of a nerve trunk has not proven too success-ful. In the center of the graft fibrosis develops, which im-pairs neurotization ( Bielschowsky and Unger, 1917 ). In con-sequence, nerve trunks were transplanted as pedicled nerve grafts ( Strange, 1947 ). But this means that one of two nerve trunks have to be sacrificed in otder to reconstruct the other one. At present, vascularized trunk grafts offer optimal conditions, as far as circulation is concerned. The ischemic period is reduced to a minimum. The vascularized nerve trunks have two draw-backs. There are not always avai-lable in proper size without  sacrificing another nerve trunk. The fascicular pattern of the trunk graft does not correspond to the nerve to be repaired and it is not certain that axons which enter the trunk graft in a certain area will leave it at the distal end in an corresponding area.

Cutaneous Nerve Grafts

Based on morphologic studies by Bielschowsky and Unger ( 1917 ), demonstrating the fibrosis in trunk grafts, Foerster utilized in 1916 cutaneous nerves ( Foerster, 1916, 1927 ). The thin cutaneous nerve segment with its small diameter in relation to the surface, survives free grafting without fibro-sis ( Bielschowsky and Unger, 1917 ). Cutaneous nerve grafts were very successful to bridge defects in thin nerves, like the facial nerve ( Bunnell, 1927; Ballance and Duel, 1932).

If a thick nerve trunk has to be repaired, one cutaneous nerve is not sufficient. Seddon ( 1947 ) combined several segments of a cutaneous nerve to form a cable of the same size as the nerve to be repaired. Different methods were deve-loped to suture or glue these cutaneous nerve graft segments together. Due to the fact that these nerve grafts are - with part of their surface - in contact with another free graft, there is no optimal contact with the tissue of the recipient site. It also difficult to achieve optimal fascicular coap-tation. The technique of  Interfascicular Nerve Grafting ( Millesi et al., 1966, 1967; Millesi, 1968 ) separates pre-existant fascicle groups in a polyfascicular nerve by inter-fascicular dissection and unites corresponding fascicle

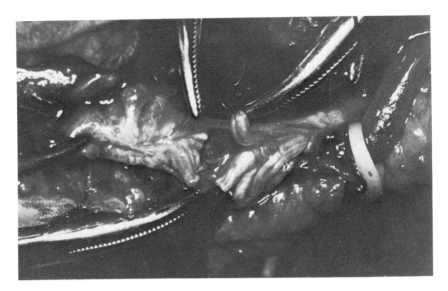

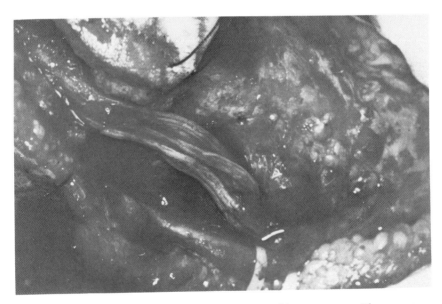

Fig. 1a,b: Bridging a defect of the median nerve. The separation of the fascicle groups of the two stumps by interfascicular dissection is demonstrated in figa 1a and fig. 1b shows the graft in place.

groups by cutaneous nerve grafts individually. The thin isolated grafts have a good chance to survive without fibrosis. Corresponding groups can united directly, if the knowledge about intraneural topography and the length of the defect permits recognition.

Fachinelli et al. ( 1981 ), Townsend et al. ( 1981 ) developed a technique to graft the sural nerve as a vascularized nerve graft. It remains to be proven whether this technique offers a real advantage.

Autografts

At present only autografts are in clinical use. For the vast majority of indications, there are sufficient donor nerves available and it is no problem to bridge defects with autografts. There are some indications ( long defects of the sciatic nerve, brachial plexus lesions with long defects ) in which additional grafts are wanted.

Allografts

Fresh allografts cause immunologic problems which up to date prevent broad clinical application. Recent studies open new prospects ( Mackinnon et al., 1982 ). In the near future the break-through in this area might be achieved and fresh allografts may become a reliable clinical tool.

Preserved Allografts

The results of utilization of preserved allografts, whether preserved by lyophilization ( Weiss, 1943; Weiss and Taylor, 1943; Jacoby et al., 1970 ) or irradiation ( Marmor, 1963, 1964, 1967; Marmor et al., 1966 ) or in cialite solution ( Afanasieff, 1967 ) were not satisfactory.

The construction of nerve grafts by expanding a Schwann cell population of the recipient patient by cell culture to populating an allograft nerve stroma might be a new way of development ( Aguayo, 1980; Bunge, 1980 ).

The present situation may be summarized as follows: Utilization of autologous cutaneous nerve grafts offer a good chance of survival and return of function, even with long defects. If microsurgical techniques are applied, reliable results can be achieved. Logically, the results are dependent on the length of the nerve defect, the age of the patient, and the time interval between transsection and repair. Microsurgery has not only proven to be very successful in the field of nerve grafting. Microsurgery makes intraneural dissections possible with maximal preservation of nerve tissue by atraumatic dissection. This fact is not only important in post-traumatic conditions, if a neurolysis is indicated, but also in surgery of benign nerve tumors. Microsurgical neurolysis has an important application in post-irradiation damage.

TUMORS OF PERIPHERAL NERVES

In benign nerve tumors ( neurinoma, neurofibroma ) or tumor-like conditions, careful excision of the tumor by microsurgical dissection with maximal preservation of nerve tissue is indicated. If individual fascicles have to be sacrificed, the continuity is restored by nerve grafts. In malignant nerve tumors ( malignant Schwannoma which may develop in a normal nerve or in a neurofibroma, malignant neurofibroma, neurofibrous sarcoma, malignant neuroepithelioma ) wide resection and restoration of contunuity by nerve grafts is attempted.

MALIGNANT TUMORS INVADING PERIPHERAL NERVES

The classical example is the facial nerve. In a malignant tumor of the parotis, the facial nerve has to be sacrificed. It is our policy to restore continuity of the nerve by nerve grafts immediately. In this case the pattern of the facial nerve can be restored much better, because the corresponding parts are still well defined. If irradiation of the tumor site is planned, the area of future irradiation is bypassed by using longer grafts. Secondary restoration of continuity of the facial nerve with its branches after tumor surgery is still possible after one or two years. The functional result might be less good but a satisfactory result with sufficient active lid closure, symmetry at rest, and the possibility to lift the upper lid, might be expected

One of the problems along with facial nerve reconstruction is the development of mass movements after regeneration. The distribution of the individual fibers for different muscle groups are not well defined. Investigations by Meissl ( 1976, 1979 ) revealed certain rules in the distribution of fibers. Within the main trunk of the facial nerve close to the foramen styleomastoideum, the fibers for the upper face muscles are located in the cranio-medial sector. The fibers for the middle face are concentrated in the cranio-lateral, and the fibers for the lower face and the neck in the caudal sector. Within the proximal third of the facial nerve trunk, there is a slight rotation. Now the fibers for the upper face are prevalent in the cranial sector, the fibers for the middle face in the caudo-lateral andfor the lower face and neck in the caudo-medial sector. Here the nerve has a mono-fascicular pattern.

Along the middle third of the main trunk distinct fas-cicle groups can be distinguished. The cranial group contains the majority of the nerve fibers to the upper face, the caudo-lateral group the fibers to the middle face, and the caudo-medial group the fibers to the lower face and the neck.

In a distal third three distinct fascicle groups are present. A cranial group which contains the fibers to the upper branch, the middle group which still contains fibers for both main branches, and the caudal group which contains fibers for the lower branch, serving the middle and the lower face muscles and the neck. In the following segment the fas-cicle group in ghe center divides. The upper half joins the cranial fascicle group, forming the upper branch, the lower half joining the caudal group, forming the lower branch.

With this pattern in mind, reconstructions can be per-formed which do not completely avoid mass movements but reduce them to a minimum. It is especially important that the mouth can be moved without simultaneous lid closure.

If a tumor can be operated radically only by resection of vast parts of the cheek, including the muscles, reconstruction is performed by a free muscle graft. The gracilis muscle ( O'Brien, 1977 ) or/pectoralis minor muscle ( Terzis 1981 ) have been used successfully.

If the facial palsy is due to a tumor operation because of atumor of the cerebello-pontine angle, neurotization of the distal branches of the paralyzed facial nerve, can be achieved by a cross-face-nerve graft ( Scaramella, 1971; Smith, 1971, 1976; Anderl, 1972, 1973, 1975 ). In about one third of the cases active motion, allowing mimic expression recovers. In a second third, the result is symmetry at rest but insufficient

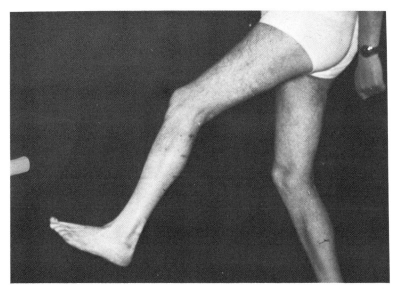

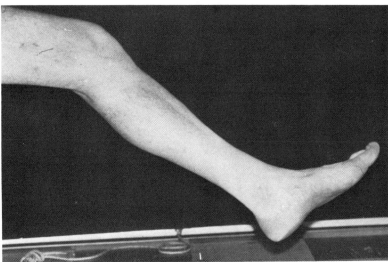

Fig.2a,b: During an operation because of a recurrent hyper —
nephroma, a segment of 15cm in length of the left femoral
nerve was resected. There was a complete palsy of the femoral
nerve innervated muscles. Four months after this operation the
the defect of the femoral nerve was bridged by four sural
nerve grafts. Fig. 2a and b show full recovery of the quadri-
ceps muscle. Note the small transverse scars at the left
leg after excision of the left sural nerve.

active innervation. One third of the cases has to be regarded as failures. The alternative is a transposition of the temporalis muscle, preferably performed with the technique of Rubin ( 1977, 1978 ).

Resection of a peripheral nerve segment to achieve radical removal of a malignant tumor was performed with several peripheral nerves of the upper and the lower extremitry, including the ulnar nerve, the femoral nerve, the sciatic nerve, and the peroneus nerve. Useful recovery was achieved in several of these cases.

SEQUELAE OF TUMOR TREATMENT

Treatment of a malignant tumor, especially irradiation, may damage peripheral nerves, making surgery necessary.

The classical example is the involvement of the brachial plexus after treatment for breast cancer. In some of the patients treated for breast cancer by irradiation, a progressive paralysis of the brachial plexus develops. Usually, the patient suffers from intolerable pain. Three particular situations have to be differentiated. The symptoms might be caused by a recurrent tumor. In other cases the symptoms are the consequence of a direct irradiation damage to the nerve tissue. In both cases the prognosis is poor. In a certain percentage of cases the brachial plexus is damaged by a constricting fibrosis, which has developed as a consequence of irradiation. The differentiation can only be achieved by exploration. If constriction by fibrosis is the cause of the problem, the situation can be improved by external and internal neurolysis. It is regarded already as a success if the progress of the paralysis is stoped and the pain controlled. The main problem in these cases is to achieve a proper soft tissue cover of the exposed brachial plexus. Usually the latissimus dorsi island flap is sufficient. In some cases we have also performed free flaps ( Tensor fascia lata flap ). Envelopment of the brachial plexus by a free transfer of omentum maius was suggested. I have no personal experience with this technique, but from other cases the tendency of the omentum maius to become fibrotic is well known, and for this reason we did not apply this technique.

Progressive paralysis of the brachial plexus due to irr-
diation in the lateral neck triangle, can be observed in
cases of neck tumors as well.

REFERENCES

Afanasieff A (1967). Premiere résultats de 20 homogreffes
de nerfs conservés par le cialite ( main et avant-bras ).
La Presse Medicale 27, 75: 1409

Aguayo AJ.(1981). In Gorio O, Millesi H, Minrgino S (Eds):
"Posttraumatic Peripheral Nerve Regeneration. Experimental
Basis and Clinical Implications," New York: Raven Press,
p. 365

Albert E (1878). Berichte der Naturwissenschaftlich- Medizi-
nischen in Innsbruck. Innsbruck,  9:97

Albert E (1885). Einige Operationen am Nerven. Wr Med Presse
26:1285

Anderl H (1973). Reconstruction of the face through cross-
face nerve transplantation in facial paralysis. Chirurgia
plastica 2:17

Ballance C, Duel AB (1932). Operative treatment of facial
palsy by the introduction of nerve grafts into fallopian
canal and by other intratemporal methods. Arch Otol
15:1

Bielschowsky M, Unger E (1916-1918). Überbrückung grosser
Nervenlücken. Beiträge zur Kenntnis der Degeneration und
Regeneration peripherer Nerven. J Physiol Neurol 22:267

Brooks D (1955). The place of nerve grafting in orthopedic
surgery. J Bone Jt Surg 37A:299

Bunge RP (1981). Construction of grafts. In Gorio O, Millesi
H, Mingrino S (eds) "Posttraumatic Peripheral Nerve Rege-
neration. Experimental Basis and Clinical Implications.
New York: Raven Press, p. 366

Bunnell S (1927). Surgery of nerves of the hand. Surg Gynecol
bstet 44:145

Bunnell S, Boyes HJ (1939). Nerve grafts. Am J Surg 45:54

Fachinelli A, Masquelet A,Restrepo J, Gilbert A (1981). The
vascularized sural nerve. Anatomy and surgical approach.
Int J of Microsurgery 3, 1:57

Foerster O (1916). Communication held at the ausserordentliche
Tagung der Deutschen Gesellschaft für Orthopaedie, Berlin
Febr. 8-9, 1916. Münch Med Wschr 63:283

Foerster O (1927). Leitungsbahnen des Schmerzgefühles und die
chirurgische Behandlung der Schmerzzustände. Berlin-Wien:
Urban & Schwarzenberg

Jacoby W, Fahlbruch R, Mackert B, Braun B, Rolie J, Schnell J. (1970). Überbrückung peripherer Nervendefekte mit lyophilisierten und desantigenisierten Transplantaten. Münchn. med.Wschr 112:586

Mackinnon S, Hudson A, Falk R, Bilbao J, Kline D, Hunter R.T. (1982). Nerve Allograft Response: A Quantitative Immunologic Study. Neurosurgery 10:1

Marmor L (1963). Regeneration of peripheral nerve defects by irradiated homografts. Lancet 1:1911

Marmor L (1964). Regeneration of peripheral nerves by irradiated homografts. J Bone Jt Surg 46A:383

Marmor L (1967) Peripheral Nerve Regeneration Using Nerve Grafts. Springfield, Ill: Charles C. Thomas, p

Meissl G (1976) In Millesi H: Facial Nerve Suture, 3rd Int Symposium on Facial Nerve Surgery Zürich. ( Fisch U ed) Amstelveen: Kugler Medical Publications BV and Birmingham Ala: Aesculapius Publishing Comp. 1977

Meissl G (1979). Die intraneurale Topographie des extrakraniellen N. facialis. Acta Chir Austr. Suppl 28; 1

Millesi H 1968). Zum Problem der Überbrückung von Defekten Peripherer Nerven. Wien Med Wschr 118:182

Millesi H, Ganglberger J, Berger A (1967). Erfahrungen mit der Mikrochirurgie peripherer Nerven. Chir Plast Reconstr 3:47

O'Brien B McC (1977). Microvascular Surgery. Edinburgh-London-New York: Churchill Livingstone, p 301

Philipeaux JM, Vulpian A (1870). Note sur les eassais de greffe d'un troncon de nerf lingual entre les deux bouts de thypoglose. Archs Phys Norm Path 3:618

Rubin LR, Bromberg BE, van Walden RH (1969). Congenital bilateral facial paralysis. Möbius syndrome, surgical animation of the face. Transact. 4th Int Congr on Plastic and Reconstr Surgery ,Amsterdam: Excerpta Medica, p 740

Scaramella L (1971): L'Anastomosi tra i due nervi facciali. Arch Otologica 82:209

Seddon HJ (1947). The use of autogenous grafts for the repair of large gaps in peripheral nerves. Br J Surg 34:423

Smith JW (1971). Fnew technique of facial animation. Transact. 5th Int Congr of Plastic and Reconstr Surgery, Melbourne Chatswood, NSW: Butterworths Pty Ltd, p 83

Smith JW (1976). Facial nerve paralysis and microsurgery. Proc. Symp. Microsurgery New York Oct 14-18, 1974. St.Louis: The CV Mosby Company

Strange FGStC (1947). An operation for nerve pedicle grafting. Preliminary comm. Br. J Surg 34:423

Terzis J (1981). Personal communication at the Int Symposium Int Society of Reconstructive Microsurgery, Melbourne, 1981

Townsend P (1981). Personal communication at the 4th Congr of the European Sect of the Int Confed for Plastic and Reconstr. Surgery, Athens, May 10-14, 1981

Weiss P (1943). Functional nerve regeneration through frozen dried nerve grafts in cats and monkeys. Proc  Soc exp Biol Med 54:277

Weiss  P, Taylor AC (1943). Repair of peripheral nerves by grafts of frozen-dried nerves. Proc Soc exp Biol Med 52:326

**13th International Cancer Congress, Part D**
**Research and Treatment, pages 399–405**
© 1983 Alan R. Liss, Inc., 150 Fifth Avenue, New York, NY 10011

SKELETAL RECONSTRUCTION FOLLOWING TUMOR SURGERY:
VASCULARIZED BONE GRAFTS

Joseph A. Buckwalter, M.S., M.D.

Orthopaedic Department
Veterans Administration and University of Iowa
Iowa City, Iowa 52242

Wide excision of selected locally aggressive and malignant bone tumors appears to provide effective local control of the lesions (Mankin et al. 1982). These procedures spare the limb but leave a large skeletal defect. Inadequate reconstruction of this defect severely limits function raising questions about the value of the limb sparing operation. In contrast, if reconstruction successfully restores the integrity of the limb the result is far more functional than an amputation. A number of possible methods of reconstructing large skeletal defects have been proposed including prosthetic implants, allografts and autografts. Occasionally these methods have been combined, such as joint prostheses combined allografts (Mankin et al. 1982) or joint prostheses combined with autografts (Imbriglia et al. 1978). Each method has advantages and limitations.

Customized implants can replace almost any segment of the skeleton including joints and entire bones (Marcove 1981). They can be implanted in a one stage operation and provide immediate stability and function. Unfortunately segmental skeletal implants may present a number of problems including loss of fixation, implant fracture, late infection, lack of soft tissue attachment to the implant and inability to remodel in response to stress. The frequency of implant failure may be especially high in young patients with reasonable expectation of a normal life span and the desire to participate in physically demanding activities. In an attempt to solve some of these problems, implants have been developed that allow fibrous or bony ingrowth of host tissue (Anderson et al. 1978) Long term results of these implants in patients remain

unknown, but theorectically by providing fixation through
bone or fibrous ingrowth they may be less prone to loosening
and mechanical failure. However, solid implant fixation to
bone may have a disadvantage. Should the implant need to be
removed because of fracture or infection an extensive operation may be necessary to retrieve it.

Allografts also can replace almost any part of the
skeleton including entire bones and joints and they can unite
with the host bone, and allow attachment of ligaments,
tendons and muscles. However, early experimental work with
allografts showed an initial host inflammatory reaction to
the grafts, demonstrated poor healing of allograft fractures
and questioned whether the host tissues will completely
incorporate an allograft (Bonfiglio 1958; Bonfiglio and
Jeter 1972). Clinical experience demonstrated high rates
of graft fracture with nonunion, partial resorption of the
grafts, infections and graft host nonunions (Ottolenghi 1972).
More recent clinical reports describe greater success with the
use of non-vascularized osteoarticular and intercalary
allografts to replace skeletal segments resected for treatment of tumors. Mankin et al. (]982), reported that 74% of
their patients had successful transplants and achieved good
or excellent function of the affected part after wide resection and allograft replacement for malignant bone tumors.
Infections, 13%, and pathologic fractures, 10%, were still
frequent. The high rate of success in this series may be
due, in part, to improved methods of harvesting and storing
allografts. Use of allografts currently is limited to those
centers equipped to procure and store large numbers and
various sizes of sterile allografts. Theoretically
vascularized allografts might have the advantage of more
rapid healing and incorporation and thus a more rapid gain
in mechanical strength. Unfortunately animal experiments
reveal short survival of vascularized allografts even with
immunosuppression (Moore et al. 1982; Phillips, Weiland 1982;
Yaremchok et al. 1982). In these grafts donor vessels show
severe intimal damage predisposing to vessel thrombosis and
loss of blood supply to the graft. For these reasons it
does not appear that vascularized autografts will be clinically applicable in the near future.

Autografts unite, incorporate and hypertrophy more pre-
dictably and more rapidly than allografts but available donor
sites limit their size and shape. Despite this limitation
reconstruction of segmental defects with large non-vascular-

ized autogenous bone grafts remains the traditional method
of providing a stable limb (Wilson 1972). Vessels from the
soft tissues grow into these large autografts and cells
accompaning the invading vascular buds resorb dead bone
replacing it with living bone as callus envelopes and re-
inforces the graft externally. The resorption significantly
weakens the bone graft but eventually it gains normal
strength and will hypertrophy in response to mechanical
loads (Enneking et al. 1975). Harvesting the autograft may
produce donor site morbidity and although large autografts
revascularize, incorporate completely and hypertrophy this is
a slow process which predisposes them to nonunion and
fracture. The techniques of vascularized bone grafting
have been developed in an attempt to avoid the prolonged
revascularization and resorption necessary for incorporation
of conventional grafts and thereby decrease time until union
and the probability of nonunion or fracture. The vascularized bone graft is immediately viable and has the advantages
of the non-vascularized autograft as well as possibly allowing more rapid incorporation, remodeling and healing (Ostrup,
Fredrickson 1979; Weiland 1981). Vascularized autografts
potentially may produce more donor site morbidity since a
vessel must be sacrificed at the donor site and a cuff of
soft tissue surrounding the graft must be dissected from
the donor site. Furthermore if the microvascular anastomoses
fail, the necrotic soft tissue impedes ingrowth of new
vessels and formation of new bone on the dead graft. Thus,
the failed vascularized graft may be slower to heal and
remodel than a non-vascularized graft (Berggren et al. 1982).

Compared with conventional autografts, vascularized
grafts increase the expense and expose the patient to greater
risk by increasing potential donor site morbidity and the
length of the operation. To justify the risk and cost
vascularized grafts must have significant advantages. Reported series of patients document the feasibility of the operation and that vascularized grafts remain viable (Berggren
et al. 1982; Berggren et al. 1982; Coleman et al. 1982; Pho
1979; Pho 1981; Taylor 1977; Taylor et al. 1975; Weiland
1981; Weiland and Daniel 1979; Weiland et al. 1977; Weiland
et al. 1979). These studies do not allow comparison of
vascularized and non-vascularized grafts. However, two
recent investigators compared the results of vascularized
and non-vascularized autografts in dogs. Mazur et al. (1982)
created bilateral segmental defects in dog ulnae and
reconstructed them with vascularized and non-vascularized

rib grafts. All grafts united but three months after surgery the vascularized grafts were mechanically stronger. Dell and Burchardt (1982) compared the incidence and frequency of union and the strength of vascularized and conventional fibula grafts. There were no differences in incidence and frequency of union. At two weeks following surgery vascularized grafts were significantly weaker but at six weeks they were stronger. After six weeks both types of graft had equal strength. Thus, it appears that in normal tissue vascularized grafts may not unite any more frequently or rapidly. Vascularized grafts may·initially be weaker because they respond to decreased loads or possibly small areas of necrosis caused by the procedure with partial resorption. Following this initial period vascularized grafts may be stronger because they do not have to be extensively resorbed and revascularized. Once the conventional grafts have been revascularized there is no difference in strength. Since conventional grafts rely on the soft tissue vessels to invade and revascularize the graft, non-vascularized grafts might not unite and gain strength as quickly in tissues scarred by radiation or trauma or sites where the well vascularized muscle and soft tissues have been resected. In these situations, grafts that bring their own blood supply might have an important advantage.

Three types of vascularized bone grafts have been used in skeletal reconstruction: the ilium, the rib, and the fibula. The fibula has several advantages for reconstruction of long bones (Taylor 1977). It has a long straight length in the adult. The tubular shape of the fibula gives it good resistance to angulatory and rotational stresses. Its diameter fits well in replacement of segments of the radius and ulna and it can be snugly inserted in the medullary cavities of the femur, tibia, or humerus. The relatively large vessels of the fibula facilitate the vascular anastomoses. The peroneal artery in the adult has a diameter of between 1.8 and 2.5 mm. and the veins which parallel the peroneal vessel have a diameter of 2 to 4 mm.

Current applications of vascularized fibula grafts include reconstruction of segmental defects confined primarily to the diaphysis of long bones or the distal radius (Coleman et al. 1982; Pho 1979; Pho 1981; Taylor 1977; Weiland et al. 1979). Defects involving the metaphysis can make fixation and stabilization of the graft more difficult. The vascularized graft requires a prolonged procedure and thus the patient must be able to tolerate a lengthy operation. Children with significant remaining skeletal growth present a special problem. The blood supply to the proliferating cells of the growth plate enters from the epiphyseal side (Brighton 1978). However, growth plate function may be distrubed by interrupting the penetrating vessels on the metaphyseal side (Donski et al. 1979). Therefore, normal growth may require adequate blood supply from several sets of vessels and the role of vascularized grafts in skeletally immature children needs careful investigation.

There are several circumstances in which use of a vascularized fibula graft may be ill-advised. Small defects, those less than 6 ot 8 cm., may be reconstructed satisfactorily using simpler methods. Segmental defects that involve a significant portion of the metaphysis should be approached with caution because of potential problems with stabilizing the graft and joint, and candidates for the procedure must have satisfactory donor and recipient vessels. Furthermore the grade or stage of the tumor may preclude reconstruction with a vascularized graft. The surgeon's primary goal must be resection of the tumor with adequate margins of normal soft tissue and bone. This goal should not be compromised to save vessels or bone that allow reconstruction with a vascularized bone graft.

Recent experience demonstrates that vascularized fibular grafts remain viable and can successfully reconstruct large segmental defects in long bones. These grafts appear to unite and hypertrophy rapidly, however, available experimental evidence suggest that in time vascularized and non-vascularized grafts have equal strength, complete incorporation, and equal ability to hypertrophy in response to loads. Thus the potential advantages of the vascularized graft appears to lie in more rapid incorporation and achievement of mechanical strength. The vascularized graft may have special value in the reconstruction of major bone defects where soft tissue blood supply has been compromised by radiation, trauma, or surgery and vascular invasion of conventional grafts would be slow. In these circumstances the vascularized graft brings its own blood supply and potentially could unite and gain strength more rapidly. The potential advantages and appropriate applications of vascularized grafts in reconstruction of skeletal defects needs further definition, as Taylor (1977) observed "Free vascularized bone graft is recommended only when conventional bone grafting techniques are difficult or when they are unavailable. It would be a tragedy to see this exacting tehnique abused and then discarded only to be labeled a triumph of technique over reason."

Anderson GBJ, Gaechter A, Galante JO, Rostoker W (1978). Segmental replacement of long bones in baboons using a fiber titanium implant. J Bone Joint Surg 60A:31.

Berggren A, Weiland AJ, Ostrup LT (1982). Bone scintigraphy in evaluating the viability of composite bone grafts re-vascularized by microvascular anastomoses, conventional autogenous bone grafts, and free non-vascularized periosteal grafts. J Bone Joint Surg 64A:799.

Berggren A, Weiland AJ, Ostrup LT, Dortman H (1982). Micro-vascular free bone transfer and revascularization of the medullary and periosteal circulation alone. J Bone Joint Surg 64A:73.

Brighton CT (1978). Structure and function of the growth plate. Clin Orthop 136:22.

Bonfiglio M (1958). Repair of bone transplant fractures. J Bone Joint Surg 40A:446.

Bonfiglio M, Jeter WS (1972). Immunological responses to bone. Clin Orthop 87:19.

Coleman DA, Blair WF, Buckwalter JA, Weinstein SL (1982). The free autogenous fibula graft. Iowa J Ortho 2:70.

Daniel RK, Weiland AJ (1982). Free tissue transfers for upper extremity reconstruction. J Hand Surg 7:66.

Dell PC, Burchardt H (1982). Mechanical and roentgenographic evaluation of vascular segmental dog cortical autografts. Trans Ortho 7:140.

Donski PK, Carwell GR, Sharzer LA (1979). Growth in revascularized bone grafts in young puppies. Plast Reconst Surg 64:239.

Enneking WF, Burchardt H, Puhl J, Piotrowski G (1975). Physical and biological aspects of repair in dog cortical-bone transplants. J Bone Joint Surg 57A:237.

Imbriglia JE, Neer CS, Dick HM (1978). Resection of the proximal one half of the humerus in a child for chondro-sarcoma. J Bone Joint Surg 60A:262.

Mankin HJ, Doppelt SH, Sullivan Tr, Tomford WW (1982). Osteoarticular and intercalary allograft transplantation in the management of malignant tumors of bone. Cancer 50:613.

Marcove RC (1981). Therapeutic procedures. In Marcove: The surgery of tumors of bone and cartilage. New York: Grune and Stratton, p 23.

Mazur JM (1982). Torsional testing of vascularized and non-vascularized autogenous bone grafts. Trans Ortho Res Soc 7:138.

Moore Jr, Phillips TW, Weiland AJ, McDonald DF (1982). Influence of immunotherapy on allogenic transplants of bone revascularized by microvascular anastomoses. Trans Ortho Res Soc 7:175.

Ostrup LT, Frederickson JM (1979). Distant transfer of a free living bone graft by microvascular anastomoses. Plast Reconst Surg 54:274.

Ottolenghi GE (1972). Massive osteo and osteo-articular bone grafts. Clin Ortho 87:156.

Phillips TW, Weiland AJ (1982). Microsurgically revascular-ized allografts of bone - An animal model to assess their effectiveness in bridging a large bone defect. Trans Ortho Res Soc 7:139.

Pho RWH (1979). Free vascularized fibular transplant for replacement of the lower radius. J Bone Joint Surg 61B:362.

Pho RWH (1981). Malignant giant cell tumors of the distal end of the radius treated by a free vascularized fibular transplant. J Bone Joint Surg 63A:877.

Taylor GI, Miller GOH, Hamm FJ (1975). The free vascularized bone graft. A clinical extension of microvascular tech-niques. Plast Reconst Surg 55:533.

Weiland AJ (1981). Current concepts review. Vascularized free bone transplants. J Bone Joint Surg 63A:166.

Weiland AJ, Daniel RK (1979). Microvascular anastomoses for bone graft in the treatment of massive defects in bone. J Bone Joint Surg 61A:98.

Weiland AJ, Daniel RK, Riley RH (1977). Application of the free vascularized bone graft in the treatment of malignant or aggressive bone tumors. Johns Hopkins Med J 140:385.

Weiland AJ, Kleinert HE, Kutz JE, Daniel RK (1979). Free vascularized grafts in surgery of the upper extremity. J Hand Surg 4:129.

Wilson PD (1972). A clinical study of the biomechanical behavior of massive bone transplants used to reconstruct large bone defects. Clin Orthop 87:81.

Yaremchuk MJ, Sedecca T, May JW (1982). Vascularized knee allograft transplantation in a rabbit model. Trans Ortho Res Soc 7:174.

13th International Cancer Congress, Part D
Research and Treatment, pages 407–420
© 1983 Alan R. Liss, Inc., 150 Fifth Avenue, New York, NY 10011

MYOCUTANEOUS FLAPS TUMOR SURGERY OF THE HEAD AND NECK

Charles W. Cummings, M.D.

University of Washington   RL-30
1959 NE Pacific Street
Seattle, WA   98195

INTRODUCTION

Nowhere in the sphere of surgical reconstruction has the need for imagination and innovation been more apparent than in the surgical treatment of head and neck malignancies. The ability to reconstruct has lagged behind the ability to resect tumor and create large defects. Primary closure or resurfacing of the defects by complicated, marginally successful, multistaged procedures was the norm. The development of the axial flap, such as the deltopectoral flap based on the internal mammary arterial system was a major step in reconstruction. The use of local, well vascularized tissue, specifically from the tongue, increased success with resurfacing the oral cavity, yet contributed added disabilities as well, such as impairing deglutition and articulation. The use of split thickness skin grafts initially found favor and then fell into relative disrepute because of the contracture and compromise of the oral cavity. However, a rekindling of interest in the split thickness graft has ensued with the realization that one must overcompensate for the contracture at the time of development. The last five years has allowed for a new wave of reconstructive fervor associated with the development of the myocutaneous flap. At no time in the span of head and neck surgery has enthusiasm run as rampant as that which is associated with this new reconstructive technique.

General Design and Mechanics

The myocutaneous flap is based on the anatomical fact that with most major muscle groups there are vessels running perpendicular to the skin which provide a sustaining blood supply. In general, the body is provided with two broad groups of muscles--those that are round in configuration, such as the sternocleidomastoid muscle and those that are flat in configuration, such as the trapezius or pectoralis muscles. The flat muscles have a segmental blood supply which is a named artery, such as the pectoralis artery or the transverse cervical artery. These vessels lie beneath the muscle groups. From these emanate perforating vessels which supply the muscles themselves. Cutaneous vessels course from the muscle to the skin. The round muscles do not possess a segmental blood supply as such, and possess a less defined system. Recognition of this anatomical fact has allowed for the development of a family of flaps which are based on the named segmental vessels of the flat muscles. Pertinent to head and neck reconstruction are the pectoralis, trapezius, and latissimus dorsi myocutaneous flaps. Lesser myocutaneous flaps can be developed from the platysma and sternocleidomastoid muscle. However, the success rate for these flaps is more guarded because of a random blood supply. The myocutaneous flaps to be discussed in this paper are the pectoralis, upper and lower trapezius flaps. In general, the advantages of the myocutaneous flaps are: 1) there is a defined vascular supply which the surgeon can readily identify and preserve, thereby assuring transport of well vascularized tissue to the recipient site; 2) bulk may be provided on the basis of transported muscle when needed; 3) ease of transport; 4) a significant length of scope allowing for resurfacing of areas distant from the source of the flap; 5) the capability of these flaps to resurface oral and oral pharyngeal defects with ease without the creation of additional intraoral defects; and 6) the singular most significant advantage is that these flaps usually are nondelayed and are unassociated with the need for second-stage procedures. The surgeon is, therefore, allowed to achieve the ultimate goal of a single-stage extirpative/reconstructive procedure. Let us turn to the previously cited flaps.

The Pectoralis Myocutaneous Flap

This flap utilizes the arterial system afforded by the pectoralis artery as it courses underneath the pectoralis major muscle. The skin may be harvested at a level as low as the fifth rib and the inferior-most portion of the flap may in fact be extended below the lower limits of the pectoralis muscle by approximately 4 cm without need for delay or impairment of cutaneous perfusion. The skin to be harvested may extend from the lateral border of sternum to the nipple, thus insuring transport of a large surface area of skin, should it be required.

Advantages. The advantages of the pectoralis flap are: 1) it may provide bulk to fill in significant defects surgically created in the neck as well as those which are created by partial mandibular resection; 2) the skin is supple and, as previously mentioned, may be of large surface area; 3) there is sufficient scope provided by the pectoralis artery to allow transport of the skin to resurface areas as high as the nasopharynx; 4) the flap is extremely durable and because of this attribute, has become the workhorse in this family of vascularized pedicle flaps; and 5) it, as with others, is a one-stage procedure and may incorporate an osseous component to the flap--either the fifth rib or the outer portion of sternum, should mandibular reconstruction be an added requisite.

Disadvantages. The disadvantages of the pectoralis flap are: 1) there are occasions when the bulk of the pectoralis flap is disadvantageous, such as the anterior floor of the mouth; 2) a donor site deformity is created, not significant in the male as a rule, however, in the female this loss of symmetry becomes a consideration; 3) when a radical neck dissection is incorporated as a portion of the procedure (implying that the spinal accessory nerve must be sacrificed), additional functional disability is created at the shoulder by compromise of pectoralis muscular function; and 4) (a minor disadvantage) in the hirsute individual transfer of hair bearing skin introduces a problem.

Indications for Use. This flap may be utilized wherever there is a need for bulk in the oral cavity or oropharynx and wherever there is a need for closure of large surgical defects. It is especially advantageous in those patients requiring subtotal glossectomies or total tongue resections as well as those patients undergoing

composite resections involving the retromolar trigone
tonsillar fossa, including the angle of the mandible.
Resection of the hypopharynx and cervical esophagus has
heretofore been handled surgically by multi-staged reconstructed procedures. A single-stage reconstruction with
re-establishment of continuity from the oral cavity to the
lower cervical esophagus may be achieved with this method.

Construction of Flap. The desired paddle of skin is
outlined and the scope of the pedicle determined prior to
any incision. Subsequently, the lateral aspect of a deltopectoral flap is raised to preserved potential for use
of this valuable flap, should postoperative or intraoperative complications with the pectoralis flap ensue (Fig. I,
Sec. 1). The pectoralis artery may be found in one of
several ways--either by identification of the sternal and
clavicular heads of the pectoralis muscle and separation
of these two heads at the mid-clavicular level. The pectoralis artery will be found in the underlying soft
tissue. Dissection may then be carried along a medial
inferior plane with the pectoralis artery in view to avoid
inadvertent transection. An alternative method is to outline the medial aspect of the paddle of the pectoralis
flap, dissect to the level immediately overlying the peri-
osteum of the ribs, and then proceed laterally. This also
will enable visualization of the pectoralis artery. It is
mandatory that the paddle be sutured to the underlying
muscle to avoid accidental shearing or avulsion of the
fine cutaneous vessels emanating from the muscle. The
vessel is then followed superiorly with a division of the
pectoralis muscle being tailored to the surgical needs.
The lateral portion of the pedicle is then developed by
incision of the pectoralis muscle. After completion of
flap development, should it become obvious that there is
need for slightly greater scope, the clavicular head of
the pectoralis muscle may be incised. Tethering and traction of the vascular pedicle over the clavicle will even-
tuate in vascular compromise and flap necrosis, however.
Introduction of pedicle into the oral or oropharyngeal
defect should be accomplished without tension and water-
tight mucosal to cutaneous approximation achieved (Fig. I,
Sec. 2-3). Additional support for the pedicle may be
accomplished by suturing the muscular component of the
pedicle to the underlying cervical musculature. It is
mandatory as well to avoid any constricting dressing post-
operatively which may compromise the vascular supply.

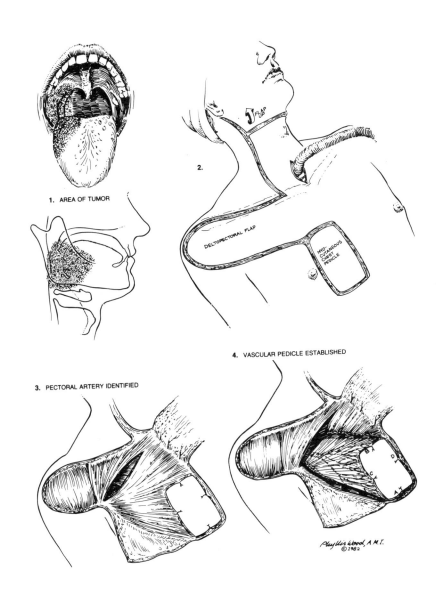

1. AREA OF TUMOR

2.

DELTOPECTORAL FLAP

MYO-CUTANEOUS CHEST PEDICLE

3. PECTORAL ARTERY IDENTIFIED

4. VASCULAR PEDICLE ESTABLISHED

Phyllis Wood, A.M.I.
©1982

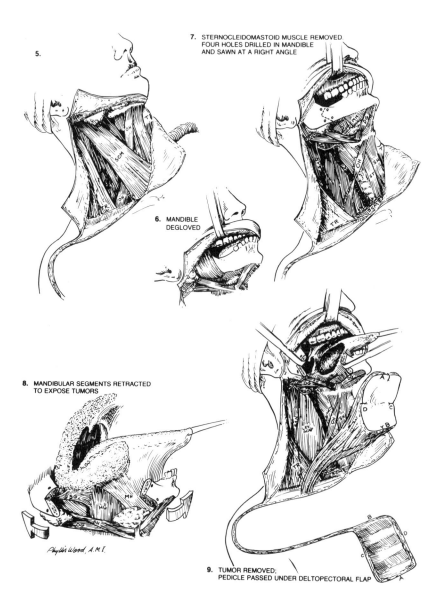

**5.**

**6.** MANDIBLE DEGLOVED

**7.** STERNOCLEIDOMASTOID MUSCLE REMOVED.
FOUR HOLES DRILLED IN MANDIBLE
AND SAWN AT A RIGHT ANGLE

**8.** MANDIBULAR SEGMENTS RETRACTED
TO EXPOSE TUMORS

Phyllis Wood, A.M.I.

**9.** TUMOR REMOVED;
PEDICLE PASSED UNDER DELTOPECTORAL FLAP

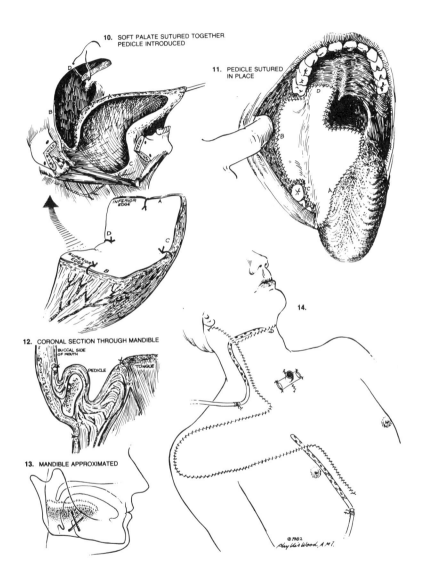

10. SOFT PALATE SUTURED TOGETHER. PEDICLE INTRODUCED

11. PEDICLE SUTURED IN PLACE

12. CORONAL SECTION THROUGH MANDIBLE

13. MANDIBLE APPROXIMATED

14.

Trapezius Myocutaneous Flap

The trapezius muscle and its vascular supply provide three separate exceptionally useful methods for resurfacing. The upper trapezius flap may be based on the transverse cervical artery as an island flap or on the occipital artery as a more standard segmental artery myocutaneous flap.

Advantages. The advantages of these two flaps are: 1) they may be used in females without introduction of breast asymmetry; 2) they provide thin supple cutaneous lining; and 3) they are relatively surgically accessible.

Disadvantages. The disadvantages of these two flaps are: 1) donor site will require skin grafting, thus another step is introduced into the procedure; 3) one may incur a compromised shoulder function on the basis of muscular disruption and spinal accessory nerve division; 3) the island trapezius flap has a rather short vascular pedicle and is therefore easily compromised. The integrity of the transverse cervical artery must be assured prior to creation of the island flap; 4) the upper trapezius flap based on the occipital artery has a gradually increasing bulky pedicle, as the base of the flap extends more medially; and 5) if the cutaneous portion of the upper flap extends beyond the lateral border of the trapezius muscle by greater than 3 cm, a delaying procedure is required to optimize chances for flap viability. Both of these flaps require minor intraoperative position changes to optimize unimpaired access to the shoulder.

Indications for Use. The indications for use of the upper trapezius flaps are: 1) pharyngocutaneous fistulae; 2) through-and-through cheek defects; and 3) posterior oral cavity, and oropharyngeal mucosal defects.

Construction of Flap (Island). The transverse cervical artery must be identified prior to creating the cutaneous paddle. The pedicle length must be assessed prior to creating the cervical paddle. The lateral most margin of the cutaneous paddle is outlined and the dissection is carried medially to incorporate the trapezius muscle in the flap (Fig. II, Sec. 1). The medial portion of the cutaneous paddle cannot be incised until the transverse cervical vessel is seen to enter that portion of the

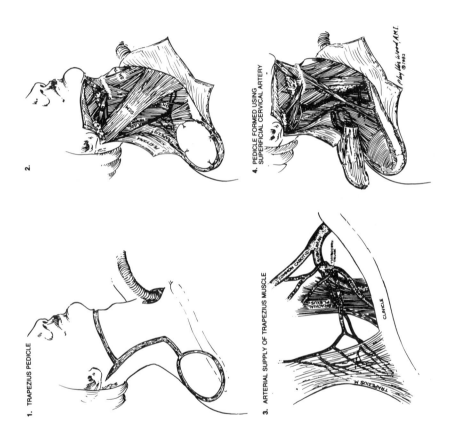

2.

4. PEDICLE FORMED USING SUPERFICIAL CERVICAL ARTERY

1. TRAPEZIUS PEDICLE

3. ARTERIAL SUPPLY OF TRAPEZIUS MUSCLE

trapezius muscle which underlies the cutaneous paddle.
Once the paddle is developed, care should be taken to
avoid tension or kinking of the vascular pedicle. The
paddle with pedicle is then transfered to the surgical
defect and a saliva-tight closure is accomplished. The
donor site is then covered with split thickness skin
graft.

Construction of Upper Trapezius Flap (Occipital).
The lateral limit of the flap is defined initially and may
extend beyond the lateral border of the trapezius muscle
by 3 cm without meriting a delay procedure (Fig. 2, Sec.
2). The anterior border of the trapezius muscle
represents the anterior incision between developing the
cutaneous pedicle. The dissection is carried medially and
includes the trapezius muscle as a pedicle. The flap is
then rotated medially to resurface the posterior oral
cavity, oropharyngeal, or upper cervical defect. If the
proximal tissue overlying the muscle pedicle is preserved
with the pedicle, this will create a rather broad dog ear
at the superior portion of the root of the pedicle.
Before excision, the dog ear must be preserved for at
least four weeks to assure revascularization of the flap
in its new surroundings. A split thickness graft is
applied to the donor defect. Physiotherapy, both active
and passive, is beneficial to those patients undergoing
trapezius myocutaneous flaps to eliminate as best as
possible the secondary defects associated with the loss of
the spinal accessory nerve, such as shoulder drop, etc.


Lower Trapezius Myocutaneous Flap (Descending Transverse
Cervical)

General: This flap is based upon the descending
branch of the transverse cervical artery which courses
underneath the trapezius muscle from the root of the neck
inferiorly.

Advantages. The advantages of this flap are: 1)
that this flap provides the thinnest skin of all of the
herein described myocutaneous flaps. The vascular pedicle
underlining the trapezius muscle is very identifiable and
mirrors the architecture found in the pectoralis flap; 2)
the spinal accessory nerve may be preserved along with the
function of the upper portion of the trapezius muscle; 3)

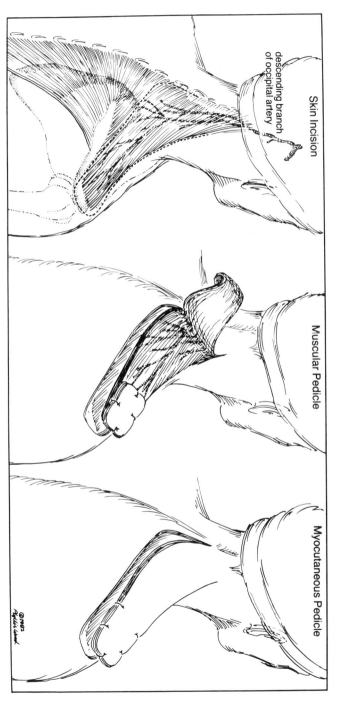

UPPER TRAPEZIUS MYOCUTANEOUS FLAP

Skin Incision

descending branch
of occipital artery

Muscular Pedicle

Myocutaneous Pedicle

a narrow pedicle may be developed which is sufficiently
long to traverse the neck and to resurface an oral cavity
defect, therefore, the scope of the pedicle is great; 4)
the cutaneous paddle of the pedicle is usually hairless
which is a distinct advantage in intraoral resurfacing;
and 5) the resultant donor site defect is minimal and may
be used advantageously in the female. The donor site may
be closed primarily, therefore split thickness skin
grafting is not required.

Disadvantages. The disadvantages of this flap are:
1) that because the flap is based on the descending
portion of the transverse cervical artery, the integrity
of this vascular system is a requisite to flap success,
necessitating care during a radical or conservation neck
dissection; and 2) that there is a mandatory intraoperative position change in that the patient must be placed in
the prone position during harvesting of the flap and then
reversed to the supine position for the definitive surgical procedure.

Indications for Use. This flap is most useful when
reconstructing: 1) through-and-through cheek defects; 2)
large defects in the posterior pharyngeal, oropharyngeal
wall; 3) the floor of the mouth; 4) the tonsillar and
retromolar trigone region. Resurfacing of orbital antral
defects is also distinctly feasible considering the length
of the vascular pedicle.

Construction of Flap. With the patient in the prone
position, the paddle of the flap is outlined subsequent to
assessment of the length of vascular pedicle needed (Fig.
IV, Sec. 1). The cutaneous paddle is then created and an
ascending incision is placed in the paravertebral region
up to the root of the neck. The overlying skin is then
undermined to expose the trapezius muscle. The paddle is
then sutured to the underlying trapezius. The inferor-
medial aspect of the trapezius is then separated from the
underlying rhomboid muscle and is rotated laterally to
expose the easily identifiable descending branch of the
transverse cervical artery (Fig. III, Sec. 1). The
vascular pedicle is then created with inclusion of some of
the overlying trapezius muscle for protection. At the
root of the neck, the junction of the descending portion
of the transverse superior artery with the main artery
will be identified. The paddle (with pedicle) will then

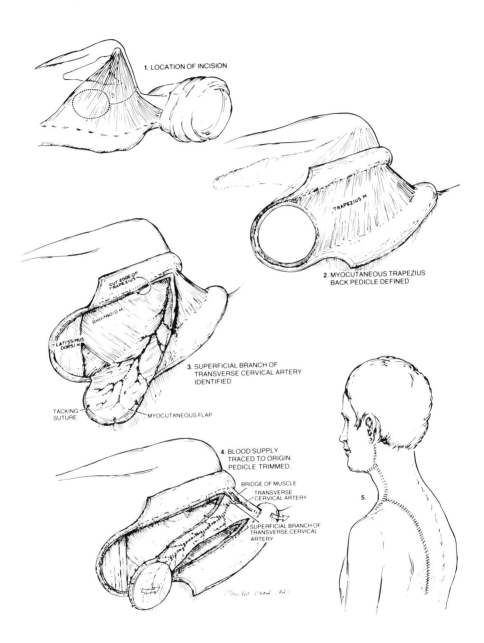

1. LOCATION OF INCISION

TRAPEZIUS M.

2. MYOCUTANEOUS TRAPEZIUS
BACK PEDICLE DEFINED

CUT EDGE OF
TRAPEZIUS

RHOMBOID M.

LATISSIMUS
DORSI M.

3. SUPERFICIAL BRANCH OF
TRANSVERSE CERVICAL ARTERY
IDENTIFIED

TACKING
SUTURE — MYOCUTANEOUS FLAP

4. BLOOD SUPPLY
TRACED TO ORIGIN.
PEDICLE TRIMMED.

BRIDGE OF MUSCLE

TRANSVERSE
CERVICAL ARTERY

SUPERFICIAL BRANCH OF
TRANSVERSE CERVICAL
ARTERY

5.

be delivered into the anterior neck region underneath the upper portion of the trapzius muscle, thereby protecting the spinal accessory nerve and muscle. Resurfacing is accomplished as previously described after primary closure of the donor defect and repositioning of the patient.

CONCLUSIONS

The development of the myocutaneous flap procedures has eased the dilemma created by major extirpation of oral and oropharyngeal tumors as well as the inadvertent development of large cutaneous defects and oropharyngeal fistulae created by postoperative infection or necrosis. The exuberance created by this advance in reconstruction should not blind the therapist to consideration of lesser, yet as effective, surgical measures for resurfacing defects. The advantage of single-stage reconstruction is patently the most attractive factor in consideration of myocutaneous flap reconstruction.

**13th International Cancer Congress, Part D**
**Research and Treatment, pages 421–428**
© **1983 Alan R. Liss, Inc., 150 Fifth Avenue, New York, NY 10011**

MYOCUTANEOUS FLAP RECONSTRUCTION OF THE TRUNK AND EXTREMITIES
IN CANCER SURGERY

David L. Larson, M.D.

M. D. Anderson Hospital and Tumor Institute
University of Texas System Cancer Center
Houston, Texas   77030

Tissue morbidity always results from the effective
treatment of cancer, regardless of the modality of that
therapy.  In most patients, the regenerative reserve of
normal tissue is sufficient to allow the patient satisfactory rehabilitation.  But some methods of treatment result
in severe debilitation and death if the tissue defect is not
reconstructed, either immediately or after a reasonable delay.  It is in these particularly difficult wounds that the
plastic and reconstructive surgeon's skill is most valuable.

Recent investigations into the anatomy of skin flaps
have resulted in revolutionary advances in plastic and reconstructive surgery.  A myocutaneous flap differs from previous skin flaps in that the muscle underlying the skin is
included in the flap.  This entire unit is rotated on a
single vascular pedicle.  With this new flap, a large mass
of skin and muscle can be safely introduced into a soft
tissue or bony defect in a one-stage reconstruction immediately following ablation or as a delayed procedure.  Not
only does this provide safe, predictable wound coverage, but
it also introduces an additional fresh blood supply into an
area in which the blood vessels may have been damaged by
chemotherapy, radiation, or surgery.  If the overlying skin
is not required for reconstruction, the muscle may be used
alone (Figure 1).

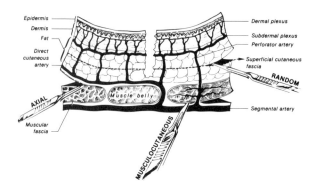

Figure 1

The most effective illustration of the use of these flaps can be seen in the following examples:

Case 1:   A 43-year-old woman who had had a right mastectomy three years previously for breast cancer developed recurrent local disease, which continued to increase in size despite radiotherapy and chemotherapy.  This resulted in total destruction of the sternum by a wound that intermittently bled, required transfusions and was a constant source of pain and potential sepsis (Figure 2).

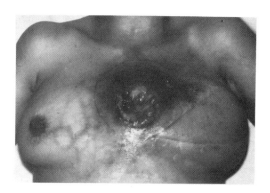

Figure 2

Treatment consisted of resection of her entire sternum (Figure 3).

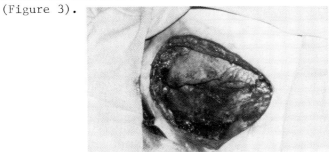

Figure 3

The wound was covered with a latissimus dorsi myocutaneous flap (Figure 4) taken from the left posterior trunk.

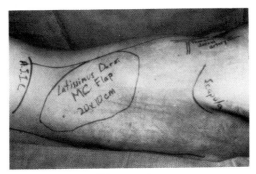

Figure 4

The patient made an uneventful recovery and was ready to resume chemotherapy with a painless wound within ten days (Figure 5).

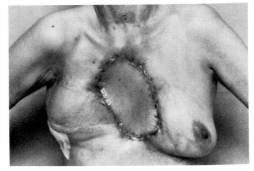

Figure 5

Case 2: A 49-year-old patient had a large necrotic mass in the right anterior chest wall following failure of standard treatment modalities for recurrent breast cancer (Figure 6).

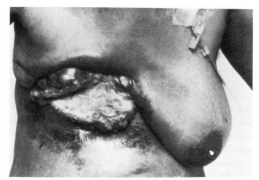

Figure 6

Surgical resection resulted in exposed thoracic and abdominal cavities (Figure 7).

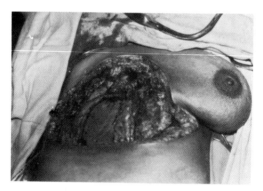

Figure 7

A contralateral rectus abdominus myocutaneous flap based on the superior epigastric artery was rotated into place (Figure 8), while the donor defect was closed primarily.

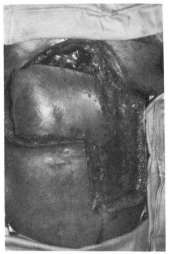

Figure 8

Follow-up at two weeks showed good flap viability (Figure 9).

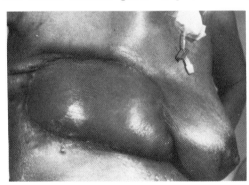

Figure 9

Case 3: A 54-year-old patient with a malignant fibrous histiocytoma of the right groin (Figure 10) required resection of the lower half of the right anterior abdominal wall (Figure 11).

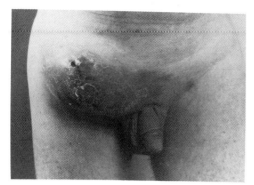

Figure 10

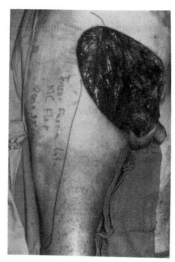

Figure 11

Safe reconstruction was obtained by the use of a tensor
fascia lata myocutaneous flap taken from the lateral surface
of the right leg (Figure 12). The flap is based on the lateral circumflex artery, a branch of the profunda femoral artery.

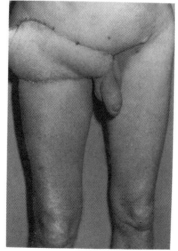

Figure 12

Case 4: A 70-year-old black man with a level V melanoma of the heel required resection and concomitant limb perfusion combined with groin dissection. The treatment resulted in exposed calcaneous (Figure 13) that, in the past, might have been covered with a skin graft, resulting in an unstable wound.

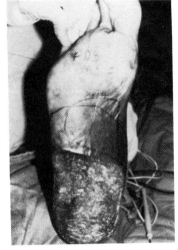

Figure 13

However, the flexor digitorum brevis myocutaneous flap was harvested from the non-pressure bearing area of the instep and rotated posteriorly to provide sensate coverage with the same highly specialized tissue of the plantar surface of the foot (Figure 14).

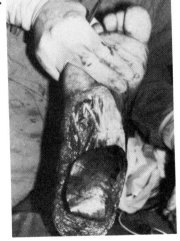

Figure 14

The late results at nine months show good take of the flap, skin graft in a non-pressure bearing area, and a totally functional foot (Figure 15).

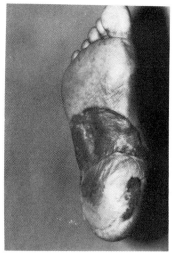

Figure 15

The value of myocutaneous flaps is obvious from these few examples. Not only do these flaps extend the ablative capabilities of the surgeon, but they can also reduce tumor bulk and infection, which aides the clinical oncologist and results in more effective care of the cancer patient.

Larson DL, McMurtrey M, Irish E, Howe HJ (1982). Major chest wall reconstruction after chest wall irradiation. CANCER 49:1286.

Mathes SJ, Nahai F (1982). "Clinical applications for muscle and musculocutaneous flaps". St. Louis: C.V. Mosby.

McCraw J, Gibbell D, Carraway J (1977). Clinical definition of independent myocutaneous vascular territories. Plast Reconstr Surg 60:3.

CONGRESS SYMPOSIA

ACUTE LYMPHOBLASTIC LEUKEMIA Pavlovsky, S.,
Argentina, Chairman; Pinkel, D., USA,
Co-Chairman; Arena

Immunobiological Classification of Acute
Lymphoblastic Leukaemia (ALL). *Gavosto, F.
and Ferrarini, M., Turin, Italy and Genova, Italy.

Prognosis of Acute Lymphoblastic Leukemia Related
to Initial Findings and Treatment.
*Henze, G., Lampert, F., Langermann, H-J.,
Schellong, G. and Riehm, H-J., Giessen, W. Germany
and Munster, W. Germany.

Treatment of Acute Lymphoblastic Leukemia.
*Pinkel, D., Los Angeles, CA USA. (By Title Only)

Extramedullary Leukaemia. *Kay, H. E. M.,
London, England.

Late Effects of Treatment for Acute Lymphoblastic
Leukemia (ALL): Adverse Sequellae of Central
Nervous System (CNS) Preventive Therapy.
*Poplack, D. G. and Moss, H., Bethesda, MD USA.
(By Title Only)

Please note: Papers that are listed as "By Title
Only" were presented at the 13th International
Cancer Congress, but are not included in these
volumes.

13th International Cancer Congress, Part D
Research and Treatment, pages 431–444
© 1983 Alan R. Liss, Inc., 150 Fifth Avenue, New York, NY 10011

IMMUNOBIOLOGICAL CLASSIFICATION OF ACUTE LYMPHOBLASTIC
LEUKAEMIA (ALL)

Felice Gavosto^, Manlio Ferrarini¨,
Federico Caligaris Cappio^, Robin Foa^
^Ist.Medicina Interna, I Catt.Patologia Sp.Medica
 Università di Torino, Italy
¨Catt.Immunologia, Università di Genova, Italy

The use of immunological techniques has allowed the definition of a number of cell surface markers specific for
lymphocytes or for their subsets specialized in particular
functions. For example, normal lymphocytes can be recognized
as T or B cells according to the presence of receptors for
sheep erythrocytes (E-rosettes) (Jondal et al 1972) or of sur
face immunoglobulins (SmIg) (Preud'homme, Labaume 1976), respectively. The identification of T and B cells (or of their
subsets) can be also carried out by the use of heterologous
antisera or, more recently, of monoclonal antibodies directed
against specific cell surface molecules. The above and other
cell surface markers together with the use of conventional
cytochemical methods and the possibility of detecting the
nuclear enzyme terminal deoxynucleotidyl transferase (TdT),
have enabled to distinguish lymphoid cells at all levels of
maturation from the cells of the other hemic lineages. The
application of these methods to the study of human acute
lymphoblastic leukaemia (ALL) has led to a more precise clas
sification of this disease.

Initially, three major subgroups of ALL were identified
and namely :T-ALL, B-ALL and non-T, non-B-ALL according to
the presence of E receptors or of SmIg or to the absence of
both (Borella, Sen 1973). Statistical analysis indicated that
approximately 20% of all ALL were of T-cell origin, whilst on
ly 1-2% were of B-cell type, the remaining being negative for

both markers. Clinical evaluations suggested a correlation between the immunological data and the clinical course of the disease, showing that patients with B- and T-ALL had a worse prognosis (Sen, Borella 1975 ; Tsukimoto et al 1976; Bel pomme et al 1977).

The production of a heterologous antiserum recognising an antigen present on the blasts of a large proportion of non-T, non-B-ALL (called common ALL antigen or cALLA), has led to the identification of a new subset of ALL (common-c-ALL) (Greaves et al 1975). The clinical relevance of this finding has been confirmed by longitudinal studies showing that patients with cALLA positive ALL had a relatively low WBC count and a more benign clinical course (Chessels et al 1977) On the contrary, B and T-ALL at presentation generally have a higher WBC count than c-ALL. Therefore, the B and T phenoty pe does not represent an independent prognostic factor( as demonstrated by multivariate statistical analysis) and does not express per se an initial prognostic parameter. Approximately 25% of cALLA positive ALL contain a variable proportion of lymphoblasts with cytoplasmic Ig (CyIg) and no evidence of SmIg (Vogler et al 1978; Brouet et al 1979). This finding may indicate that cALLA positive cells represent very early B cells, some of which can mature into pre-B cells (characterised by the presence of intracytoplasmic $\mu$ chains). Preliminary data seem to suggest that patients with CyIg positive blasts may have a significantly worse prognosis. Clini cal studies are currently underway on large series of ALL ca ses to confirm whether the presence or absence of CyIg positive cells truly represents an important prognostic marker.

The role of the nuclear enzyme TdT (present only in the thymus —Chang 1971— at high levels and in the bone marrow at lower levels —Coleman et al 1974—), although less relevant in terms of subclassification and prognosis of ALL, represents nonetheless an important tool in the differential diagnosis between ALL and acute myeloblastic leukaemia (AML), in that the great majority of ALL are TdT positive, while this is an exceptional finding in AML (McCaffrey et al 1975; Hutton, Cole man 1976). Further correlations between TdT and the surface phenotype of ALL blasts,indicate that practically all cases of cALL and T-ALL have increased levels of TdT,the highest values being observed in cALL (Hoffbrand et al 1977;Coleman et al 1978).Of the non-B,non-T-ALL and/or unclassified acute leukaemias, about half of the cases are TdT positive (Hoffbrand et al 1977). The rare cases of B-ALL tested have revealed near-normal TdT values (Coleman et al 1978). Unlike TdT, adenosine deaminase (ADA) activity,which is present in many lymphoid tissues (Huang et al 1976),is higher in T-ALL than in non-B,non-T-ALL (Coleman et al 1978;Smyth et al 1978 ); as TdT, ADA appears low in B-ALL (Coleman et al 1978). Rather than from a diagnostic point of view, findings on the levels of ADA in ALL may be relevant with respect to treatment. A potent inhibitor of ADA, 2'-deoxycoformycin-lymphotoxic in experimental models (Smyth et al 1978)-,may have a role in the management of individual cases of refractory ALL (Prentice et al 1981). At the same time, the importance of acid phosphatase for the recognition of T-ALL has been well established (Catovsky et al 1978).

Recent cytogenetic studies have revealed that the most frequent abnormality in ALL is the presence of a Ph' chromosome. Although little information is available on large series of ALL, it appears that the incidence of this abnormality is in the order of 15-25% in adult ALL (Bloomfield et al 1978; Catovsky et al 1979),whilst only of 2-3% in childhood ALL (Chessels et al 1979). Banding techniques have shown that a 9;22 translocation,similar to that found in 90 % of patients with chronic myeloid leukaemia (CML),occurs also in ALL, although in several cases other cytogenetic abnormalities have been reported mainly in non-B,non-T-ALL (Cimino et al 1979;Arthur et al 1982). The question of whether Ph' positive ALL represents an individual disorder or simply the acute presentation of Ph' positive CML has still to be fully clarified (Catovsky et al 1979).Nonetheless, the presence of the Ph' chromosome and of other cytogenetic abnormalities seems to correlate with a more aggressive disease (Catovsky et al 1979;Arthur et al 1982) and a worse prognosis,thus stressing the importance of further cytogenetic (and kinetic) studies associated with modern immunological classifications.

Several authors have reported a 8;14 translocation in B-ALL (Mitelman et al 1979;Berger et al 1979), identical to that reported as a marker chromosome in Burkitt lymphoma (Manolov,Manolova 1972). The prognosis appears consistently extremely unfavourable.

The recent availability of monoclonal antibodies has considerably improved the possibility of a more precise cha racterization of the malignant cells.Monoclonal antibodies are homogeneous reagents which recognize specific epitopes and can be produced in potentially unlimited quantity (Kohler,Milstein 1975),thereby allowing the standardization of the results obtained in different laboratories. Monoclonal antibodies are particularly useful in identifying antigenic determinants on the membrane of lymphoid cells,and utilized in combination with conventional markers (Janossy et al, 1980) such as anti-SmIg,anti cALLA,anti-HLA-Dr (Ia-like),an ti-TdT, have permitted a better understanding of the matura tion of normal and pathological cells.

The combined use of several monoclonal antibodies has been of particular relevance in the identification of the differentiation pathway of normal T lymphocytes(Reinherz et al 1980;Tidman et al 1981).For example, the use of monoclonal antibodies of the OKT series (Ortho Diagnostics) has demonstrated that early prothymocytes are recognized by the OKT9, OKT10 (Which however is not T-lineage specific) and OKT1 rea gents (the latter antibody detects T-cells at all levels of differentiation) (Reinherz et al 1980;Reinherz et al 1979 ). In the course of maturation, the cells acquire another antigen detected by the OKT6 monoclonal antibody (Reinherz et al 1980).Subsequently, the cells express other antigens,recognized by the OKT4,OKT5-OKT8 and OKT3 monoclonals,which characterize mature T-cell subsets in the peripheral blood and lymphoid organs,OKT3 recognizing the majority of T cells (pan-T),OKT4 T cells with helper/inducer activity and OKT5-OKT8 T cells with suppressor/cytotoxic activity (Kung et al

1979;Reinherz et al 1979;Kung et al 1980). Finally,OKT11 re
cognizes structures associated with the E-rosette receptor
(Verbi et al 1982) and therefore reacts with thymocytes as
well as with circulating T lymphocytes (Kung et al 1980).
The overall pattern of T-cell differentiation, as demonstra
ted by the OKT reagents (plus E-rosettes and TdT determination), is illustrated in Table 1.

THYMUS

| Reagent | Precursors | Cortical | Medullary | Circulating |
|---------|------------|----------|-----------|-------------|
| OKT1 | + | + | + | + |
| OKT3 | − | − | + | + |
| OKT4 | − | +a | +b | +b |
| OKT6 | − | +a | −b | −b |
| OKT5/8 | − | +a | +b | +b |
| OKT9 | + | − | − | − |
| OKT10 | + | + | ± | − |
| OKT11 | ± | + | + | + |
| E Ros. | ± | + | + | + |
| TdT | + | + | − | − |

Table 1:Phenotypic expression of thymic and circulating T
lymphocytes; a:simultaneously expressed;b:individually expressed.

The application of monoclonal antibodies to the study
of ALL lymphoblasts has confirmed the initial subclassifica
tion based on conventional immunological techniques and iden
tified a previously unrecognized heterogeneity of T-ALL.
Thus, monoclonal antibodies have shown that the large majority of T-ALL,unlike neoplastic lymphoid cells from chronic
T-lymphoproliferative disorders (Greaves et al 1981),dis -
play an immature ,thymic -like phenotype (Reinherz et al
1980). The expression of more mature T-cell antigens(e.g.
those recognised by the OKT3,OKT4,OKT8 monoclonals)is present in variable combinations only in a minority of T-ALL
(Greaves et al 1981).The most frequent T-ALL phenotype appears to be E ros[+],OKT1[+] (Leu1-Engleman et al 1981-,RFA1 -
Caligaris Cappio et al 1982-)[+],OKT6[+],OKT10[+] (A10-Malavasi et

al 1982)[+],OKT11[+] with a variable degree of positivity for the OKT3,OKT4 or OKT8 reagents (Greaves et al 1981).

A further point revealed by monoclonal antibodies is that a large proportion of cALLA positive and null ALL (i.e. non-T non-B,non-cALLA positive) share a number of antigens with the cells of the B lineage,indicating a possible B-lymphocyte origin of the malignant cells (Kersey et al 1981).Recently, it has been shown that part of the immunoglobulin heavy chain variable region is coded for by a set of genes that , although located on the same chromosome, are far apart from the other H chain genes (i.e. those coding for the remaining part of the V region or for the constant region)(reviewed by Vogler 1982). The distance between these two gene clusters is lower in B-cells (or in their precursors)than in other somatic cells, indicating that a process of gene rearrangement takes place during B-cell maturation (reviewed by Vogler 1982). The finding that many cALLA positive ALL have a H chain gene rearrangement suggests that the malignant transformation may have occurred when they were already committed to B-cell differentiation (Korsmeyer et al 1981).

An appropriate analysis with monoclonal antibodies allows a better characterization of cases, which otherwise would probably have been classified as undifferentiated acute leukaemias or null ALL. While some may well belong to the B-cell lineage , several data indicate that others are of T-cell origin (Sondel et al 1981;Gobbi et al 1982). In our experience, rare cases of adult acute leukaemia E-rosette negative, SmIg negative,cALLA negative,TdT positive,acid phosphatase positive (Sudan Black and peroxidase negative), were considered of T-cell origin only on the basis of more extensive cellular analysis ( Table 2 ). Evidence of the true T cell nature of the leukaemic cells, suspected on the basis of the acid phosphatase and TdT positivities, was in fact obtained with the unequivocal reactivity with RFA1 (OKT1,Leu1) and (generally) with OKT6 (Foa et al 1982). They were also A10 (OKT10) positive, but OKT3,OKT4,OKT8,OKT11 consistently negative.Taken together the above observations stress the importance of monoclonal antibodies as a valuable tool for a

|  | Pt.1 | Pt.2 | Pt.3 |
|---|---|---|---|
| WBC x $10^3/mm^3$ | 13 | 112 | 6,5 |
| PBL | 80 | 98 | 40 |
| % Blasts | | | |
| BM | 98 | 99 | 98 |
| E-Ros. | 5 | 10 | 8 |
| RFA1 | 85 | 89 | 91 |
| OKT3 | 12 | 11 | 12 |
| OKT4 | 0 | 0 | 3 |
| OKT6 | 2 | 53 | 90 |
| OKT8 | 0 | 9 | 5 |
| A10 | 75 | 69 | 53 |
| OKT11a | 7 | 9 | 0 |
| OKIa | 0 | 0 | 82 |
| OKM1 | 3 | 0 | -- |
| cALLA | 0 | 0 | 0 |
| TdT | 90 | 90 | 90 |
| Ac.Phosph. | +++ | ++ | + |

Table 2: Main haematological and immunological features of the patients studied. WBC = white blood cells; PBL = peripheral blood lymphocytes; BM = bone marrow.The numbers indicate the percentage of positive cells with the markers utilized.

more extensive characterization of the leukaemic lymphoblasts
Based on this evidence, we propose a simplified scheme of
characterization of newly diagnosed cases of non-myeloid (
sudan black and peroxidase negative) acute leukaemias,which
should allow the recognition of cALL,B-ALL,pre-B-ALL and T-
ALL at different stages of maturation (Table3 ).

| Marker | Diagnosis |
| --- | --- |
| E ros | T-ALL |
| SmIg | B-ALL |
| Ac.Phosph. | T-ALL |
| CyIg | pre-B-ALL |
| TdT | pre-B,c-,T-ALL |
| cALLA^ | cALL |
| OKT1 | T-ALL |
| OKT6 | T-ALL |

Table 3:Scheme of characterization for newly diagnosed non-
myeloid acute leukaemias. ^Two monoclonal antibodies directed against the cALLA have been described,J5 (Ritz et al
1980) and VIL-A1 (Knapp et al 1982).

     In conclusion, the use of conventional immunological
techniques together with the advent of monoclonal antibodies
has dramatically improved our knowledge on the neoplastic
cells of ALL and led to at least three major achievements:
1)the recognition of the heterogeneity of ALL,specially of
T-ALL ;2) the recognition of the normal counterpart of the
cells of each major subgroup of ALL. At present, no surface
marker appears leukaemia-related, and in all cases the markers expressed by the malignant cells are detected on normal
cells at particular stages of differentiation;3) the definition of a putative site of origin of the cells from each ma
jor subgroup of ALL:e.g. cALL appears to originate in the
bone marrow (Janossy et al 1979) and the different forms of
T-ALL in the thymus (Reinherz et al 1979;Bradstock et al
1980). In addition, the uniformity of surface markers found
on the cells from each individual case suggests that ALL,
like other hemic malignancies, may be of clonal origin.For-
mal proof for this possibility, obtained with markers of clo

nality,is this far scanty owing to technical difficulties.

A note of caution seems however realistic.All the recent important achievements have been relevant to the clarification of the processes of human lymphoid ontogeny and
differentiation,but have had limited implications in terms
of prognosis and treatment of patients with ALL. On the o-
ther hand,the possibility of utilizing monoclonal antibodies directed against specific antigens offers exciting new
prospects towards the in vitro modulation of leukaemic and
immunocompetent cells (Granger et al 1982;Ritz et al 1982).

Arthur DC,Bloomfield CD,Lindquist LL,Nesbit ME Jr(1982).
   Translocation 4;11 in acute lymphoblastic leukemia.Clini-
   cal characteristics and prognostic significance.Blood 59:
   96.
Belpomme D,Mathé G,Davies AJS(1977). Clinical significance
   and prognostic value of the T-B immunological classification of human primary acute lymphoid leukaemias.Lancet I:
   555.
Berger R,Bernheim A,Brouet JC,Daniel MT,Flandrin G (1979).
   t (8;14) translocation in a Burkitt's type of lymphoblastic leukaemia (L3).Br J Haematol 43:87.
Bloomfield CD,Linquist LL,Brunning RD,Yunis JJ,Coccia PF
   (1978).The Philadelphia chromosome in acute leukemia.Vir-
   chow Archives B 29:81.
Borella L,Sen L (1973).T cell surface markers on lymphoblas
   ts from acute lymphocytic leukemia.J Immunol 111:1257.
Bradstock KF,Janossy G,Pizzolo G,Hoffbrand AV,McMichael A,
   Pilch JR,Milstein C,Beverley P,Bollum FJ (1980).Subpopula
   tions of normal and leukemic human thymocytes:analysis
   with the use of monoclonal antibodies. J Natl Canc Inst
   65:33.
Brouet JC,Preud'homme JC,Penit C,Valensi F,Rouget P,Selig-
   mann M (1979).Acute lymphoblastic leukemia with pre-B cell
   characteristics.Blood 54:269.
Caligaris Cappio F,Gobbi M,Bofill M,Janossy G (1982).Infre-
   quent normal B lymphocytes express features of B-chronic
   lymphocytic leukaemia.J Exp Med 155:623.
Catovsky D,Cherchi M,Greaves MF,Janossy G,Pain C,Kay HEM

(1978).Acid-phosphatase reaction in acute lymphoblastic leukaemia. Lancet 1:749.

Catovsky D,Pittman S,o'Brien M,Cherchi M,Costello C,Foa R, Pearse E,Hoffbrand AV,Janossy G,Ganeshaguru K,Greaves MF (1979). Multiparameter studies in lymphoid leukemias.Am J Clin Path 72:736.

Chang LMS (1971).Development of terminal deoxynucleotidyl transferase activity in embryonic calf thymus gland.Biochim Biophys Res Comm 44:124.

Chessels JM,Hardisty RM,Rapson NT,Greaves MF (1977).Acute lymphoblastic leukaemia in children:classification andpro gnosis. Lancet II:1307.

Chessels JM,Janossy G,Lawler SD,Secker Walker LM (1979).The Ph' chromosome in childhood leukemia.Br J Haematol 41 :25.

Cimino MC,Rowley JD,Kinnealey A,Variakojis D,Golomb HM (1979) Banding studies of chromosomal abnormalities in patients with acute lymphoblastic leukemia.Canc Res 39:227.

Coleman MS,Hutton JJ,De Simone P,Bollum FJ (1974).Terminal deoxynucleotidyl transferase in human leukemia. Proc Natl Acad Sci USA 71:4404.

Coleman MS,Greenwood MF,Hutton JJ,Holland P,Lampkin B,Krill C,Kastelic JE (1978).Adenosine deaminase,terminal deoxynucleotidyl transferase and cell surface markers in childhood acute leukemia. Blood 52:1125.

Engleman E,Warnke R,Fox RI,Dilley J,Benike CJ,Levy R (1981). Studies of a human T lymphocyte antigen recognized by a monoclonal antibody. Proc Natl Acad Sci USA 28:1791.

Foa R,Caligaris Cappio F,Campana D,Fierro MT,Bergui L,Giubel lino MC,Lusso P (1982).Relevance of monoclonal antibodies in the diagnosis of unusual T-cell acute lymphoblastic leu kaemia. Submitted to Scand J Haematol.

Gobbi M,Lauria F,Raspadori D,Bandini G,Tura S (1982).Diagno sis with monoclonal antibodies of "T acute lymphoblastic leukaemia" expressing an unusual phenotype.Haematologica 67:487.

Granger S,Janossy S,Francis G,Blacklock H,Poulter LW,Hoffbrand AV (1982).Elimination of T lymphocytes from human bone marrow with monoclonal T-antibodies and cytolytic com plement. Br J Haematol 50:367.

Greaves MF,Brown G,Lister TA,Rapson N (1975).Antisera to acute lymphoblastic leukaemia cells.Clin Immunol Immunopa thol 4:67.

Greaves MF,Rao J,Hariri G,Verbi W,Catovsky D,Kung P,Gold - stein G (1981). Phenotypic heterogeneity and cellular o- rigins of T cell malignancies.Leuk Res 5:281.

Hoffbrand AV,Ganeshaguru K,Janossy G,Greaves MF,Catovsky D, Woodruff RK (1977).Terminal deoxynucleotidyl-transferase levels and membrane phenotypes in diagnosis of acute leu- kaemia.Lancet,II:520.

Huang AT,Logue GL,Engelbrecht HL (1976).Two biochemical mar kers in lymphocyte subpopulations.Br J Haematol 34:631.

Hutton JJ,Coleman MS (1976).Terminal deoxynucleotidyl tran- sferase measurements in the differential diagnosis of ad- ult leukaemias. Br J Haematol 34:447.

Janossy G,Bollum FJ,Bradstock KF,McMichael A,Rapson N,Grea- ves MF (1979).Terminal deoxynucleotidyl transferase-posi- tive human bone marrow cells exhibit the antigenic pheno- type of common acute lymphoblastic leukemia.J Immunol 123: 1525.

Janossy G , Bollum FJ,Bradstock KF,Ashley J (1980).Cellular phenotypes of normal and leukemic hemopoietic cells deter mined by analysis with selected antibody combinations. Blood 56:430.

Jondal M,Holm G,Wigzell H (1972).Surface markers on human T and B lymphocytes.I.Large population of lymphocytes for- ming non-immune rosettes with sheep red blood cells.J Exp Med 136:207.

Kersey JH,LeBien TW,Gajil-Peczalska K,Nesbit M,Jansen J,Kung P,Goldstein G,Sather H,Coccia P,Siegel S,Bleyer A,Hammond D (1981).Acute lymphoblastic leukemia/lymphoma:cell mar- kers define phenotypic heterogeneity.In Knapp W (ed):"Leu kemia Markers",New York:Academic Press,p 453.

Knapp W,Majdic O,Bettelheim P,Liszka K (1982).VIL-A1,a mono clonal antibody reactive with common acute lymphatic leu- kemia cells.Leuk Res 6:137.

Kohler G,Milstein C (1975).Continuous cultures of fused cells secreting antibody of predefined specificity.Nature 256: 495.

Korsmeyer SJ,Hieter PA,Ravetch JV,Poplack DG,Leder P,Waldmann TA (1981).Patterns of immunoglobulin gene arrangement in human lymphocytic leukemias.In Knapp W (ed):"Leukemia Markers",New York:Academic Press,p 85.

Kung PC,Goldstein G,Reinherz EL,Schlossman SF (1979).Monoclonal antibodies defining distinctive human T cell surface antigens. Science 206:347.

Kung PC,Talle MA,De Maria M,Butler M,Lifter J,Goldstein G (1980). Strategies for generating monoclonal antibodies defining human T lymphocyte differentiation antigens. Transplant Proc ,Suppl 12:141.

Malavasi F,Caligaris Cappio F,Janossy G,Richiardi P,Carbonara A (1982).Monoclonal antibody specific for early hemopoietic stem cells.XXX Coll Prot Biol Fluids.

Manolov G,Manolova Y (1972). Marker band in one chromosome 14 from Burkitt lymphomas.Nature 237:33.

McCaffrey R,Harrison TA,Parkman R,Baltimore D (1975).Terminal deoxynucleotidyl transferase activity in human leukemic cells and in normal human thymocytes.N Engl J Med 292: 775.

Mitelman F,Andersson-Anvret M,Brandt L,Catovsky D,Klein G, Manolov G,Manolova Y,Mark-Vendel E,Nilsson PG (1979).Reciprocal 8;14 translocation in EBV-negative B-cell acute lymphocytic leukemia with Burkitt type cells.Int J Canc 24:27.

Prentice HG,Russel NH,Lee N,Ganeshaguru K,Blacklock H,Piga A,Smyth JF,Hoffbrand AV (1981).Therapeutic selectivity of and prediction of response to 2'-deoxyxoformycin in acute leukaemia.Lancet II:1250.

Preud'homme JL,Labaume S (1976). Detection of surface immunoglobulins on human cells by direct immunofluorescence. In Bloom BR,David JR (eds):"In vitro methods in cell mediated and tumour immunity",New York:Academic Press,p 155.

Reinherz EL,Kung PC,Goldstein G,Schlossman SF (1979).A monoclonal antibody with selective reactivity with functionally mature thymocytes and all peripheral T cells.J Immunol 123:1312.

Reinherz EL,Kung PC,Goldstein G,Schlossman SF (1979).Further characterization of the human inducer T cell subset defined by monoclonal antibody.J Immunol 123:2894.

Reinherz EL,Nadler LM,Sallan SE,Schlossman SF (1979).Subset derivation of T-cell acute lymphoblastic leukemia.J Clin Invest 64:362.

Reinherz EL,Kung PC,Goldstein G,Levey RH,Schlossman SF (1980). Discrete stages of human intrathymic differentia tion: analysis of normal thymocytes and leukemic blasts of T lineage.Proc Natl Acad Sci USA 77:1598.

Ritz J,Pesando JM,Notis-McConarty J,Lazarus H,Schlossman S F (1980).A monoclonal antibody to human acute lymphoblas tic leukaemia antigen.Nature 283:583.

Ritz J,Schlossman SF (1982).Utilization of monoclonal anti- bodies in the treatment of leukemia and lymphoma.Blood 59:1.

Sen L,Borella L (1975).Clinical importance of lymphoblasts with T markers in childhood acute leukemia.N Engl J Med 292:828.

Sondel PM,Borcherding W,Shahidi NT,Ganik DJ,Schultz JC,Hong R (1981).Recategorizing childhood acute lymphoblastic leu kemia with monoclonal antibodies to human T cells.Blood 57:1135.

Smyth JF,Young RC,Young DM (1978).In vivo toxicity to lym- phoid tissue by 2'-deoxycoformycin.Canc Chemot Pharmac 1: 49.

Smyth JF,Poplack DG,Holiman BJ,Leventhal BG,Yabro G (1978). Correlation of adenosine deaminase activity with cell sur face markers in acute lymphoblastic leukemia.J Clin Invest 62:710.

Tsukimoto I,Wong KY,Lampkin BC (1976). Surface markers and prognostic factors in acute lymphoblastic leukemia. N Engl J Med 294:245.

Tidman N,Janossy G,Bodger M,Granger S,Kung PC,Goldstein G (1981).Delineation of human thymocyte differentiation path ways utilizing double-staining techniques with monoclonal antibodies. Clin exp Immunol 45:457.

Verbi W,Greaves MF,Schneider C,Koubek K,Janossy G,Stein H, Kung P,Goldstein G (1982).Monoclonal antibodies OKT11 and OKT11A have panT reactivity and block sheep erythrocyte " receptors".Eur J Immunol 12:81.

Vogler LB,Crist WM,Lawton AR,Bockman DE,Pearl ER,Cooper MD

(1978). Pre-B cell leukemia. N Engl J Med 298:872.

Vogler LB (1982). Bone marrow B cell development.In Janossy G (ed):"The lymphocytes",Clin Haematol,London:Saunders W B,in the press.

Acknowledgements: This work was supported by CNR,ROME,PFCCN grants N. 81.01313.96 and N. 81.01367.96.

13th International Cancer Congress, Part D
Research and Treatment, pages 445–449
© 1983 Alan R. Liss, Inc., 150 Fifth Avenue, New York, NY 10011

# PROGNOSIS OF ACUTE LYMPHOBLASTIC LEUKEMIA RELATED TO INITIAL FINDINGS AND TREATMENT

Günter Henze[+], Fritz Lampert[++], Hans-Joachim Langermann[+], Günther Schellong[+++], Hans-Jörg Riehm[+]

Department of Pediatrics
Universities of West-Berlin[+], Giessen[++], Münster[+++]
Federal Republic of Germany

Progress in the treatment of childhood acute lymphoblastic leukemia (ALL) and disappearance of adverse prognostic factors can readily be demonstrated in 3 German therapy studies. This improvement was achieved by prolongation and intensification of induction therapy and by adding an intensive reinduction course in patients with high risk.

In the Federal Republic of Germany over the last 12 years, more than 700 children were involved in 3 cooperative clinical trials. The main difference in these 3 studies was the mode of treatment during the first half year after diagnosis.

The therapy of the nation-wide DAL-study 71/74 (495 patients; Lampert 1977, Henze, Langermann, Lampert et al. 1979) was closely adapted from the St. Jude protocol VII i.e. prednisone-vincristine induction; followed by CNS prophylaxis with cranial irradiation and intrathecal methotrexate; and further maintenance therapy for 28 months with 6-mercaptopurine, methotrexate (and cyclophosphamide).

In the BFM-study 70/76 (119 patients; Riehm, Gadner, Henze, et al. 1980), the induction therapy was prolonged, intensified and included CNS prophylaxis. This West Berlin protocol consisted of an intensive 8-week multi-drug regimen in which remission induction was obtained with prednisone, L-asparaginase, vincristine and daunorubicin (given for 4 weeks), and consolidation (for another 4 weeks) was performed with cyclophosphamide, cytosine arabinoside, 6-mercaptopurine, and craniospinal or cranial irradiation and intrathecal methotrexate. Maintenance treatment including vincristine/ prednisone reinduction pulses was carried out with 6-mercaptopurine and methotrexate (and cyclophosphamide). The total duration of therapy was 21 - 36 months.

In the BFM-study 76/79 (158 patients; Henze, Langermann, Gadner, et al. 1981), the same therapy protocol (I) for remission induction was used for all patients. A risk index, however, was established for definition of high risk patients. Children and adolescents with a risk index over 3 received, in addition to the former therapy, a reinforced reinduction protocol (II) within the first 6 months after diagnosis. This intensive reinduction treatment consisted of dexamethasone, vincristine, adriamycine, L-asparaginase (given for 4 weeks), followed by cyclophosphamide, cytosine arabinoside, intrathecal methotrexate, and 6-thioguanine (given for 2 weeks). Total duration of treatment was 104 weeks (2 years) in the standard risk group and 128 weeks (2 1/2 years) in the high risk group.

Our long-term treatment results expressed in actual numbers are shown in the table. The number of patients in continuous complete remission (CCR) including all patients from the

Treatment results

| Groups | DAL 71/74 n (%) | BFM 70/76 n (%) | BFM 76/79 n (%) |
|---|---|---|---|
| Total | 495 (100) | 119 (100) | 158 (100) |
| Non-responders | 7 (1.4) | 1 (0.8) | 1 (0.6) |
| Died during remission induction | 14 (2.8) | 5 (4.2) | 4 (2.5) |
| Achieved remission | 474 (95.8) | 113 (95.0) | 153 (96.9) |
| Died in CCR | 37 (7.5) | 8 (6.7) | 6 (3.8) |
| Relapses | 268 (54.1) | 39 (32.8) | 36 (22.8) |
| BM (isolated) | 175 (35.4) | 26 (21.8) | 11 (7.0) |
| CNS(isolated) | 36 (7.3) | 6 (5.0) | 8 (5.1) |
| Testes (isolated) | 20 (4.0) | 6 (5.0) | 5 (3.2) |
| BM/CNS | 16 (3.2) | 1 (0.8) | 3 (1.9) |
| BM/Testes | 16 (3.2) | 0 (0.0) | 7 (4.4) |
| Others | 5 (1.0) | 0 (0.0) | 1 (0.6) |
| In CCR | 167 (33.7) | 66 (55.5) | 111 (70.3) |

beginning of therapy rose from 33.7 % to 55.5 %, and now to
70.3 %. This improvement was mainly due to the reduced incidence of bone marrow relapses which decreased from over 35 %
in the DAL-study to 22 % and now 7 % in the BFM-studies.
There was no increase in non-leukemia related fatalities
due to the intensification of therapy in the induction
period as death rates in CCR decreased from 7.5 % in the
DAL-study to 6.7 % and now 3.8 % in the BFM-studies.

Treatment results can be even better demonstrated by life
table analysis: The propability of survival in these 3 German ALL therapy studies increased from 39 % to 58 %, and
now to 83 %; and relapse-free survival from 33 % to 55 %,
and now to 69 %.
The effects of more aggressive induction therapy were specifically analysed with respect to factors considered to be
associated with a poor prognosis:

1. High initial white blood count (WBC): In patients with
   WBC over 25.000/µl, the proportion of p-CCR increased
   from 0.21 in the DAL-study to 0.40 and now 0.68 in the
   BFM-studies.

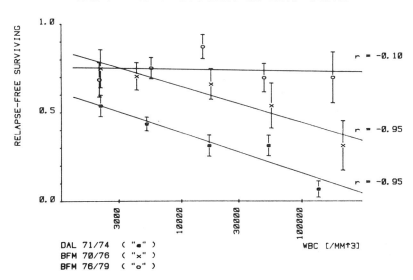

INFLUENCE OF THE INITIAL WBC ON 5 YEAR RELAPSE-FREE SURVIVAL
RATES IN PATIENTS FROM 3 GERMAN ALL THERAPY STUDIES

As shown in the figure, the consideration of high initial WBC as an adverse prognostic factor can be completely eliminated through the concept of stratified therapy (Study BFM 76/79).

2. Mediastinal mass at diagnosis: The p-CCR for patients with initial mediastinal mass increased from 0.13 in the DAL 71/74 study (n = 47) to 0.47 in the BFM 70/76 study (n = 15) and to 0.79 in the BFM 76/79 study (n = 14). Only in the DAL 71/74 study in which only prednisone-vincristine was used for induction, there was a highly significant difference in outcome between children with (p-CCR = 0.13; n = 47) and those without (p-CCR = 0.35; n = 448) mediastinal mass. Thus, as also proposed by Hann, Lustbader, Evans, et al. 1981, patients with mediastinal masses need special therapy. With more intensive induction treatment, these patients do not have a poorer prognosis compared with patients without mediastinal mass.

3. T-cell characteristics: In the BFM 76/79 study, there was no difference in the p-CCR between children with and those without immunologically identifiable T-ALL characteristics when the former group was stratified to the more intensive treatment group (in most cases because of the high concomitant WBC).

4. Male sex: The sex-related difference in outcome found by analysis of over 3000 children with ALL (Sather, Miller, Nesbit, et al. 1981), was only seen in our DAL 71/74 study: The p-CCR for girls (0.39; n = 231) was better than that for boys (0.28, including testicular relapses; 0.33, excluding testicular relapses; n = 264). No influence of sex on outcome, however, was seen in the BFM-studies. The incidence of testicular relapse in these trials was below 5 %.

5. Age: In neither the DAL 71/74 nor the BFM 70/76 study were there significant differences among the groups (younger vs. older than 2 vs. older than 10 years at diagnosis). However, in the BFM 76/79 study, a lower p-CCR (0.51; n = 37) was found in the age group older than 10 years compared with younger age groups ($<$ 2 years: 0.67; $>$ = 2 and $<$ 10 years: 0.76).

In summarizing the long-term results of these 3 therapeutic trials in Germany, we conclude that prognosis in ALL can be most strikingly altered by the mode of treatment. Most of the high risk factors, excepting possibly B-cell characteristics and possibly higher age, can be overcome by intensification of treatment. Thus, about 70 % of all children with ALL can now expect a relapse-free survival.

Hann HL, Lustbader ED, Evans AE, Toledano SR, Lilli PD, Jasko LB (1981). Lack of influence of T-cell marker and importance of mediastinal mass on the prognosis of acute lymphocytic leukemias of childhood. JNCI 66:285.

Henze G, Langermann HJ, Lampert F, Neidhardt M, Riehm H (1979): ALL therapy study 1971-1974 of the German Working Group for leukemia research and therapy in childhood: Prognostic significance of initial features and different therapeutic modalities. Klin Paediat 191:114.

Henze G, Langermann HJ, Gadner H, Schellong G, Welte K, Riehm H (1981). Results of study BFM 76/79 in children and adolescents treated for acute lymphoblastic leukemia. Klin Paediat 193:28.

Lampert F (1977). Combination chemotherapy and cranial irradiation in 530 children with acute lymphoblastic leukemia. Dtsch med Wschr 102:917.

Riehm H, Gadner H, Henze G, Langermann HJ, Odenwald E (1980). The Berlin childhood acute lymphoblastic leukemia study. 1970-1976. Am J Pediatr Hematol Oncol 2:299.

Sather H, Miller D, Nesbit M, Heyn R, Hammond D (1981). Differences in prognosis for boys and girls with acute lymphoblastic leuaemia. Lancet 1:739.

**13th International Cancer Congress, Part D**
**Research and Treatment, pages 451–457**
© **1983 Alan R. Liss, Inc., 150 Fifth Avenue, New York, NY 10011**

# EXTRAMEDULLARY LEUKAEMIA

Humphrey E.M. Kay,

Professor of Haematology

Institute of Cancer Research, London, S.W.3.

Although ALL is essentially a neoplastic disorder originating in a cell which is normally resident in the bone marrow, the biological significance of extramedullary disease is not quite the same as that of metastatic disease in other forms of neoplasia. For one thing the stem cells of the bone marrow normally have a capability for migrating via the blood stream to other sites, and proliferation of such cells and their differentiated progeny can occur either normally or in a response to a stimulus in organs such as the spleen, lymph nodes, liver etc. Even the central nervous system which is clinically the most important site of extramedullary infiltration may be affected in this form of physiological metastasis since both B and T lymphocyte activity and proliferation can occur there in response to stimulus (e.g. as in subacute sclerosing panencephalitis) and such a process is presumably preceded by the migration of appropriate precursor cells, B, T, pre-B, pre-T etc. Indeed now that ALL is recognised to comprise different diseases with the predominant cell at different stages of ontogeny, is probable that many cases of T-cell and B-cell ALL initially originate in the thymus and lymph nodes respectively with retrograde metastasis to the bone marrow. However other sites of extramedullary disease such as the kidney or the gonads may represent a true pathological form of metastasis and hence perhaps a more malignant type of neoplasm.

## Central Nervous System

The clinical importance of the Central Nervous System

(CNS) is that special therapy is needed to deal with cells
beyond the blood-brain barrier. Whether the invasion of
the CNS occurs mainly by migration of cells through the walls
of blood vessels as suggested by Price and Johnson (1973)
or is at least sometimes attributable to small haemorrhages
of blood in which leukaemic blasts are prevalent is uncertain
and of no great concern. For practical purposes it must be
assumed that invasion may have already occurred when the
diagnosis of ALL is first made and that the more aggressive
the type of disease the earlier will be the manifestations
of CNS leukaemia. In this respect T-cell ALL (which is
usually associated with high blood blast counts) more often
results in meningeal leukaemia and it may be that this is
a property of T-ALL as such (Lilleyman and Sugden 1981).

The symptomatology and diagnosis of extramedullary
leukaemia are, on the whole, well understood but it
remains to be seen whether certain manifestations e.g.
cranial nerve palsies are more often the consequence of
T-ALL whereas the commoner symptoms of vomiting, headache
and polydipsia occur more often in C-ALL, as was suggested
in one reported series (Lilleyman and Sugden 1981).
Occasional difficulties may be found when virus meningitis
is an alternative diagnosis, and the morphology of the
cells in the C.S.F. is ambiguous. In such cases the
identification of Tdt-containing cells is a very useful
diagnostic test indicating the leukaemic rather than
inflammatory nature of lymphoid cells. (Bradstock et al
1981). Similarly in testicular biopsies the presence of
a sparse intertubular infiltrate may be difficult to
interpret and Tdt demonstration may give conclusive
evidence of leukaemia (Thomas et al 1982).

With the exception of the CNS (and possibly the gonads)
special treatment measures are not needed for extramedullary leukaemia and this applies also to the putative
primary site of some T-ALL in the thymus, which responds
to treatment of the disease as a whole and is seldom the
site of recurrence.

In the case of the CNS although perhaps a third of
all cases do not have involvement at the time of diagnosis
and although the condition when it does occur can sometimes
be cured it is the general consensus that all cases should
receive 'prophylaxis' that is to say treatment of early
pre-symptomatic disease.

It has been made quite clear from various trials that such prophylaxis is effective both in preventing CNS leukaemia and in thereby prolonging disease free remissions.

Nevertheless there seems to be some controversy concerning the ultimate benefit of CNS prophylaxis in prolonging survival. Thus Nesbit et al (1981b) pointed out that in their study CCG.101 an inadequate form of prophylaxis (I.T. MTX 12 mg 6 times in 3 weeks) was associated with a higher incidence of CNS leukaemia but no greater rate of bone marrow relapse and hence - for low count cases at least - no difference in long-term survival, one inference being that reseeding of cells from CNS to marrow is not a significant occurrence. Data from St. Jude (Simone 1981) with a longer follow-up are in contrast and the M.R.C. figures for UKALL I show a smaller difference for the ten-year survivals.

Such differences in survival may be partly attributed to chance partly to length of follow-up and partly perhaps to effectiveness of therapy of CNS leukaemia when it has occurred. Certainly some patients, it seems, can be cured if spinal as well as cranial irradiation is given after the C.S.F. has been cleared of cells by I.T. MTX (Willoughby 1976, Frankel et al 1982). However where CNS leukaemia occurs after prophylaxis with cranial radiation and methotrexate then the disease is seldom fully controlled. Thus the emphasis returns to the optimum form of prophylaxis not only for ALL as a whole but for different categories of disease. On the one hand it can be shown that cranial irradiation combined with continued intrathecal methotrexate e.g. up to one year, can totally prevent CNS relapse (MRC 1973) but this may be attended by some degree of neurotoxicity and may not combine with systemic treatment to give optimum disease free remissions. Less frequent I.T. MTX, on the other hand, e.g. 3-monthly, does not significantly alter the incidence in the long run (Sackmann-Muriel et al 1978). Irradiation by itself is not completely effective and because of its toxicity the trend has been to lower the dose of cranial irradiation from 24 Gray to 18 Gray which does not appreciably impair effecitveness of the prophylaxis (Nesbit et al 1981a).

A most interesting comparison between three methods of prophylaxis has been made by the CCSG, CALGB and the Boston paediatric group. Their results were reported in 1980

(Green et al 1980) and are being updated by Dr. Green. As yet he reports that the only change from those published in 1980 is that there is no longer a significant difference in disease-free survival of standard risk patients treated with methotrexate infusions compared to those treated on the Boston protocol. The conclusion to be drawn is that for increased risk patients cranial irradiation plus at least six doses of IT MTX is needed and that the same schedule is probably as good as any for standard risk ALL also.

One set of circumstances which needs special consideration is that of very poor risk ALL for which a marrow transplant in first remission is intended. This group of cases is small, particularly as the results for BMT in second remission are becoming reasonably good, but most centres would include all B-ALL, cases with 4:11, 8:14 and 9:22 chromosome translocations, perhaps some high count cases e.g. over 100,000/ml, and perhaps those with CNS leukaemia at the first diagnosis. In these patients standard treatment, including cranial irradiation, if followed by T.B.I., runs the high risk of severe encephalopathy. The best procedure, therefore, is to prevent or reduce CNS disease as much as possible by intrathecal therapy continued up to the time of T.B.I. which one may hope would be eradicative: whether further intrathecal therapy should be given is as yet undecided and more experience is needed.

## Testicular and Ovarian Disease

Turning to the other main site of extramedullary relapse that needs separate consideration - the gonads - on can, for practical purposes ignore the ovary since overt and isolated relapse there is very uncommon - in the M.R.C. series three cases in over 800 girls and young women. The testis, on the other hand, can be a relatively frequent site of relapse without evidence of disease elsewhere: whether that is because of a blood testis barrier (Dym and Fawcett 1970) or because the testis is relatively cool and cells are thereby protected from the action of cytotoxic drugs (Van Eys and Sullivan 1976) or for any other reason is uncertain. In some series of cases this is a frequent complication, in others not (Kay 1983) and, as we have heard from the German group (Henze et al 1982) with intensive early treatment it does not seem to be a serious problem. The evidence certainly suggests that testicular disease occurs when consolidation treatment is not intensive: one interesting observation is that intermediate dose methotrexate in a CALGB trial prevented testicular relapse in all but one case out of 129 compared to 10 out of 140 in the control group (Freeman et al 1982). The incidence was also zero in the series of Moe et al (1981) and in a current M.R.C. study after the same dose of methotrexate the incidence was 0/27 compared to 4/18 in the controls of children under 14 (M.R.C. unpublished).

Previously, alarmed by our high incidence of testicular disease we had resorted to prophylactic irradiation which has, indeed, prevented relapse in the testis in all 71 patients who were irradiated compared to 11 out of 105 who were not. The question then is: does this also prevent bone marrow relapse which could be attributed to reseeding of cells from the testis? The answer is, so far, 'no' since the marrow relapse rates have been 25/71 and 39/105 respectively (M.R.C. unpublished). We must hope that the widespread adoption of intensive consolidation regimes will eliminate the problem of testicular relapse since, when it does occur, the long-term results are poor although a few are successfully treated (Eden et al 1982). Such treatment must include both irradiation to the opposite testicle of at least 20 Gy and the resumption of intensive systemic chemotherapy as well as the renewal of some intrathecal methotrexate as a further prevention of CNS leukaemia.

Extramedullary disease will continue to be seen in conjunction with marrow relapse and, occasionally as an isolated problem, especially perhaps after B.M.T. When that occurs it must be treated vigorously with removal, radiation and the resumption of systemic chemotherapy with a reasonable hope that it may, indeed, represent isolated disease which can be totally eradicated.

Bradstock KF, Janossy G, Pizzolo G and 6 others (1980) Subpopulations of normal and leukemic human thymocytes: An analysis with the use of monoclonal antibodies. J Nat Cancer Inst 65:33.

Dym M and Fawcett DW (1970). The blood-testis barrier in the rat and the physiological compartmentation of the seminiferous epithelium. Biology of Reproduction 3:308

Eden OB, Rankin A, Kay HEM (1982). Isolated testicular
    relapse in acute lymphoblastic leukaemia of childhood.
    Arch Dis Child - in press.
Frankel LS, Hockenberry MJ, Johnston DA (1982). The
    curative potential of central nervous system (CNS)
    relapse in childhood acute lymphocytic leukemia (ALL).
    Proceedings of the Amer Soc of Clin Oncol 1:124.
Freeman AI, Weinberg VE, Brecher ML, Jones B, Glicksman A
    (1982). Comparison of intermediate dose methotrexate
    (IDM) with cranial irradiation (CRT) in acute
    lymphocytic leukemia (ALL). Proceedings of the Amer Soc
    of Clin Oncol 1:130.
Green DM, Freeman AI, Sather HN, Sallan SE, Nesbit Jr ME,
    Cassady JR, Sinks LF, Hammond D, Frei III E, (1980).
    Comparison of three methods of central-nervous-system
    prophylaxid in childhood acute lymphoblastic leukaemia.
    The Lancet 1:1398.
Henze G, Lambert F, Langermann H-J, Schellong G, Riehm H
    (1982). Prognosis of acute lymphoblastic leukemia (ALL)
    as related to initial findings and treatment.
    Proceedings of the Amer Soc of Clin Oncol - in press
Kay HEM (1983). Testicular infiltration in ALL. Brit J
    Haem - in press.
Lilleyman JS, Sugden PJ (1981). T lymphoblastic leukaemia
    and the central nervous system. Br J Cancer 43:320.
Moe PJ, Seip M, Finne PH (1981). Intermediate dose
    methotrexate (IDM) in childhood acute lymphocytic
    leukemia in Norway. Acta Paediatr Scand 70:73.
M.R.C. Working Party (1973). Treatment of acute
    lymphoblastic leukaemia: effect of "prophylactic"
    therapy against central nervous system leukaemia. Brit
    Med J II:381.
Nesbit Jr ME, Robison LL, Littman PS, Sather HN, Ortega J,
    D'Angio GJ, Hammond GD (1981). Presymptomatic central
    nervous system therapy in previously untreated childhood
    acute lymphoblastic leukaemia: comparison of 1800 rad
    and 2400 rad. A report for children's cancer study group.
    The Lancet 1:461.
Nesbit ME, Sather HN, Ortega J, D'Angio GJ, Robison LL,
    Donaldson M, Hammond GD (1981). Effect of isolated
    central nervous system leukaemia on bone marrow
    remission and survival in childhood acute lymphoblastic
    leukaemia. The Lancet 1:1386.
Price RA, Johnson WW (1973). The central nervous system in
    childhood leukemia. I. The arachnoid. Cancer 31:320.

Sackmann-Muriel F, Svarch E, Eppinger-Helft M, Braier JL, Pavlovsky S, Guman L, Vergara B, Ponzinibbio C, Failace R, Garay GE, Bugnard E, Ojeda FG, De Bellis R, De Sijvarger SR, Saslavsky J (1978). Evaluation of intensification and maintenance programs in the treatment of acute lymphoblastic leukemia. Cancer 42:1730.

Simone JV (1981). Leukaemia Remission and Survival. The Lancet 1:531.

Thomas JA, Janossy G, Eden OB, Bollum FJ (1982). Demonstration of nuclear terminal deoxynucleotidyl transferase (TdT) in leukaemic infiltrates of testicular tissue. Br J Cancer- in press.

Van Eys J, Sullivan MP (1976). Testicular leukaemia and temperature. The Lancet II:256.

Willoughby MLN (1976). Treatment of overt meningeal leukaemia in children: results of second MRC meningeal leukaemia trial. BMJ 1:864.

CONGRESS SYMPOSIA


VIRUSES AND POSSIBLE RELATIONSHIPS TO HUMAN
CANCER Bentvelzen, P., Netherlands, Chairman;
Pagano, J., USA, Co-Chairman; Flag Pavilion A

Herpes Simplex Type 2 and Cervical Cancer:
Immunological and In Situ Hybridization Studies.
*Simard, R., Kessous, A., Mansour, M.,
Camonis, J. and Rawls, W. E., Montreal, Quebec,
Canada and Hamilton, Ontario, Canada.

EBV and Human Malignancies. *Klein, G.,
Stockholm, Sweden. (By Title Only)

Retroviruses Associated with Human Leukemias and
Lymphomas. * Kaplan, H. S., Stanford, CA USA.

BK Virus and Its Variants: Association with
Tumors and Transormed Cells. *Pater, M. M.,
Pater, A. and diMayorca, G., Newark, NJ USA.

Hepatitis B Virus DNA and Human Hepatocellular
Carcinoma. *Brechot, C., Wain-Hobson, S.,
Pourcel, C., Dejean, A., Hadchouel, M., Scotto, J.
and Tiollais, P., Paris, France and Bicetre,
France.

Please note: Papers that are listed as "By Title
Only" were presented at the 13th International
Cancer Congress, but are not included in these
volumes.

**13th International Cancer Congress, Part D**
**Research and Treatment, pages 461–469**
© **1983 Alan R. Liss, Inc., 150 Fifth Avenue, New York, NY 10011**

HERPES SIMPLEX TYPE 2 AND CERVICAL CANCER:   IMMUNOLOGICAL
AND IN SITU HYBRIDIZATION STUDIES

Rene Simard, Allegria Kessous, Michael Mansour,
Jacques Camonis and William E. Rawls*
Institut du Cancer de Montreal, Centre Hospita-
lier Notre-Dame, Montreal, H2L 4M1, Canada and
*Department of Pathology, McMaster University,
Hamilton, Canada

INTRODUCTION

The association of herpes simplex virus type 2 (HSV-2)
to cervical carcinoma has received support from several investigations ranging from oncogenic in vitro transformation
(Rapp, Duff 1973; MacNab 1974; Kessous et al. 1979), to
seroepidemiological studies and demonstration of viral products in cervical tumors.  Seroepidemiological studies have
shown a higher frequency or titer of HSV-2 antibodies in
women with cervical carcinoma when compared to normal population (Thomas, Rawls 1978; Rawls et al. 1980; Graham et al.
1982).  The presence of viral antigens in tumor cells has
been demonstrated by different methods (Aurelian 1973;
Dreesman et al. 1980).  Recently, Gilman et al. (1980) have
shown that sera from patients with cervical carcinoma immu-
noprecipitate two HSV-2 polypeptides with molecular weights
38,000 and 118,000.  The search for viral nucleic acids has
led to controversial findings: all attempts to detect viral
DNA in cervical tumors have yielded negative results (Zur
Hauzen et al. 1974; Cassai et al. 1981) except in one case
(Frenkel et al. 1972).  However, the use of $^3$H-labelled
HSV-2 DNA as a probe to detect viral RNAs on tissue sections, demonstrated the presence of HSV-2 RNAs in a signi-
ficative percentage of cervical carcinomas and dysplasias
(Jones et al. 1978; McDougall et al. 1980; Eglin et al. 1980;
Maitland et al. 1981).  These studies, except for one recent
publication (McDougall et al. 1982), tried to produce evi-
dence for the presence of one viral product - could it be
DNA, RNA or protein - in cervical carcinoma tissues.

In an attempt to verify if the presence of viral RNAs could be correlated with that of HSV-2 antibodies, we have examined by in situ hybridization cervical tissues obtained from 189 women (including normal tissues, cervical intraepithelial neoplasia (CIN), dysplasias and other pathological conditions), of which 86 sera have been tested blindly for the presence of HSV-2 antibodies using microneutralization and radioimmunoassay methods.

MATERIALS AND METHODS

Tissue Samples:

Biopsies of pathological cervices were taken from patients attending the colposcopy clinic for various conditions. Biopsies of normal cervices were obtained from individuals referred to the gynecology clinic for problems unrelated to the pathology of the cervix. All samples were immediately frozen and stored in liquid nitrogen until further manipulation. Blood samples, when obtained, were left to clot and sera were decanted and stored at -70°C.

Virus and DNA Probes:

HSV-2 virus was grown for 36 to 48 hr on primary rabbit kidney cells and the DNA was purified from the virions on CsCl gradient as described elsewhere (Kessous et al. 1979). The purity of the viral DNA was checked after complete digestion of a sample by EcoRI and Hind III restriction enzymes. DNA controls ($\lambda$ and SV40 DNA) were purchased from Bethesda Research Laboratories (Bethesda, Maryland). The labelling of HSV-2 and control DNAs was done using the nick translation method (Maniatis et al. 1976) and $^3$H-labelled deoxyribonucleoside triphosphates (dTTP 80 Ci/mmol, dATP, dGTP, dCTP 20-30 Ci/mmol). Unincorporated triphosphates were removed by gel filtration on Sephadex G-50. The specific activity thus obtained was around $2 \times 10^7$ cpm/µg DNA.

In Situ Hybridization:

Cytological sections from the biopsies were obtained in a cryostat and mounted on extensively washed and heat-sterilized slides. They were fixed in Carnoy fixative (ethanol, chloroform, acetic acid, 6V/3V/1V) at 4°C for 15 min, dehydrated in increasing concentration of ethanol and vacuum-dried for several hours. The hybridization conditions have been described elsewhere (Fournier et al. 1982): briefly, the reaction was carried out in a 15 μl mixture containing 50% formamide, 10 mM Tris-HCl, pH 7.5 1 mM EDTA, 600 mM NaCl, 0.02% ficoll, 0.02% polyvinylpyrrolidone, 1 μg/ml bovine serum albumin and finally 1 x $10^5$ cpm/slide of labelled DNA previously denatured at 100°C for 15 min. The reaction mixture was sealed under a coverslip and the sections were incubated at 37°C for 36 hr. The slides were then unsealed in a 2 x SSC buffer and twice washed in the hybridization buffer (10 mM Tris-HCl, pH 7.5, 1 mM EDTA, 600 mM NaCl) at 4°C. They were further washed twice in the same buffer supplemented with 50% formamide, twice more without formamide and incubated for 1 hr at 55°C. After a final wash overnight in 2 x SSC at 4°C, they were dehydrated through an ethanol serie.

For serology, the samples were assayed for antibodies to HSV-1 and 2 with two methods. The microneutralization test was carried out as described by Rawls et al. (1980). The neutralizing antibodies titers were determined against each virus type and a 2/1 index calculated from the titers. The sera with a 2/1 index of 85 or greater were considered positive for HSV-2. The radioimmunoassay was performed using conditions described by Rawls et al. (1980) with a modification: the counts per minute (cpm) bound to HSV-1 antigen were substracted from the cpm bound to HSV-2 antigen to obtain cpm attributed to HSV-2 specific antibodies; thus, sera were considered positive for HSV-2 antibodies when they exhibited 60 or more HSV-2 specific cpm.

RESULTS

All the specimens examined in this study were processed blindly and the code for diagnoses was deciphered after compiling the results. Each biopsy was tested by in situ hybridization in two different experiments totalizing at least four sections. The criteria for positivity were the number of sections with a significant level of labelling as determined for each serie of biopsies treated similarly, and the localization of the labelling on different sections. Figure 1 (a-d) illustrates the results observed with HSV-2 DNA probe on normal, dysplastic, neoplastic and cervicitis biopsies. The autoradiographic grains are evenly spread over the malignant tissue in the cervical intraepithelial neoplasia (fig. 1c) with occasional clusters over some cells. In other cases,

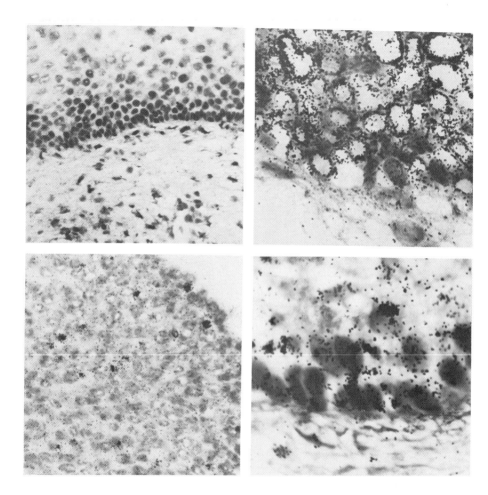

Fig. 1. In situ hybridization of ³H-labelled HSV-2 DNA to
frozen cervical biopsies. a) Normal cervical epithelium showing a complete absence of silver grain (x 700); b) severe
dysplasia with a large amount of silver grains over epithelial cells and little activity in the underlying submucosa
(x 2800);c) Intraepithelial cervical neoplasia showing an
evenly spread radioactivity with few scattered clusters
(x 700); d) Recurrent chronic cervicitis with a large amount
of silver grains over the basal layer of the malpighian epithelium: note the absence of radioactivity in the submucosa
(x 2800).

particularly in cervicitis (fig. 1d), the labelling is associated with the epithelium mostly at the level of the basal
layer. Negative biopsies such as the normal epithelium in
figure 1a, display scattered silver grains approximating the
background level. Figure 1b shows a severe dysplasia where
radioactivity is important over the epithelial cells. In
general, even in highly positive cases, the labelling was
located over the epithelium except in herpes lytic infection
where stromal cells are also positive.

A total of 189 biopsies have been examined by in situ
hybridization including 67 normals, 54 dysplasias (mild: 25;
moderate: 11; severe: 18), 38 CIN and 30 various pathological conditions (cervicitis: 12; chronic inflammation: 4;
prior or present HSV-2 infection: 3; acanthosis: 2; condyloma: 1; hyper- and metaplasia: 3; non-functional endometrium:
2; atypia: 1; polyposis: 1; placenta: 1). As reported in
table 1, positive scores with in situ hybridization have been
observed in 32.8% of normal tissues, 57.4% of dysplasia, 71%
of CIN and 60% of the other pathological conditions. In
parallel experiments, λ DNA bounded to 16% of cases in any
group of patients, and no cases were scored as positive with
SV40 DNA.

Table 1: Occurrence of HSV RNAs and antibodies

| Diagnosis | In situ hybridi-zation (% posi-tive) | HSV-antibodies | | |
|---|---|---|---|---|
| | | % positive type 2 | % positive type 1 | % negative type 1 & 2 |
| Normal | 32.8 | 26.3 | 43.2 | 32.5 |
| Dysplasia | 57.4 | 18.8 | 54.5 | 27.2 |
| Epithelioma | 71 | 53.8 | 38.4 | 7.6 |
| Others* | 60 | 35.7 | 28.5 | 35.7 |

* See text for diagnosis

Immunological tests have led to the following data (table 1). HSV-2 antibodies were found in 9/37 normals, 2/22
dysplasia, 7/13 CIN and 5/14 patients with diseases other
than CIN and dysplasia. Those results, when expressed in %,
amount respectively to 26.3%, 18.8%, 53.8% and 35.7%. Antibodies to HSV-1 are observed in 16/37 (43.2%) normals, 12/22
(54.4%) dysplasia, 5/13 (38.4%) CIN and 4/14 (28.5%) in various other conditions.

Table 2: Occurrence of HSV-antibodies among cases with positive and negative scores for in situ hybridization

| Diagnoses | Cases positive by in situ hybridization | | | | | Cases negative by in situ hybridization | | | | |
| | HSV-antibodies | | | | | HSV-antibodies | | | | |
| | ND* | HSV-2 | HSV-1 | None | Total | ND* | HSV-2 | HSV-1 | None | Total |
|---|---|---|---|---|---|---|---|---|---|---|
| Normal | 8 | 5 | 4 | 5 | 22/67 | 22 | 4 | 12 | 7 | 45/67 |
| Dysplasia | 19 | 4 | 6 | 2 | 31/54 | 13 | 0 | 6 | 4 | 23/54 |
| CIN | 18 | 4 | 4 | 1 | 27/38 | 7 | 3 | 1 | 0 | 11/38 |
| Others | 9 | 4 | 1 | 4 | 18/30 | 7 | 1 | 3 | 1 | 12/30 |

* ND   Not determined

The examination of the results when the data obtained by the two approaches are combined led to the following observations (table 2): 5/14 normal, 4/12 dysplasia, 4/9 CIN and 4/9 various conditions exhibited positive hybridization as well as antibodies to HSV-2; among cases with negative scores for hybridization, 4/23 normal, 3/4 CIN and 1/5 various conditions were found bearing antibodies to HSV-2.

DISCUSSION

In situ hybridization has proved to be a powerful mean for detection of nucleic acids on material such as cultured cells or tissue sections: indeed, several investigators have searched for the presence of HSV-2 RNAs in carcinoma of the cervix. However the sensitivity and reliability of the technique on human cervical biopsies are difficult to assess for several reasons dealing not only with patient and control samplings and follow up, but also with tissue biopsies on which repeated experiments are not always possible. Thus the coupling of immunological and cytological tests was indicated to allow a better correlation between HSV-2 and cervical carcinoma. The data collected from our study led us to the following observations:
      a) As seen by other investigators (McDougall et al. 1980; Eglin et al. 1981; Maitland et al. 1981), there is an increased number of cases with positive scores for in situ hybridization among patients with dysplasia and CIN. The per-

centages observed, 57.4% for dysplasia and 71% for CIN, are
in good agreement with those published in other studies
(Maitland et al. 1981; Eglin et al. 1981) but appear somewhat higher than the ones reported by McDougall et al.
(1982). The proportion of positive controls is also higher
as compared to the studies of Eglin et al. (1981) and
McDougall et al. (1980), but rather close to the percentage
reported by Maitland et al. (1981). This increased positivity in our study might be explained by the fact that the
controls were considered normal on the basis of a normal
histology, regardless of the clinical and serological status.
In fact, 26% of the normal controls were found positive for
HSV-2 antibodies at the time of the study.

   b) 60% of the patients with pathological conditions
other than dysplasia and carcinoma were found positive by
hybridization. This high proportion might be due to the fact
that 5/12 cervicitis cases, 3/3 herpes infection and 3/3
hyper- and metaplasia showed positive scores for hybridization. Interesting enough, these three pathological conditions have been mentioned as predisposing to cervical
carcinoma, although no correlation between cervicitis, hyper-/
metaplasia and HSV-2 has been reported.

   c) Concerning the data obtained by serology, HSV-2
antibodies were found in 9/37 (24%) normal cases, a prevalence which is in good agreement with a previous study
(McDonald et al. 1974) on Montreal women. This prevalence
increased to 54% (7/13) in cervical carcinoma as previously
observed by Rawls et al. (1980).

   d) Finally, when the two approaches were compared in
situ hybridization was found positive in 68% (17/25) of the
HSV-2 antibody carriers, in 40.5% (15/37) of the HSV-1 antibody carriers, and in 44.4% (12/27) of non HSV carriers.
The positivity in cases that should be negative according to
serology can be explained in several ways: Firstly HSV-1 and
2 display a 50% homology and genital infections have been
reported with HSV sero type 1; it is therefore not surprising
to find a positive hybridization in HSV-1 antibody carriers.
Secondly HSV-2 antibodies present in unsufficient amount are
probably not detectable by the methods available. Thirdly
positive hybridization reactions in negative antibody carriers or negative reaction in positive carriers could result
from artefactual procedures previously discussed (McDougall
et al. 1980; Maitland et al 1981).

   Nevertheless, the correlation between serology and in
situ hybridization is such that further studies using the

two approaches should be actively persued.

REFERENCES

Aurelian L (1973). Virions and antigens of Herpes virus type 2 in cervical carcinoma. Canc Res 33:1539.

Cassai E, Rotola A, Meneguzzi G, Milanesi G, Garsia S, Remotti G, Rizzi G (1981). Herpes simplex virus and human cancer. I. Relationship between human cervical tumours and Herpes simplex type 2. Europ J Cancer 17:685.

Dreesman GR, Burek JA, Kaufman E, Melnick RH, Powell KL, Purifoy DJ (1980). Expression of Herpes virus-induced antigens in human cervical cancer. Nature 283:591.

Eglin RP, Sharp F, MacLean AB, MacNab JCM, Clements JB, Wilkie NM (1981). Detection of RNA complementary to Herpes simplex virus DNA in human cervical squamous cell neoplasms. canc Res 41:3597.

Fournier JG, Kessous A, Richer G, Brechot C, Simard R (1982). Detection of hepatitis B viral RNAs in human liver tissues by in situ hybridization. Biol Cell 43:225.

Frenkel N, Roizman B, Cassai E, Nahmias A (1972). A Herpes simplex 2 DNA fragment and its transcription in human cervical cancer tissue. Proc Natl Acad Sci USA 69:3784.

Gilman SC, Docherty JJ, Clarke A, Rawls WE (1980). The reaction patterns of Herpes simplex virus type 1 and type 2 proteins with the sera of patients with uterine cervical carcinoma and matched controls. Canc Res 40:4640.

Graham S, Rawls W, Swanson M, McCurtis J (1982). Sex partners and Herpes simplex virus type 2 in the epidemiology of cancer of the cervix. Ann J Epidemiol 115:729.

Jones KW, Fenoglio CM, Shevchuck-Chaban M, Maitland NJ, McDougall JK (1978). Detection of Herpes virus-2 mRNA in human cervical biopsies by in situ hybridization. In de The G, Henle W, Rapp F (eds): "Oncogenesis and Herpes virus III," Lyon, France: International Agency for Research on Cancer, p 917.

Kessous A, Bibor-Hardy V, Suh M, Simard R (1979). Analysis of chromosomes, nucleic acids and polypeptides in hamster cells transformed by Herpes simplex virus type 2. Canc Res 39:3225.

MacNab JCM (1974). Transformation of rat embryo cells by temperature-sensitive mutants of Herpes simplex virus. J Gen Virol 24:143.

Maitland NJ, Kinross JH, Busuttil A, Ludgate SM, Smart GE, Jones KW (1981). The detection of DNA tumour virus-specific RNA sequences in abnormal human cervical biopsies by in situ hybridization. J Gen Virol 55:123.

Maniatis T, Gee SG, Efstradiadis A, Kafatos FC (1976). Amplification and characterization of a α-globulin gene synthesized in vitro. Cell 8:163.

McDougall JK, Crum CP, Fenoglio CM, Goldstein LC, Galloway DA (1982). Herpes virus-specific RNA and protein in carcinoma of the uterine cervix. Proc Natl Acad Sci USA 79: 3853.

McDougall JK, Galloway DA, Fenoglio CM (1980). Cervical carcinoma detection of Herpes simplex virus RNA in cells undergoing neoplastic change. Int J Cancer 25:1.

Rapp F, Duff R (1973). Transformation of hamster embryo fibroblasts by Herpes simplex viruses type 1 and 2. Canc Res 33:1527.

Rawls WE, Clarke A, Smith KO, Docherty JJ, Gilman SC, Graham S (1980). Specific antibodies to Herpes simplex virus type 2 among women with cervical cancer. In Essen M, Todaro E, zur Hausen H (eds): "Viruses in naturally occurring cancers," New York: Cold Spring Harbor Laboratories, p 117.

Thomas DB, Rawls WE (1978). Relationship of Herpes simplex virus type 2 antibodies and squamous dysplasia to cervical carcinoma in situ. Cancer 42:2716.

zur Hausen H, Schulte-Holtehausen H, Wolf H, Dorres K, Egger H (1974). Attempts to detect virus-specific DNA in human tumours. II. Nucleic acid hybridization with complementary RNA of human herpes group viruses. Int J Cancer 13:657.

13th International Cancer Congress, Part D
Research and Treatment, pages 471–484
© 1983 Alan R. Liss, Inc., 150 Fifth Avenue, New York, NY 10011

RETROVIRUSES ASSOCIATED WITH HUMAN LEUKEMIAS AND LYMPHOMAS

Henry S. Kaplan, M.D.

Cancer Biology Research Laboratory, Department of
Radiology, Stanford University School of Medicine,
Stanford, California 94305

INTRODUCTION

The fact that type C retroviruses are the etiologic
agents of leukemias and lymphomas in a spectrum of avian and
mammalian species (Kaplan, 1978) has suggested that the human
leukemias and lymphomas may also be induced by retroviruses.
This hypothesis was made more plausible by the fact that the
morphologic characteristics and clinical manifestations of
the leukemias and lymphomas of mice, cats, cattle, and gibbon
apes closely resemble those in man (Kaplan, 1974). However,
a decade of intensive and arduous effort to detect such
viruses in human leukemias and lymphomas, using molecular
probes and immunologic reagents derived from murine, feline,
and subhuman primate retroviruses, proved fruitless (Aaronson
and Schlom, 1975; Gardner et al., 1977; Nicolson et al.,
1978; Hogg et al., 1979). Although the initial reaction of
many investigators was to conclude that leukemogenic human
retroviruses may not exist, a few groups persisted in the
search, using improved cell culture techniques. These continuing efforts now appear to have been rewarded.

When the search for retroviruses in human leukemias and
lymphomas first began about a decade ago, evidence began to
emerge suggesting the presence, in subcellular fractions
prepared from human tumor cells, of reverse transcriptase-
like activity and/or DNA or RNA sequences complementary to
those of murine or subhuman primate retroviral cDNA probes.
Those early studies, which are summarized elsewhere (Kaplan,
1980), are no longer widely credited because it is now recognized that the assays and probes available at that time were

not sufficiently specific. This review is therefore limited
to retroviruses produced in culture by human leukemia and
lymphoma cells.

## HUMAN LEUKEMIA-LYMPHOMA CANDIDATE RETROVIRUSES

### HL-23V and Related Retroviruses

Particles with the properties of a mammalian retrovirus
were detected in supernatant culture fluids of cultures
from a patient (HL-23) with acute myelogenous leukemia
(Gallagher and Gallo, 1975). The virus (HL-23V) was reiso-
lated 14 months later from bone marrow cells of the same
patient (Gallagher et al., 1975). It was observed to bud
from the plasma membranes of the leukemic cells and had
typical type C morphology by electron microscopy (Hall and
Schidlovsky, 1976). Several other cell lines were found to
be permissive for its sustained replication (Teich et al.,
1975). However, further analysis yielded the surprising and
puzzling conclusion that HL-23V preparations contained two
viruses indistinguishable by immunologic and molecular
hybridization techniques from two unrelated subhuman primate
viruses, the baboon endogenous virus (BaEV) and the woolly
monkey sarcoma virus complex (SSV-1/SSAV) (Chan et al.,
1976; Okabe et al., 1976; Reitz et al., 1976).

Other groups have reported the detection of particles
with the properties of type C retroviruses in short-term
cultures of bone marrow or peripheral blood cells from patients with lymphomas and leukemias (Klucis et al., 1976;
Mak et al., 1974, 1975; Vosika et al., 1975; Kotler et al.,
1977; Yaniv et al., 1980). Nooter et al. (1975) used the
co-cultivation technique to propagate a type C virus, initially detected in short-term culture of bone marrow cells
from a child with lymphoblastic leukemia, on human embryo
fibroblasts and canine thymus cells. Later, Nooter et al.
(1977, 1978) used this isolate to rescue a pseudotype of the
Kirsten murine sarcoma virus. However, the transforming
activity of the pseudotype could be inhibited by antibody to
SSV-1/SSAV, and the viral nucleic acid, reverse transcriptase, and major internal core protein were indistinguishable
from those of SSV-1/SSAV (Smith et al., 1979). Thus,
although these early studies were undoubtedly of great
interest, it ultimately proved impossible to exclude the

possibility that contamination with subhuman primate
retroviruses such as BaEV or SSV-1/SSAV had occurred.

## SU-DHL-1 Virus

The SU-DHL-1 human histiocytic lymphoma cell line was
established from the malignant pleural effusion of a child
with diffuse histiocytic lymphoma (Epstein and Kaplan,
1974). Reverse transcriptase activity was detected in
particles with a density of 1.15 g/ml in pelleted culture
fluids, and electron micrographs revealed particles resem-
bling mammalian type C retroviruses (Kaplan et al., 1977).
When SU-DHL-1 cells were co-cultivated with rat XC cells,
syncytial microplaques similar to those induced by other
mammalian type C retroviruses were observed. Antibody
prepared against the purified envelope glycoprotein of the
gibbon ape leukemia virus (GaLV) yielded positive membrane
immunofluorescence reactions with SU-DHL-1 cells (Kaplan
et al., 1979).

The polymerase displayed the template-primer characteristics expected of a viral reverse transcriptase, and
appeared to be distantly related antigenically to the
enzymes of the subhuman primate retroviruses. After purification by affinity chromatography on poly(rC).agarose,
the enzyme was radioiodinated and subjected to tryptic
digest peptide mapping. The maps revealed 5 or 6 peptides
similar to those of the reverse transcriptases of SSV-1/SSAV,
GaLV, and BaEV, but one or two unique peptides were also
detected (Goodenow and Kaplan, 1979; Goodenow et al., 1980).
The antigenic relatedness of SU-DHL-1 viral reverse trans-
ciptase to the enzymes of the subhuman primate viruses was
further documented with the aid of a monoclonal hybridoma
antibody (Goodenow et al., 1980, 1982). Another monoclonal
antibody reactive with the 28 kilodalton (kd) major core
protein (p28) cross-reacted with and immunoprecipitated
the p28 of SSV-1/SSAV (Goodenow et al., 1980, 1982).

The SU-DHL-1 virus had little or no infectivity when
tested with a spectrum of human and nonhuman cell lines.
Normal human hematopoietic cells sometimes exhibited striking changes in growth behavior and morphology suggestive of
abortive transformation when co-cultivated with the SU-DHL-1
virus, but their growth could not be sustained, and they
failed to take when heterotransplanted in congenitally athy-

mic nude mice (Kaplan et al., 1979). It proved impossible
to obtain enough high molecular weight RNA to permit the
molecular cloning and genomic characterization of the
virus. An effort was made to circumvent this difficulty by
using the molecularly cloned genome of $GaLV_{SF}$ (Scott et al.,
1981) as probe, but no evidence of homology could be detected
in SU-DHL-1 cell DNA, even under relaxed hybridization conditions.

## HTLV and ATLV

In the last two years, Gallo and his colleagues have
described a number of type C retroviral isolates, collec-
tively designated human T cell leukemia/lymphoma virus (HTLV),
which differ significantly from all previously known avian
or mammalian retroviruses. The first such isolate, $HTLV_{CR}$,
was detected in the culture fluids of a cell line, HUT-102,
established from the neoplastic T-lymphocytes of a lymph
node biopsy from a 28 year old black male patient with a
diagnosis of cutaneous T-cell lymphoma (CTCL; mycosis
fungoides). The production of virus particles by HUT-102
cells required induction with 5-iodo-2-deoxyuridine (IUdR)
from passage 4 through passage 50; constitutive production of
virus began by passage 56 and continued thereafter (Poiesz et
al., 1980). Virus particles were again detected when fresh
peripheral blood mononuclear cells from the same patient were
placed in culture one year later. A new cell line, CTCL-3,
established from this peripheral blood sample, continues to
produce virus constitutively. Electron microscopy revealed
typical type C virus particles budding from the cell membrane
and immature and mature type C particles in clumps of extracellular debris (Poiesz et al., 1980). Soon thereafter, a
new isolate, $HTLV_{MB}$, was isolated from another cell line,
CTCL-2, established from the peripheral blood of patient
MB, a 64 year old black female with Sézary syndrome
(the leukemic phase of CTCL; Poiesz et al., 1981). The
properties of $HTLV_{MB}$ and of several additional HTLV isolates
(Popovic et al., 1982) have been similar to or identical
with those of $HTLV_{CR}$. C-type virus-like particles have
also been seen by electron microscopy in Langerhans cells
and related cells of skin and lymph nodes of 7 patients with
mycosis fungoides and 2 with Sézary syndrome (van der
Loo et al., 1979).

Assay of doubly banded HTLV preparations revealed the

presence of reverse transcriptase activity in fractions with a density of 1.16 g/ml. The enzyme had a molecular weight of about 95 kd and utilized the same template primers as other viral reverse transcriptases, but exhibited an unusual preference for magnesium over manganese as the divalent cation. Antibody inhibition tests revealed that the reverse transcriptase of HTLV is immunologically distinct from the reverse transcriptases of all known type C, type B, and type D retroviruses (Rho et al., 1981).

The structural proteins of $HTLV_{CR}$ had molecular weights of approximately 10, 12, 19, 24, 42, and 52 kd. The 24 kd protein (p24), identified as the major internal core protein of HTLV, was precipitated by a rabbit antiserum raised against disrupted $HTLV_{CR}$. This precipitation reaction was competed for by unlabeled $HTLV_{CR}$ and by cytoplasmic proteins from cells producing the virus, but not by proteins from normal human cells. Proteins from several mammalian type B, type C, and type D retroviruses failed to compete in this immunological reaction, and $HTLV_{CR}$ did not react in inter-species assays for the core protein antigens of several mammalian type C and type D viruses (Kalyanaraman et al., 1981 b). A monoclonal hybridoma antibody raised against the 19 kd protein (p19) also yielded positive indirect immuno-fluorescence reactions with the HUT-102, CTCL-2, and CTCL-3 cell lines but not with an extensive series of other human B cell and T cell lines or normal peripheral blood lymphocytes (Robert-Guroff et al., 1981). The amino acid composition, the COOH-terminal amino acid and the $NH_2$-terminal amino acid sequence of the first 25 residues of the HTLV p24 have been determined (Oroszlan et al., 1982). HTLV p24 differs from the major internal core proteins of all other animal retroviruses, except that it shares the same $NH_2$-terminal amino acid (proline) and the same COOH-terminal amino acid (leucine). Alignment of the amino acid sequence of HTLV p24 with those of several other retrovirus core proteins revealed statistically significant, though limited, sequence homology only with the p24 of bovine leukemia virus.

$HTLV_{CR}$ and $HTLV_{MB}$ were found to contain high molecular weight (~70S) RNA, from which [3]H-cDNA was synthesized by reverse transcription. In liquid molecular hybridization experiments, this cDNA hybridized almost completely to the 70S RNA of $HTLV_{CR}$, but showed little capacity to hybridize to the RNAs of GaLV, BaEV, or avian myeloblastosis virus. Nucleic acid sequences related to [3]H-cDNA or [125]I-70S

RNA of $HTLV_{CR}$ were present in HUT-102 cells, but were not detected in the DNA of normal human tissues, indicating that $HTLV_{CR}$ is not an endogenous human retrovirus (Reitz et al., 1981).

Recently, a new type of lymphoid neoplasm, adult T-cell leukemia-lymphoma (ATL), has been described (Uchiyama et al., 1977; Takatsuki et al., 1979). A striking feature is its clustering in Southwestern Japan, particularly on the islands of Kyushu and Shikoku (Takatsuki et al., 1979; Matsumoto et al., 1979; Ichimaru et al., 1979). Sera from patients with ATL revealed an antigen (ATLA) in the cytoplasm of 1-5% of the cells of a T cell line, MT-1, established from the peripheral blood of a patient with ATL (Miyoshi et al., 1980; Hinuma et al., 1981). Antibodies against this antigen were detected in the sera of all of 44 patients with ATL and in those of 32 of 40 patients with malignant T cell lymphomas, as well as in the sera of 26% of healthy adults from ATL-endemic areas of Japan (Hinuma et al., 1981). Electron microscopy revealed extracellular type C virus particles associated with MT-1 cells cultured in the presence of IUdR. Virus particles, as well as ATLA, were also detected in a permanently established T cell line, MT-2, derived from male umbilical cord blood leukocytes transformed by co-cultivation with peripheral blood leukocytes of a female patient with ATL (Miyoshi et al., 1981 a,b). These two viral isolates, designated adult T-cell leukemia virus (ATLV), have a density of ~ 1.15 g/ml and contain high molecular weight RNA and structural proteins with molecular weights of ~ 11, 14, 17, 24, and 45 kd (Yoshida et al., 1982 a). HTLV p24 and p19 are serologically indistinguishable from the corresponding proteins of the MT-1 isolate, and the proviral DNA sequences in MT-1 cell DNA have more than 80% homology to HTLV cDNA in liquid hybridization assays (Reitz et al., 1982) indicating that ATLV is closely similar to and may well be identical with HTLV.

Seroepidemiologic studies, though still incomplete, have yielded striking results. The coded sera of 17 American patients with CTCL and 55 normal donors were tested for the presence of natural antibodies to $HTLV_{CR}$ structural proteins, using competition RIA and radioimmune precipitation (RIP) assays (Posner et al., 1981). The sera of two patients, CR and CTCL-4, bound strongly to $HTLV_{CR}$, and the serum of patient patient CR also reacted strongly with $HTLV_{MB}$. These reactions were remarkably specific; they could be competed only by HTLV$_{CR}$ or HTLV$_{MB}$, and not by a number of other solubilized retroviral preparations. The sera of most of the other patients with CTCL showed limited reactivity or were negative, as were the sera of the 55 normal donors. Interestingly, however, serum from the wife of patient CR was strongly reactive (Kalyanaraman et al., 1981 a).

Regional and national seroepidemiologic studies (Shimoyama et al., 1982; Hinuma et al., 1982) have confirmed and extended the association of anti-ATLA antibodies with the ATL endemic area in Japan. In a study of 278 patients with hematological malignancies, positive sera were obtained from 10 of 29 (34.5%) born in the endemic area, and in only 8 of 249 (3.2%) born in other parts of Japan. Preliminary evidence is suggestive of horizontal transmission of the virus (Tajima et al., 1982). Natural antibodies to HTLV were also detected in the sera in 6 of 7 Japanese patients with ATL, and in 6 of 32 with other types of leukemia, but in none of 39 healthy donors from the ATL endemic region of Japan and none of 41 random normal donors from other regions of Japan (Robert-Guroff et al., 1982 b). Using quantitative RIP assays high titers of natural antibody to HTLV p24 were detected in 12 of 12 Japanese patients with untreated ATL (Kalyanaraman et al., 1982). All of 79 sera from normal Japanese donors, including 39 individuals from the endemic area, were negative.

T-lymphosarcoma cell leukemia (T-LCL), a neoplastic condition very similar to Japanese ATL, occurs endemically in black individuals inhabiting the West Indies and neighboring countries of South America (Catovsky et al., 1982). HTLV isolates have been obtained from cell lines established from the malignant T cells of these patients (Popovic et al., 1982), and natural antibodies to the HTLV p24 have been detected in their sera (Robert-Guroff et al., 1982 a). Seroepidemiologic studies of other populations are currently in progress.

Although HTLV$_{CR}$ and HTLV$_{MB}$ had little or no infectivity, other HTLV and ATLV isolates have shown infectivity for normal human cord blood and adult peripheral blood T-lymphocytes (Yamamoto et al., 1982; Popovic et al., 1982). Moreover, some of these isolates have shown the remarkable property of immortalizing normal cord blood T-lymphocytes, transforming them into permanent cell lines which then became virus producers (Miyoshi et al., 1981; Yamamoto et al.,

1982). Of 14 healthy family members of an ATL patient who were tested for antibodies to ATLA antigen, 5 proved to be seropositive; short-term cultures of phytohemagglutinin-stimulated peripheral blood lymphocytes from 4 of these 5 expressed both ATLV and ATLA (Miyoshi et al., 1982). ATLV and/or ATLA were also detectable in clonal lines of T-cells established, in the presence of TCGF, from the peripheral blood lymphocytes of 5 ATLA seropositive healthy adults (Gotoh et al., 1982). T-cell lines established from the lymphocytes of 6 seronegative adults expressed neither the virus nor its associated antigen. Thus, the normal T-cells of healthy individuals whose sera contain natural antibodies to ATLA may be carriers of the virus. A recent report describes the later development of typical ATL in two individuals whose sera were anti-ATLA positive 5 and 10 years before clinical onset of disease (Kinoshita et al., 1982). That the virus may be transmitted by blood transfusion is suggested by the seroconversion of 3 of 6 recipients of formed blood elements from healthy seropositive donors (Okochi et al., 1982).

The molecular cloning of ATLV and HTLV has recently been reported (Wong-Staal et al., 1982; Yoshida et al., 1982 b). This achievement opens the way to "molecular" epidemiologic studies (Kaplan, 1982). Radiolabelled probes prepared from these cloned genomes may also detect the presence of defective retroviral genomes in apparently virus-negative human leukemias and lymphomas. It is thus not unlikely that evidence for the retroviral etiology of a broad spectrum of human leukemias and lymphomas will unfold in the years immediately ahead.

Aaronson SA, Schlom J (1975). The search for RNA tumor viruses in human cancer. In Ariel IM (ed): "Progress in Clinical Cancer," New York: Grune and Stratton, Vol. 6, p 51.

Catovsky D, Greaves MF, Rose M, Galton DAG, Goolden AWG, McCluskey DR, White JM, Lampert I, Bourikas G, Ireland R, Brownell AI, Bridges JM, Blattner WA, Gallo RC (1982). Adult T-cell lymphoma-leukemia in blacks from the West Indies. Lancet 1:639.

Chan E, Peters WP, Sweet RW, Ohno T, Kufe DW, Spiegelman S, Gallo RC, Gallagher RE (1976). Characterization of a virus (HL 23V) isolated from cultured acute myelogenous leukaemic cells. Nature 260:266.

Epstein AL, Kaplan HS (1974). Biology of the human malignant lymphomas. I. Establishment in continuous cell culture and heterotransplantation of diffuse histiocytic lymphomas.

Cancer 34:1851.

Gallagher RE, Gallo RC (1975). Type C RNA tumor virus isolated from cultured human acute myelogenous leukemia cells. Science 187:350.

Gallagher RE, Salahuddin SZ, Hall WT, McCredie KB, Gallo RC (1975). Growth and differentiation in culture of leukemic leukocytes from a patient with acute myelogenous leukemia and re-identification of type-C virus. Proc Acad Natl Acad Sci USA 72:4137.

Gardner MB, Rasheed S, Shimizu S, Rongey RW, Henderson BE, McAllister RM, Klement V, Charman HP, Gilden RV, Heberling RL, Huebner RJ (1977). Search for RNA tumor virus in humans. In Hiatt HH, Watson JD, Winsten JA (eds): "Origins of Human Cancer," New York: Cold Spring Harbor Laboratory, p 1235.

Goodenow RS, Brown S, Levy R, Kaplan HS (1980). Partial characterization of the virion proteins of a type-C RNA virus produced by a human histiocytic lymphoma cell line. In Essex M, Todaro G, zur Hausen H (eds): "Viruses in Naturally Occurring Cancers," New York: Cold Spring Harbor Laboratory, p 737.

Goodenow RS, Kaplan HS (1979). Characterization of the reverse transcriptase of a type C RNA virus produced by a human lymphoma cell line. Proc Natl Acad Sci USA 76:4971.

Goodenow RS, Liu S-L, Fry KE, Levy R, Kaplan HS (1982). Expression of C-type RNA viral proteins by a human lymphoma cell line. In Rosenberg SA, Kaplan HS (eds): "Malignant Lymphomas - Etiology, Immunology, Pathology, Treatment," New York: Academic Press, p 185.

Gotoh Y, Sugamura K, Hinuma Y (1982). Health carriers of a human retrovirus, adult T-cell leukemia virus (ATLV): Demonstration by clonal culture of ATLVcarrying T cells from peripheral blood. Proc Natl Acad Sci USA 79: in press.

Hall WT, Schidlovsky G (1976). Typical type-C virus in human leukemia. J Nat Cancer Inst 56:639.

Hinuma Y, Komoda H, Choba T, Kondo T, Kohakura M, Takenaka T, Kikuchi M, Ichimaru M, Yunoki K, Sato I, Matsuo R, Takiuchi Y, Hanaoka M (1982). Antibodies to adult T-cell leukemia virus-associated antigen (ATLA) in sera from patients with ATL and controls in Japan: a nation-wide seroepidemiologic study. Int J Cancer, in press.

Hinuma Y, Nagata K, Hanaoka M, Nakai M, Matsumoto T, Kinoshita K, Shirakawa S, Miyoshi I (1981). Adult T-cell leukemia: antigen in an ATL cell line and detection of antibodies to the antigen in human sera. Proc Natl Acad Sci USA 78:6476.

Hogg N, Hope J, Teich N, Wallace D (1979). A search for type-C virus expression in man. In Neth R, Gallo RC, Hofschneider P-H, Mannweiler K (eds): "Modern Trends in Human Leukemia III," Berlin: Springer-Verlag, p 401.

Ichimaru M, Kinoshita K, Kamihira S, Ikeda S, Yamada Y, Amagasaki T (1979). T-cell malignant lymphoma in Nagasaki District and its problems. Jpn J Clin Oncol 9:337.

Kalyanaraman VS, Sarngadharan MG, Bunn PA, Minna JD, Gallo RC (1981 a). Antibodies in human sera reactive against an internal structural protein of human T-cell lymphoma virus. Nature 294:271.

Kalyanaraman VS, Sarngadharan MG, Nakao Y, Ito Y, Aoki T, Gallo RC (1982). Natural antibodies to the structural core protein (p24) of the human T-cell leukemia (lymphoma) retrovirus found in sera of leukemia patients in Japan. Proc Natl Acad Sci USA 79:1653.

Kalyanaraman VS, Sarngadharan MG, Poiesz B, Ruscetti FW, Gallo RC (1981 b). Immunological properties of a type C retrovirus isolated from cultured human T-lymphoma cells and comparison to other mammalian retroviruses. J Virol 38:906.

Kaplan HS (1974). Leukemia and lymphoma in experimental and domestic animals. Ser Haematol 7:94.

Kaplan HS (1978). Etiology of lymphomas and leukemias: role of C-type RNA viruses. Leuk Res 2:253.

Kaplan HS (1980). Prospects for the etiologic involvement of RNA tumor viruses in human cancer. In Stephenson JR (ed): "Molecular Biology of RNA Tumor Viruses," New York: Academic Press, p 485.

Kaplan HS (1982). "Molecular" epidemiology of human lymphomas and leukemias: implications of non-producer retrovirus-induced avian and mammalian lymphomas. In Magrath IT, Ramot B, O'Conor GT (eds): "Influence of the Environment on Leukemia and Lymphoma Subtypes," New York: Raven Press, in press.

Kaplan HS, Goodenow RS, Epstein AL, Gartner S, Declève A, Rosenthal PN (1977). Isolation of a C-type RNA virus from an established human histiocytic lymphoma cell line. Proc Natl Acad Sci USA 74:2564.

Kaplan HS, Goodenow RS, Gartner S, Bieber M (1979). Biology and virology of the human malignant lymphomas: 1st Milford D. Schulz Lecture. Cancer 43:1.

Kinoshita K, Hino S, Amagasaki T, Momita S, Yamada Y, Ikeda S, Samihira S, Ichimaru M, Munehisa T, Hinuma Y (1982). Development of adult T-cell leukemia from two anti-ATLA antibody-positive apparently healthy adults. Gann, in press.

Klucis E, Jackson L, Parsons PG (1976). Survey of human lymphoblastoid cell lines and primary cultures of normal and leukemic leukocytes for oncornavirus production. Int J Cancer 18:413.

Kotler M, Balabanova H, Ben-Moyal Z, Friedman A, Becker Y (1977). Properties of the oncornavirus particles isolated from P3HR-1 and Raji human lymphoblastoid cell lines. Isr J Med Sci 13:740.

Mak TW, Kurtz S, Manaster J, Housman D (1975). Viral-related information in oncornavirus-like particles isolated from cultures of marrow cells from leukemic patients in relapse and remission. Proc Natl Acad Sci USA 72:623.

Mak TW, Manaster J, Howatson AF, McCulloch EA, Till JE (1974). Particles with characteristics of leukoviruses in culture of marrow cells from leukemic patients in remission and relapse. Proc Natl Acad Sci USA 71:4336.

Matsumoto M, Nomura K, Matsumoto T, Nishioka K, Harada S, Furosho H, Kikuchi K, Kato Y, Utsunomiya A, Uematsu T, Iwahashi M, Hashimoto S, Yunoki K (1979). Adult T-cell leukemia-lymphoma in Kagoshima District, Southwestern Japan: clinical and hematological characteristics. Jpn J Clin Oncol 9:325.

Miyoshi I, Kubonishi I, Yoshimoto S, Akagi T, Ohtsuki Y, Shiraishi Y, Nagata K, Hinuma Y (1981 b). Type C virus particles in a cord T-cell line derived by co-cultivating normal human cord leukocytes and human leukaemic T cells. Nature 294:770.

Miyoshi I, Taguchi H, Fujishita M, Niita K, Kitagawa T, Ohtsuki Y, Akagi T (1982). Asymptomatic type C virus carriers in the family of an adult T-cell leukemia patient. Gann 73:339.

Miyoshi I, Yoshimoto S, Taguchi H, Ohtsuki Y, Kubonishi I, Shiraishi Y, Akagi T (1981 a). Transformation of normal human cord lymphocytes by co-cultivation with a lethally irradiated human T-cell line carrying type C virus particles. Gann 72:997.

Nicolson MO, Gilden RV, Charman H, Rice N, Heberling R, McAllister RM (1978). Search for infective mammalian type-C virus-related genes in the DNA of human sarcomas and leukemias. Int J Cancer 21:700.

Nooter K, Aarssen AM, Bentvelzen P, de Groot G, van Pelt FG (1975). Isolation of infectious C-type oncornavirus from human leukaemic bone marrow cells. Nature 256:595.

Nooter K, Bentvelzen P, Zurcher C, Rhim J (1977). Detection of human C-type "helper" viruses in human leukemic bone marrow with murine sarcoma virustransformed human and rat nonproducer cells. Int J Cancer 19:59.

Nooter K, Overdevest J, Dubbes R, Koch G, Bentvelzen P, Zurcher C, Coolen J, Calafat J (1978). Type-C oncovirus isolate from human leukemic bone marrow: further in vitro and in vivo characterization. Int J Cancer 21:27.

Okabe H, Gilden RV, Hatanaka M, Stephenson JR, Gallagher RE, Gallo RC, Tronick SR, Aaronson SA (1976). Immunological and biochemical characterisation of type C viruses isolated from cultured human AML cells. Nature 260:264.

Okochi K, Sato H, Hinuma Y (1982). Induction of antibody to adult T cell leukemia in recipients of blood components from donors carrying antibody to the adult T cell leukaemia antigen. Lancet, in press.

Oroszlan S, Sarngadharan MG, Copeland TD, Kalyanaraman VS, Gilden RV, Gallo RC (1982). Primary structure analysis of the major internal protein p24 of human type C T-cell leukemia virus. Proc Natl Acad Sci USA 79:1291.

Poiesz BJ, Ruscetti FW, Gazdar AF, Bunn PA, Minna JD, Gallo RC (1980). Detection and isolation of type C retrovirus particles from fresh and cultured lymphocytes of a patient with cutaneous T-cell lymphoma. Proc Natl Acad Sci USA 77: 7415.

Poiesz BJ, Ruscetti FW, Reitz MS, Kalyanaraman VS, Gallo RC (1981). Isolation of a new type C retrovirus (HTLV) in primary uncultured cells of a patient with Sézary T-cell leukaemia. Nature 294:268.

Popovic M, Sarin PS, Kalyanaraman VS, Robert-Guroff M, Sarngadharan MG, Minowada J, Aoki T, Mann D, Blattner W, Broder S, Golde D, Gallo RC (1982). New HTLV isolates from geographically different parts of the world and their infectivity of human T-cells. Proc RNA Tumor Virus Meeting, New York: Cold Spring Harbor Laboratory, p 289 (abst).

Posner LE, Robert-Guroff M, Kalyanaraman VS, Poiesz BJ, Ruscetti FW, Fossieck B, Bunn PA, Jr., Minna JD, Gallo RC (1981). Natural antibodies to the human T cell lymphoma virus in patients with cutaneous T cell lymphomas. J Exp Med 154:333.

Reitz MS, Miller NR, Wong-Staal F, Gallagher RE, Gallo RC, Gillespie DH (1976). Primate type-C virus nucleic acid sequences (woolly monkey and baboon types) in tissues from a patient with acute myelogenous leukemia and in viruses isolated from cultured cells of the same patient. Proc Natl Acad Sci USA 73:2113.

Reitz MS, Poiesz BJ, Ruscetti FW, Gallo RC (1981). Characterization and distribution of nucleic acid sequences of a novel retrovirus isolated from neoplastic human T-lymphocytes. Proc Natl Acad Sci USA 78:1887.

Reitz MS, Jr., Popovic M, Kalyanaraman VS, Sarngadharan MG, Robert-Guroff M, Nakao Y, Miyoshi I, Ito Y, Minowada J, Gallo RC (1982). HTLV is the virus of Japanese adult T-cell leukemia. Proc RNA Tumor Virus Meeting, New York: Cold Spring Harbor Laboratory, p 185 (abst).

Rho HM, Poiesz B, Ruscetti FW, Gallo RC (1981). Characterization of the reverse transcriptase from a new retrovirus (HTLV) produced by a human cutaneous T-cell lymphoma cell line. Virology 112:355.

Robert-Guroff M, Kalyanaraman VS, Sarngadharan MG, Blattner WA, Catovsky D, Merino F, Gallo RC (1982 a). Serologic studies show HTLV is associated with aggressive T-cell malignancies in various geographic locations. Proc RNA Tumor Virus Meeting, New York: Cold Spring Harbor Laboratory, p 288 (abst).

Robert-Guroff M, Nakao Y, Notake K, Ito Y, Sliski A, Gallo RC (1982 b). Natural antibodies to human retrovirus HTLV in a cluster of Japanese patients with adult T cell leukemia. Science 215:975.

Robert-Guroff M, Ruscetti FW, Posner LE, Poiesz BJ, Gallo RC (1981). Detection of human T-cell lymphoma virus p19 in cells of some patients with cutaneous T cell lymphoma and leukemia using monoclonal antibody. J Exp Med 154:1957.

Scott ML, McKereghan K, Kaplan HS, Fry KE (1981). Molecular cloning and partial characterization of unintegrated gibbon ape leukemia virus DNA. Proc Natl Acad Sci USA 78:4213.

Shimoyama M, Minato K, Tobinai K, Horikoshi N, Ibuka T, Deura K, Nagatani T, Ozaki Y, Inada N, Komoda H, Hinuma Y (1982). Anti-ATLA (antibody to the adult T-cell leukemia cell associated antigen) positive hematologic malignancies in Kanto district, Japan. Jpn J Clin Oncol, in press.

Smith RG, Nooter K, Bentvelzen P, Robert-Guroff M, Harewood K, Reitz MS, Lee SA, Gallo RC (1979). Characterization of a type-C virus produced by co-cultures of human leukemic bone-marrow and fetal canine thymus cells. Int J Cancer 24: 210.

Tajima K, Tominaga S, Suchi T, Kawagoe T, Komoda H, Hinuma Y, Oda T, Fujita K (1982). Epidemiological surveys of anti-ATLA (adult T-cell leukemia virusassociated antigens)-positive persons in an ATL-endemic area: possible horizontal transmission of ATL virus. Gann, in press.

Takatsuki K, Uchiyama T, Ueshima Y, Hattori T (1979). Adult T-cell leukemia: further clinical observations and cytogenetic and functional studies of leukemic cells. Jpn J

Clin Oncol 9:317.

Teich NM, Weiss, RA, Salahuddin SZ, Gallagher RE, Gillespie DH, Gallo RC (1975). Infective transmission and characterisation of a C-type virus released by cultured human myeloid leukaemia cells. Nature 256:551.

Uchiyama T, Yodoi J, Sagawa K, Takatsuki K, Uchino H. Adult T-cell leukemia: clinical and hematologic features of 16 cases. Blood 50:481.

van der Loo EM, van Muijen GNP, van Vloten WA, Beens W, Scheffer E, Meijer CJLM (1979). C-type virus-like particles specifically localized in Langerhans cells and related cells of skin and lymph nodes of patients with mycosis fungoides and Sézary syndroms. A morphological and biochemical study. Virchows Arch B Cell Path 31:191.

Vosika GJ, Krivit W, Gerrard JM, Coccia PF, Nesbit ME, Coalson JJ, Kennedy BJ (1975). Oncornavirus-like particles from cultured bone marrow cells preceding leukemia and malignant histicytosis. Proc Natl Acad Sci USA 72:2804.

Wong-Staal F, Mangari V, Gelmann EP, Westin E, Franchini G, Josephs S, Dalla Favera R, Gallo RC (1982). Integration and expression of human T-cell leukemialymphoma virus (HTLV) in infected cells and molecular cloning of the 5'-proximal viral sequences. Proc RNA Tumor Virus Meeting, New York: Cold Spring Harbor Laboratory, p 291 (abst).

Yamamoto N, Okada M, Koyanagi Y, Kannagi M, Hinuma Y (1982). Transformation of human leukocytes by cocultivation with an adult T-cell leukemia virus producer cell line. Science, in press.

Yaniv A, Gotlieb-Stematsky T, Vonsover A, Perk K (1980). Evidence for type-C retrovirus production by Burkitt's lymphoma-derived cell line. Int J Cancer 25:205.

Yoshida M, Miyoshi I, Hinuma Y (1982 a). Isolation and characterization of retrovirus from cell lines of human adult T-cell leukemia and its implication in the disease. Proc Natl. Acad Sci USA 79:2031.

Yoshida M, Seiki M, Hattori S (1982 b). Human retrovirus, ATLV: characterization of the viral genome and associated with adult T-cell leukemia (ATL). Proc RNA Tumor Virus Meeting, New York: Cold Spring Harbor Laboratory p 290 (abst).

13th International Cancer Congress, Part D
Research and Treatment, pages 485–494
© 1983 Alan R. Liss, Inc., 150 Fifth Avenue, New York, NY 10011

BK VIRUS AND ITS VARIANTS:   ASSOCIATION WITH TUMORS AND
TRANSFORMED CELLS.

Mary M. Pater, Ph.D., Alan Pater, Ph.D., Giampiero
di Mayorca, M.D.
UMDNJ - New Jersey Medical School, Department of
Microbiology, 100 Bergen Street, Newark, NJ
07103

The human papovavirus BKV, first isolated by Gardner et
al. (1971), is highly oncogenic in rodents and transforms rodent cells readily in vitro (Padgett, 1980).  Antibody against the virus is detected in 75-80% of adults.  The virus
is present persistently in the human population, and is
released in the urine under immunosuppressive conditions.
High antibody titer against BKV has been detected in patients
with tumors of the urinary system (Corallini et al., 1976).
In addition, high antibody titer has been associated with
lower life expectancy in patients with renal cell carcinoma
(Pyrhonen et al., 1978).

The presence of BKV DNA in human tumors was first reported
by this laboratory by reassociation kinetics (Fiori and di
Mayorca, 1976).  Using this approach for a survey of various
human tumors, BKV DNA sequences were not detected in any human cells and tissues (Wold et al., 1978).  We (Pater et al.,
1980a) and others (Israel et al., 1978) have detected sequences hybridizing to BKV probe by the Southern technique
of blotting (Southern, 1975).  In our extensive survey of
105 tumor and normal tissues and cell lines, we detected
bands hybridizing to BKV DNA probe.  A summary of the results
is shown in Table 1.  Of the 12 tumors of the urinary system
examined, 9 had bands hybridizing with BKV DNA.  Bands comigrating with specific HindIII fragments A and B of BKV DNA
were detected in 4 normal and 7 tumor tissues and cell lines.
Three out of these 7 positive tumors (42%) were from the
urinary system.  These data indicate that a more extensive
survey of tumors of the urinary system for BKV sequences is
needed.

In our survey of human tissues and cell lines we detected

TABLE 1

Summary of the Results of the Survey of Human Tissues
and Cell Lines for the Presence of BKV

| Type of tissues and cells | | Number examined |
|---|---|---|
| Normal from non-cancer patient | (+)* | 3 |
| Normal from cancer patient | (−) | 3 |
| Normal from cancer patient | (+) | 2 |
| Normal from cancer patient | (−) | 2 |
| Tumor tissue | (+) | 39 |
| Tumor tissue | (−) | 56 |
| Liver tumor | (+) | 5 |
| Liver tumor | (−) | 9 |
| Lung tumor | (+) | 6 |
| Lung tumor | (−) | 11 |
| Tumor of the urinary system | (+) | 9 |
| Tumor of the urinary system | (−) | 3 |

*The (+) and (−) indicate the presence and absence of bands
hybridizing to BKV DNA.

bands hybridizing with BK DNA in 43 out of 105 tissues and
cell lines when cellular DNA was cleaved with HindIII.
Bands comigrating with HindIII fragments A and B of BKV DNA
were detected in only 11 tissues and cell lines. This is
not surprising considering the genome organization of RF
(Pater et al., 1980b) and MG (Pater et al., 1981a), the two
isolates of BKV that we have been analyzing. Figure 1 shows
the maps of the R1 and R2, the two complementary defective
genomes of RF. As can be seen, the sizes of most restriction
enzymes are different for the R1 species as compared to that
of BKV. Figure 2 shows the restriction map of the two defective complementary genomes of MG. Most of the restriction
sites do not correspond to those of BKV DNA. While some of
the restriction sites in MG and RF are missing, others are
in MG and/or RF but not in BKV WT. There are also deletions
(Figure 3) and insertions (Figures 1 and 2) in both of the
defective molecules of MG and RF. It is thus apparent that
in surveying human tissues for BKV DNA by the blotting method one might detect bands that do not correspond exactly to
the restriction fragments of the prototype BKV.

We have been studying transformation of rodent cells by
GS, a closely related isolate of BKV (Pater, et al., 1979).
Transplantable tumors classified as undifferentiated glio-
blastomas were induced in the syngeneic host (Beth et al.,

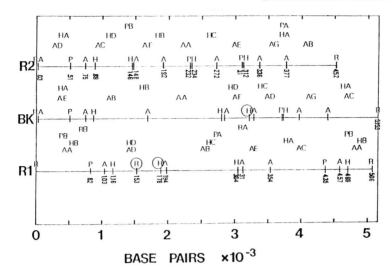

Fig. 1. The map of restriction sites for BKV DNA and R1 and R2 species of RFV DNAs. The site of cleavage for HindIII on the DNA is designated as H, for AvaII as A, for EcoRI as R, and for PvuII as P. The HindIII fragments are designated as HA, HB, HC and HD. AvaII fragments are designated as AA, AB, AC, AC, etc. (Pater et al., 1980b).

1981) when injected with the transformed hamster brain cells. Examination of cellular DNA revealed the presence of a large copy number of viral DNA (47 copies per cell) in the transformed cells. We then examined the status of viral DNA by blot-hybridization (Southern, 1975). As can be seen from the data presented in Figure 4, the majority of the viral DNA in the transformed cells is present in a free form when high molecular weight cellular DNA either uncleaved or cleaved with HincII, for which there is no cleavage site in viral DNA, is blotted and hybridized to BKV probe. Furthermore, cleavage with restriction endonucleases EcoRI, BamHI, and HpaII, which cleave viral DNA at unique but different positions on the BKV restriction map, show only one band. Extra, faint bands were detected only after digestion with HindIII which cleaves BKV DNA at four and GS DNA at 3 sites. These results indicated that although integrated viral DNA could be detected, it was possible that at least some cells in the population had viral DNA exclusively in a free form. To examine this possibility we analyzed the status of viral

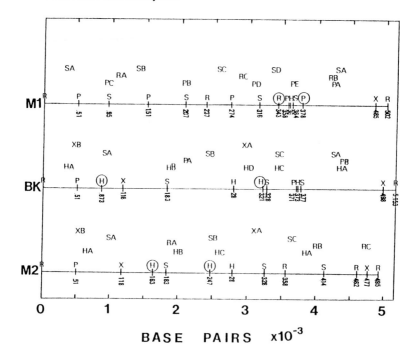

Fig. 2. The map of restriction sites for M1 and M2 species of MG DNA. The restriction map of BKV is given for comparison. Designation of the restriction sites and restriction fragments are as in Fig. 1. (Pater et al., 1981a).

DNA in 15 subclones of this transformed cell line. The results of blot-hybridization of uncleaved high molecular weight DNA from each of the subclones is presented in Figure 5. As can be seen, free and integrated viral DNA is detected in only 5 subclones. Viral DNA in the rest of subclones is present exclusively in an integrated form. The integrated state of viral DNA in the subclones was further confirmed by the cleavage of cellular DNA with HincII for which there is no cleavage site in viral DNA (Pater, et al., 1982). It is thus clear that unlike bovine papilloma viruses (Law et al., 1981), transformation by BK-type viruses requires integration. Free viral DNA was detected after mitomycin C treatment of some of the clones which contained only integrated sequences (Pater et al., 1982). These results support the postulation that free viral DNA sequences in the transformed cells are excision products

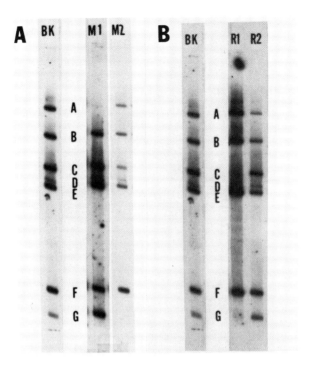

Fig. 3. Hybridization of labeled M1 and M2 (A) and R1 and R2 (B) DNAs with unlabeled BKV DNA. BKV DNA was cleaved with AvaII and separated by electrophoresis through 4/12% acrylamide gels, blotted onto nitrocellulose paper and hybridized with the various probes. (Pater et al., 1980b).

of integrated sequences. Free viral DNA sequences are present in polyoma-transformed cells and are also postulated to be excision products of integrated sequences (Zouzias et al, 1977). It is thus apparent that, although BKV is more similar to SV40 in its genome organization (Howley, 1980), it resembles polyoma in its interaction with the host genome in transformed cells.

As stated earlier, plaque-purified RFV contains two species of molecules, R1 and R2 (Figure 1). R1 has a deletion corresponding to at least 40% of the late region and R2 has a deletion corresponding to at least 50% of the early region of BKV (Figure 6). RFV is more oncogenic than the prototype BKV when injected into newborn hamsters (Dougherty, 1976) and transforms rodent cells with high efficiency

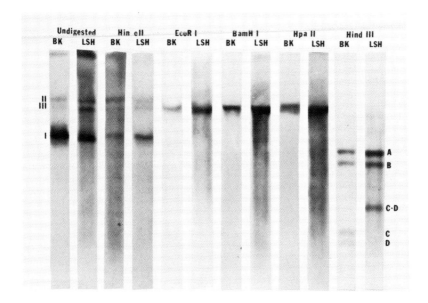

Fig. 4. Arrangement of viral DNA sequences in LSH-BR-BK cells. Cellular DNA (10 μg) was cleaved with each of the indicated restriction enzymes, and viral DNA sequences were detected by blot hybridization after electrophoresis through 1% agarose gels. (Pater et al., 1982).

(Pater et al., 1981b). Interestingly, the rodent cells transformed by this virus contain only the R1 species which has the entire early region (Figure 7). Additionally, R1 may be more oncogenic in human cells than BKV WT because it lacks late viral functions and thus may express only tumor antigens without concomitant expression of late proteins and production of virus particles. That is, R1 may be non-permissive instead of lytic in human cells and may transform instead of killing them.

The results of our tumor survey combined with our observation of the unique feature of the genome organization of BKV variants and the report of others that patients with cancer of the urinary system had higher antibody titer to BKV (Corallini et al., 1976) and that the high level of antibody to BK in patients with renal cell carcinoma was correlated with a decreased life expectancy of such patients, suggest strongly that BKV and/or its variants should be

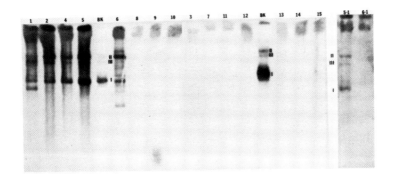

Fig. 5. Detection of viral DNA sequences in uncleaved DNA from subclones of LSH-BR-BK cells, as for Fig. 4. Resubcloning was done for subcloned 5 (5-1) and 6 (6-1) (Pater et al., 1982).

considered as strong candidates as oncogenic agents in certain types of tumors. These observations certainly call for more extensive studies of the role of BKV and its isolates in certain types of cancer in man.

Beth, E., Giraldo, G., Schmidt-Ullrich, R., Pater, M.M., Pater, A., and di Mayorca, G. (1981). BK-virus transformed inbred hamster brain cells. I. Status of viral DNA and the association of BK virus early antigens with purified plasma membranes. J Virol 40:276.

Corallini, A., Barbanti-Brodano, G., and Portolani et al. (1976). Antibodies to BK virus structural and tumor antigens in human sera from normal persons and from patients with various diseases including neoplasia. Infect Immun 13:1684.

Dougherty, R.M. (1976). Induction of tumors in Syrian hamsters by a human renal papovavirus, RF strain. J Nat Cancer Inst 57:395.

Fiori, M. and di Mayorca, G. (1976). Occurrence of BK virus DNA in DNA obtained from certain human tumors. Proc Natl Acad Sci 73:4662.

Gardner, S.D., Field, A.M., Coleman, D.V. and Hulme, B. (1971). New human papovavirus (BK) isolated from urine after renal transplantation. Lancet 1:1253.

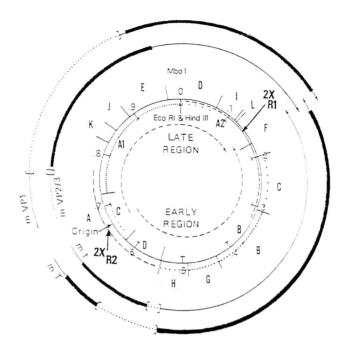

Fig. 6. Physical map of BKV DNA depicting the deletions and
insertions in R1 and R2 DNAs. The region of the genome known
to be deleted in R1 and R2 DNAs are indicated by closely
dotted circles and the regions possibly deleted are indicated
by dotted lines (Pater et al., 1980b).

Howley, P.M. (1980). Molecular biology of SV40 and human
    polyoma viruses BK and JC. In Klein G. (ed): "Viral Oncol-
    ogy", New York: Razan Press, p. 489.
Israel, M.A. et al. (1978). Evaluation of normal and neo-
    plastic human tissue for BK virus. Virology 90:187.
Law, M.-F., Lowy, D.R., Dvoretzky, I., and Howley, P.M.(1981).
    Mouse cells transformed by bovine papillomavirus contain
    only extrachromosomal DNA sequences. Proc Natl Acad Sci
    78:2727.
Pater, M.M., Pater, A., and di Mayorca, G. (1979). Compa-
    rative analysis of GS and BK virus genomes. J Virol 32:
    220.
Padgett, B. (1980). Human papovavirus. In Tooze J. (ed):

    "Molecular Biology of Tumor Viruses", 2nd ed. New York:

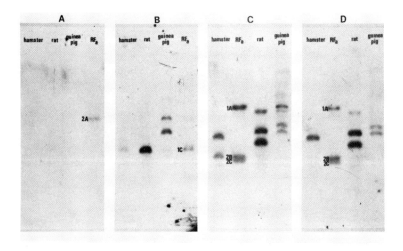

Fig. 7. Hybridization of HindIII-digested cellular DNAs
with specific MboI and HindIII fragments of labeled BKV DNA.
MboI fragment J (see Fig. 6) was used as probe in A, Fragment
G was probe in B, HindIII fragment C was used as probe in C,
and HindIII fragment D was used    in D.(Pater et al., 1981b)

Cold Spring Harbor Laboratory, p. 339.

Pater, M.M., Pater, A., Fiori, M. Slota, J. and di Mayorca,
  G. (1980a).  BK virus DNA sequences in human tumor and
  normal tissues and cell lines.  Viruses in Naturally
  Occurring Cancers.  Cold Spring Harbor Conf Cell Prol 7:329.

Pater, A., Pater, M.M. and di Mayorca, G. (1980b).  Arrangement of the genome of the human papovavirus RF virus.
  J Virol 36:480.

Pater, M.M., Pater, A., and di Mayorca, G. (1981a).  Genome
  analysis of MG virus, a human papovavirus.  J  Virol
  39:968.

Pater, A., Pater, M.M., Dougherty, R.M. and di Mayorca, G.
  (1981b).  Transformation of rodent cells by RFV, the
  human papovavirus with dual genome.  Virology 113:86.

Pater, M.M., Pater, A., di Mayorca, G., Beth, E., and
  Giraldo, G. (1982).  BK virus-transformed inbred hamster
  brain cells:  status of viral DNA in subclones.  Mol
  Cell  Biol  2:837.

Pyrhonen, S., Montyjarvi, R., Tykka, H., Sarna, S. and
  Tallberg, T. (1978).  BK and herpes simplex virus anti-

bodies in renal cell carcinoma. Med Biol 56:194.

Southern, E. (1975). Detection of specific sequences among DNA fragments separated by gel electrophoresis. J Mol Biol 98:503.

Wold, W.S.M., Mackey, J.K., Brackmann, K.H., Takemori, N., Rigden, P., and Green, M. (1978). Analysis of human tumors and human malignant cell lines for BK virus-specific DNA sequences. Proc Natl Acad Sci 75:454.

Zouzias, D., Prasad, I., and Basilico, C. (1977). State of viral DNA in rat cells transformed by polyoma virus. II. Identification of the cells containing nonintegrated viral DNA and the effect of viral mutations. J Virol 24:142.

13th International Cancer Congress, Part D
Research and Treatment, pages 495–504
© 1983 Alan R. Liss, Inc., 150 Fifth Avenue, New York, NY 10011

# HEPATITIS B VIRUS DNA AND HUMAN HEPATOCELLULAR CARCINOMA

C. Brechot, S. Wain-Hobson, C. Pourcel,
A. Dejean, M. Hadchouel[*], J. Scotto[*]
and P. Tiollais.

Unité de Recombinaison et Expression
Génétique (INSERM U.163, CNRS LA 271)
Institut Pasteur, Paris (France).

[*] Unité de Recherche d'Hépatologie Infantile
(INSERM U.56) Clinique Pédiatrique, Hôpital
d'Enfants - Le Kremlin Bicêtre (France).

Since about two hundred million people are chronic carriers of the hepatitis B virus (HBV), diseases related to this virus represent a public health problem of world-wide importance.

The association between HBV chronic infection and the development of hepatocellular carcinoma (HCC) is supported by the following epidemiologic evidence : 1) a strong geographic correlation between hepatitis B surface antigen (HBsAg) prevalence and HCC incidence (Szmuncss 1978), 2) an increase in the prevalence of HBV markers in patients with HCC (Hadziyannis 1980), 3) a very high relative risk (several hundred fold) in the development of HCC amongst HBsAg chronic carriers (Beasley et al. 1981).

Whereas the specific serologic response to HBV infection is well documented, little is known concerning the cycle of the virus during the different stages of the disease and the nature of its relationship to HCC. This is mainly for two reasons : 1) attempts to propagate HBV in cell culture have been unsuccessful and this has greatly hampered studies of the molecular biology of the virus, and 2) experimental HBV infection can only be achieved in chimpanzees, and the course of the animal disease differs from that in humans. Chimpanzees develop mainly a chronic persistent hepatitis (CPH), and HCC has not yet been observed.

The HBV-related viruses described in woodchuck, squirrel and duck constitute suitable laboratory models to study host-virus interaction (Summers et al. 1982). Nevertheless, the diseases observed for these animals also differ somewhat from the human disease. For instance, the squirrel does not seem to develop HCC and HCC observed in the woodchuck is associated with acute hepatitis or active chronic hepatitis and with a high level of viral multiplication but not with cirrhosis as observed in man.

To study further the relationship between HBV chronic infection and appearance of HCC, we used two approachs : 1) the first consisted of studying the presence and the state (free or integrated) of HBV DNA in the liver by blot-hybridization using cloned HBV DNA as a probe, 2) the second, to clone HCC cellular DNA containing integrated viral sequences and to study the structure of the cloned DNA fragments.

STATE OF HBV DNA IN HCC AND OTHER HBV-RELATED LIVER DISEASES (Bréchot et al. 1980, 1981a,b, 1982a,b)

The patients studied were separated into different groups according to two criteria : 1) the liver histology : HCC, chronic hepatitis, 2) the serological status : presence or absence of HBsAg which is a marker of current HBV infection, the hepatitis B e antigen (HBeAg) which is a marker of HBV multiplication, and antibodies to the core antigen (anti-HBc) and surface antigen (anti-HBs) which usually reflect a past and resolved HBV infection. Three main categories were considered : patients with HCC, chronic HBV carriers without tumour and patients with acute fulminant hepatitis.

1 - <u>Patients with HCC</u> : Patients were divided into three groups according to the presence or absence of HBsAg and HBeAg :

*HBsAg and/or anti-HBcAg positive, HBeAg negative patients* : Patients of different origin were studied. Bands corresponding to DNA fragments of molecular weight higher than 3.2 kb (3.2 kb is the size of the HBV genome) in the HindIII pattern and hybridization signals close to the origin of the lane in the uncut DNA pattern were observed (Fig. 1). These results demonstrated the presence and integration of HBV DNA sequences in the tumorous liver cell DNA. The

existence of several bands suggested the existence of several integration sites in the host genome. The EcoRI pattern
showed the presence of bands at different positions. When
observed the presence of a band of high intensity at the
3.2 kb position suggested the existence of two or more HBV
genomes integrated in a head-to-tail arrangement. The restriction patterns were different for the different patients
studied. Moreover, when the tumorous and non-tumorous parts
of the liver could be clearly distinguished histologically,
the restriction patterns corresponding to these two parts
were generally different. The presence of integrated HBV
DNA sequences was also demonstrated in the PLC/PRF/5 cell
line (Macnab et al. 1976), a line derived from a human HCC.

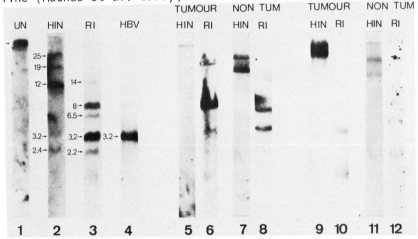

FIGURE 1 : Autoradiogram of the Southern blot analysis of
liver tissue samples of HBeAg negative patients with HCC.
Lanes 1 to 3 : tumorous part of an autopsy sample of a male
patient from Ivory Coast (patient 53 HCC). HBsAg was present in the serum but undetectable by immunofluorescence in
the tumour. Lane 4 : cloned HBV DNA. Lanes 5 to 8 and 9 to
12 : tumorous and non-tumorous samples of two other HCC.
UN : undigested DNA. Hin and RI : HindIII and EcoRI restriction patterns.

*HBsAg negative patients* : We focused on the relationship
between HBV and HCC associated with alcoholic cirrhosis.
This class of HCC is the most frequent form of HCC in
France. Two groups of alcoholic patients were studied.
Group I included 51 prospectively studied alcoholics without

apparant tumour, and Group II included 20 retrospectively studied patients with HCC and alcoholic cirrhosis (Table 1). Integrated HBV DNA sequences were detected in the 20 patients with HCC, but in only 8 of the 51 alcoholics without tumour. None of the patients with HCC had HBsAg detectable in the serum. Five had only anti-HBc, 3 had both anti-HBc and anti-HBs, 1 had only anti-HBs, and 7 had no HBV serological markers.

| Group and Patient n° | Serologic tests | | | HBV DNA in the liver | |
|---|---|---|---|---|---|
| | HBsAg | Anti-HBc | Anti-HBs | Free | Integrated |
| Group I : Alcoholics without HCC (51 cases) | 3/51 | 16/51 | 13/51 | 2/51 | 6/51 |
| Group II : Alcoholics with HCC (20 cases) | 0/16 | 8/16 | 4/16 | 0/16 | 20/20 |

TABLE 1 : State of HBV DNA in the liver and serological status of alcoholic patients with and without HCC (71 cases).

Twelve non-alcoholic European patients with HCC were studied and integrated HBV DNA sequences were also detected despite the absence of detectable HBsAg in the serum.

*HBsAg positive, HBeAg positive patients* : In these patients, the autoradiogram patterns are different from those of the two preceding groups. The first case was an early HCC (a small tumorous nodule discovered during surgery for portoclaval shunt). The HindIII patterns of the tumour and the non-tumorous part of the liver were identical and showed the presence of an intense band at the 3.2 kb position with a smear downstream (Fig. 2). This demonstrated the presence of free viral DNA. Due to the large amount of free viral DNA, integrated sequences were not clearly ascertained.

HBV DNA was also detected in the serum. The second case was an autopsy sample of an advanced HCC. Free viral DNA was present only in the non-tumorous part, whereas integrated HBV sequences were present both in the tumorous and non-tumorous tissues.

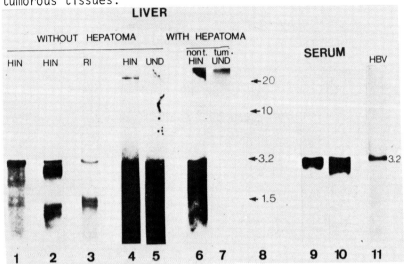

FIGURE 2 : Autoradiogram of the Southern blot analysis of liver and serum samples from HBeAg positive chronic carriers. Lanes 1and 9 : patient with slight inflammatory changes. Lanes 2, 3 and 10 : patient with chronic active hepatitis. Lanes 4 and 5 : patient with chronic active hepatitis, showing integrated sequences. Lanes 6 and 7 : patient with HCC. Lane 11 : cloned HBV DNA. Sizes are in kilobase pairs.


2 - HBV chronic carriers without appearant tumour : Patients were divided into two groups according to the presence or the absence of HBeAg.

HBeAg negative patients : The histology ranged from normal liver to chronic active hepatitis (CAH) and cirrhosis. The presence of integrated HBV DNA sequences was observed. In some cases, the EcoRI pattern suggested the existence of tandem integration. Integrated sequences were detected even for short-term chronic carriers.

HBeAg positive patients : The histological status of these patients ranges from slight inflammatory changes to CPH or

CAH. An intense band at the 3.2 kb position and a long intense smear below with few bands superimposed were observed both in the uncut DNA and the HindIII restriction patterns. HBV DNA was also detected in the serum. These results demonstrated the presence of free viral DNA in the liver and production of Dane particles. In some cases, integrated HBV DNA sequences associated with free HBV DNA were also observed.

3 - Acute fulminant infection : In the four patients with acute fulminant hepatitis studied, sharp bands corresponding to integrated viral sequences were also demonstrated. All these patients were HBeAg negative.

## CLONING OF HCC CELLULAR DNA CARRYING HBV DNA

To investigate the molecular nature of HBV DNA integration, we constructed two genomic libraries of HCC DNA. One from the liver of a serum HBsAg-positive patient (53 HCC) who died from liver failure due to HCC (Bréchot et al.1980), the other from the HBsAg secreting, hepatoma derived, cell line PLC/PRF/5 (Macnab et al. 1976).

Genomic libraries were constructed by partial cleavage of the cellular DNA with MboI and ligation into the BamHI vector λL47-1 (Loenen et al. 1980). HBV carrying recombinants were isolated by screening the libraries with nick-translated cloned HBV DNA. The restriction and structural maps of two clones, one from the patient (λIA22) and one from the cell line (λA3) are presented in Fig. 3 along with the corresponding genomic map of the virus (Tiollais et al. 1981). For λIA22 approximately 3.8 kb of DNA hybridizes to HBV probes, whereas for λA3, about 4.6 kb hybridizes. While the two clones share several features in common, they differ significantly : 1) Whereas clone λIA22 contains at least one complete unrearranged HBV genome, as evidenced by heteroduplex analysis with cloned HBV DNA, clone λA3 contains two subgenomic fragments inverted with respect to one another. 2) The left sites of integration for both clones are both located ($\pm$ 150 bp) within the gene C (the gene for HBcAg). The right site of integration for λIA22 is again within the gene C whereas for λA3 it is before the pre-S region. 3) For λIA22, the open reading frames P, X and S are complete as well as part of C. For λA3, only the pre-S region is complete. 4) When λIA22 DNA was coconvected into mouse Ltk⁻ cells with the cloned HSV tk gene, HBsAg was detected in a number of tk[+] clones demonstrating that λIA22 carries a complete functional gene S (Dejean et al. 1982). The patient from whom the clone was derived was negative by immunofluorescence for liver HBsAg. 5) The flanking sequences of these and 12 other independently derived HBV carrying clones - from both tissue and cell liver DNAs - do not carry sequences homologous to the following retroviral oncogenes : abl, fps, ras, myc, myb and src. 6) Both clones contain highly repeated DNA sequences flanking HBV genomes. In the case of λA3, there are a number of inverted sequences capable of forming multiple 'snap-back' structures when viewed by the electron-microscope.

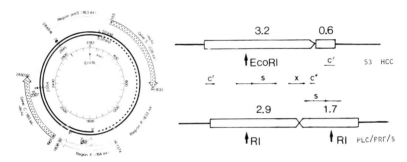

GENETIC ORGANIZATION OF THE INTEGRATED HBV DNA SEQUENCES

FIGURE 3 : Genetic map of the HBV genome and genetic orga-nization of the cloned integrated HBV DNA sequences. Clone λIA22 was obtained from patient 53 HCC, whereas λA3 was isolated from the PLC/PRF/5 cell line. Open bars represent HBV DNA. Sizes of HBV fragments are in kb. C, S and X above the arrows correspond to the open reading frames of the HBV genome.


DISCUSSION

Since the hybridization assay is a very sensitive and reproducible technique which can be performed on a needle biopsy, HBV DNA is now a new viral marker. This assay is useful for HCC epidemiology especially when studying patients with few or no HBV antigen or antibody markers either in the serum or in the liver.

We have analysed liver samples from patients from different races, from different regions (Africa, Europe, China
and the Middle East), with positive and negative serological status and with alcoholism. In all cases, we observed
the presence of HBV DNA sequences integrated in the host
cellular DNA. The case of the French alcoholic patients is
particularly striking since only a minority of alcoholics
without HCC had detectable HBV DNA in the liver, whereas
the 20 patients with HCC were HBsAg negative in the serum,
all had integrated viral sequences (Bréchot et al. 1982a).
These observations provide strong epidemiological evidence
for HBV as a carcinogenic factor in human HCC. Since a few
cases of HCC without detectable HBV DNA in the liver have
been reported more studies in countries with different
rates of HBV infection are necessary to firmly establish
these epidemiological results.

The presence of a few discrete bands on the autoradiogram is consistent with the existence of a limited number
of integration sites in the host DNA. Similar observations
have been reported by Shafritz et al. 1981a,b. Although not
surprising in a tumour which is a mono or oligoclonal
disease, this finding is amazing in chronic carriers
without tumour. The existence of a few host-DNA integration
sites leads to the question of their specificity and their
relationship with the viral multiplication since they can
be observed at an early stage of HBV infection. Such specificity has not been reported for other DNA viruses.

At the molecular level analysis of two recombinant
phages clones shows that the sites of integration are
within or close to gene C. Similar results were described
in the case of woodchuck hepatitis virus (Ogston et al.
1982). Together, this suggests that this region of the
viral genome may be involved in viral integration. For both
clones at least one copy of gene S is present and in case
of λIA22, the gene is functional. This is interesting
because the shutting of HBsAg expression parallels the evolution of the tumour (Nazarewicz-de-Mezer et al. 1981).

The assumption that HBV is involved in the development
of HCC raises the question of the mechanism of HBV carcinogenesis. By analogy with oncogenic DNA viruses (Topp et al.
1982), expression of a HBV gene could be necessary to
induce the transformed phenotype, integration would maintain the transforming gene. Alternatively, as proposed for

some retroviruses (Varmus 1982), HBV sequences could activate a cellular oncogene (promoter insertion model). The development of a tumour from a chronically infected cell either could be a direct consequence of the integration event or could necessitate action of a promoting factor. The long delay - generally more than ten years - between the HBV infection and the appearance of the tumour is an argument in favour of the later hypothesis.

Further structural analysis of the cloned HCC cellular DNA and in vitro studies of the transforming properties of HBV or HCC cellular DNA could provide better understanding of the role of HBV in liver cancer.

This work was supported by grant CR 22R29 from the Faculté de Médecine Lariboisière Saint-Louis, Université de Paris VII, grant 338C from the Délégation Générale à la Recherche Scientifique et Technique, grants ATP 72.79.104/029 and Convention 124036 from the Institut National de la Santé et de la Recherche Médicale, and a grant from the Fondation pour la Recherche Médicale (subvention triennale).

## REFERENCES

Beasley RP, Hwang LY, Lin CC, et al. (1981). Hepatocellular carcinoma and hepatitis B virus - a prospective study of 22707 men in Taiwan. Lancet 2:1129.

Bréchot C, Pourcel C, Louise A, Rain B, Tiollais P (1980) Presence of integrated hepatitis B virus DNA sequences in cellular DNA of human hepatocellular carcinoma. Nature 286:533.

Bréchot C, Hadchouel M, Scotto J, Fonck M, Potet F, Vyas GN, Tiollais P (1981a). State of hepatitis B virus DNA in hepatocytes of patients with HBsAg positive and HBsAg negative liver diseases. Proc. Natl. Acad. Sci. USA 78:3906.

Bréchot C, Hadchouel M, Scotto J, Degos F, Charnay P, Trépo C, Tiollais P (1981b). Detection of hepatitis B virus DNA in liver and serum : a direct appraisal of the chronic carrier state. Lancet 2:765.

Bréchot C, Nalpas B, Couroucé AM, Duhamel G, Callard P, Carnot F, Tiollais P, Berthelot P (1982a).Evidence that hepatitis B virus has a role in liver-cell carcinoma in alcoholic liver disease. New Engl. J. of Med. 306:1384.

Brechot C, Pourcel C, Hadchouel M, Dejean A, Louise A, Scotto J, Tiollais P (1982b). State of hepatitis B virus DNA in liver diseases. Hepatology 2:27S.

Dejean A, Carloni G, Brechot C, Tiollais P, Wain-Hobson S (1982) Organization and expression of hepatitis B sequences cloned from hepatocellular carcinoma tissue DNA. J. Cell. Biochem. in press.

Hadziyannis SJ (1980). Hepatocellular carcinoma and type B hepatitis. Clin. Gastroenterol. 9:117.

Loenen WAM, Brammar WJ (1980). A bacteriophage lambda vector for cloning large DNA fragments made with several restriction enzymes. Gene 10:249.

Macnab GM, Alexander JJ, Lecatsas G et al. (1976). Hepatitis B surface antigen produced by a human hepatoma cell line. Brit. J. Cancer 34:509.

Nazarewicz-de-mezer T, Slusarczyk J, Krawczynski K et al. (1980). Localization of hepatitis B virus antigens in hepatocellular carcinoma. Prog. Med. Virol. 27:66.

Ogston CW, Jonak GJ, Rogler CE et al. (1982). Cloning and structural analysis of integrated woodchuck hepatitis virus sequences from hepatocellular carcinomas of woodchucks. Cell 29:385.

Shafritz DA, Kew MC (1981a). Identification of integrated hepatitis B virus DNA sequences in human hepatocellular carcinomas. Hepatology 1:1.

Shafritz DA, Shouval D, Sherman HI, Hadziyannis SJ, Kew MC (1981). Integration of hepatitis B virus DNA into the genome of liver cells in chronic liver disease and hepatocellular carcinoma. New Engl. J. Med. 305:1067.

Summers J, Mason WS (1982). Properties of hepatitis B-like viruses related to their toxonomic classification. Hepatology 2:61S.

Szmuness W (1978). Hepatocellular carcinoma and the hepatitis B virus : evidence for a causal association. Prog. Med. Virol. 24:40.

Tiollais P, Charnay P, Vyas GN (1981). Biology of hepatitis B virus. Science 213:406.

Topp W, Hightower MJ, Ramundo MB et al. (1982). Common features of transformation and tumour induction by DNA viruses. Hepatology 2:51S.

Varmus HE (1982). Form and function of retroviral proviruses. Science 216:812.

# Index